Stop Fi¿ Cancer

and Start Treating the Cause

3rd Edition

DR. KEVIN CONNERS

Fellowship in Integrative Cancer Therapy

Fellowship in Anti-Aging, Regenerative, and Functional Medicine

American Academy of Anti-Aging Medicine

Pastoral Medical Association

Conners Clinic

Phone Consults Available: (651) 739-1248

Cancer is…

a symptom,

an expression of dis-ease,

an outcome,

an end product,

an effect,

a survival instinct,

an autoimmune disorder,

a compensation,

a warning sign,

a wake-up call.

It's time to wake up and change your life!

Conners Clinic

(651) 739-1248
ConnersClinic.com
shop.ConnersClinic.com

Disclaimer

CONTENTS

FOREWORD

I stepped out of my car and closed the driver's side door. Taking a moment to glance at the other businesses situated along the strip mall, I recognized restaurants and salons from previous excursions this side-of-town. The familiarity was comforting. Especially since everything else about this trip was new territory.

I focused my gaze back on my destination. A friend referred me to this place, The Upper Room Wellness Center (now Conners Clinic), owned by a doctor who said he helped people get to the "root cause" of their health conditions.

I had never heard a physician speak about getting to the "root cause." Fundamentally it made sense. Finally, *something* made sense. As if I just might find answers to questions I had been asking for an incredibly long time.

* * * * * * * * *

I was about 15 years old when I first perceived my body changing for the worse. As an active individual from a lean, athletic family, I had assumed I was healthy. But when my physical progression started to differ from other "active" and "healthy" teens I naturally became concerned.

I wanted to understand what was happening and why. I asked individuals I perceived to be in authority (parents, mentors, relatives, coaches, teachers, trainers, friends, etc.) what they thought might be happening. They were older than me, they had experience, so they should have an idea, right?

1

Unfortunately, the typical responses I received were fairly canned:

It's just your developing hormones.

I had the same stomach problems when I was your age.

Feeling bloated after you eat is normal.

Bad skin is just a sign of puberty.

A lot of people are prone to recurrent infections.

The extra weight around your waist is probably exercise related.

The loss of muscle mass is a lack of protein.

Sweating through the night is a sign you have too many blankets on.

What are you talking about, you look great!

I've never heard of a tongue feeling swollen.

Are you sure you aren't imagining things?

You're just like Grandma.

You're just like your father.

You'll grow out of it.

Just talk to the doctor about antibiotics.

Just take an Advil/Ibuprofen/Tylenol/Aspirin…

You should do more sit-ups.

You should lift more weights.

You should do more cardio.

You should eat more protein.

You should cut out fats.

It's probably nothing.

This too shall pass.

It went on like this to ad nauseum. Even doctors had vague, disappointing theories, then prescribed drugs that may have made sense in the short term but did nothing to satisfy my deepest desire to know *why*.

In hindsight I realize those answers weren't *intentionally* misleading. Vague answers simply deflect questions which would otherwise reveal that individual's ignorance or make them feel helpless. They weren't *trying* to keep me sick, they were trying to pacify my distress. However, feeling frustrated at each pacifying dead-end was a gross understatement.

By the time I was 26 it could no longer be denied that my condition was not normal. This was *not* going away on its own. I needed professional help and I deeply desired *real* answers. I had enough sense to know symptom-chasing was a lost cause; I did that for too long. I had reached a point where I was willing to make whatever sacrifice was necessary in order figure this out.

* * * * * * * *

I reached the front entrance and pulled on the handle, hearing the pleasant jingling of the doorbell overhead. The tiny clinic bustled with patients receiving chiropractic adjustments and other natural therapies. I finished signing my initial paperwork and found a place to sit so I could watch the activity until the time of my case review. I was nervous. I was emotional. But I had hope.

It was the first day of the rest of my life.

I would have never imagined my illness would ultimately lead me to finding my life's purpose. But it did. I write this foreword while sitting behind my desk, a practitioner at the very clinic with which I became a patient more than a decade ago.

Although my healing journey is certainly not complete, I would say I am healthier now than I have ever been. Some days are still rough (such is the recovery timeline for chronic illness) and I spend hours in the quiet sanctuary of my home, gently nursing my body back into balance.

Thankfully, situations like that are slowly becoming less common, a testament to the natural medicine which has given me a second chance.

I never had a formal diagnosis (also known as a medically accredited title to encompass a specific set of symptoms.) I can, however, tell each of my patients that as it pertains to dis-ease, I have walked in their shoes. Whether those shoes are treading through autoimmunity, chemical or heavy metal toxicities, acute or chronic infections, cancer, food intolerances, failing organs, and more, I have been there. I get it. I see you.

If there is a message I can impart to those picking up this book, it's this: wherever you are along your journey, don't give up.

Don't give up hope.

Don't give up believing in a bigger purpose or plan.

Don't give up on your body's ability to heal.

Don't give up on the power of forgiveness.

Don't give up your voice.

Don't give up your freedom to choose.

Don't give up the good fight.

Don't give up pursuing truth.

Don't give up asking why.

Don't give up seeking wisdom.

Don't give up praying.

Don't give up loving.

Don't give up laughter.

Don't give up the cleansing presence of tears.

Don't give up on God.

Don't give up on yourself.

I use "don't give up" because a true healing journey is nothing short of arduous. When a person begins to follow a protocol that is natural, holistic, "alternative", counterculture, unfamiliar, he or she is literally choosing The Narrow Path.

The Narrow Path will *not* be easy. Progress will often be perceived as so much slower than desired. But that is because we are healing at the speed of nature rather than forcing our bodies to bend to the brutal will of invasive medical procedures and chemical interventions.

Every second, minute, and hour of each day, week, and year throughout our entire lives our cells are working to heal us. Even when we do things in absolute opposition to our natural biology, our body fights back to try and correct itself. Our physical encasement *truly* is one of the most forgiving, adaptive, and constant gifts that we will ever be awarded in this life.

The very moment we begin to care for our earthly temple in a manner that honors our biology, our interconnectedness to the environment, and our spirit, our cells will begin to respond *in tandem* with our actions. Instead of having to work *against us*, our body now has the opportunity to work *with us*. It is a cooperative miracle taking place; a miracle to "never give up" hoping comes to fruition.

It is said that hindsight is 20/20. For the most part I would agree with that statement. I would, however, go one step further and say the interpretation of that hindsight is what allows 20/20 vision to be made manifest.

We can either interpret our history to define *who we are*, or we can use our history to make greater sense of present circumstances and redefine *the trajectory* of our future. It's choosing between permanent victimhood or a permanent focus on sanctification. And it is a choice. The former represents The Wide Path, paved flat and traveled by many, heading toward the exact same destination as everyone else. The latter is The Narrow Path, crooked and winding, slippery and steep, dotted with flowers, and heading (with purpose) toward a worldview that is unrivaled by the greatest of earthly achievements.

Your history and your present circumstances are the reasons you are reading this book. As you turn the following pages, I encourage you to imagine yourself at a fork in the road: The Wide Path to one side, The Narrow Path to the other. The choice is yours; the hard work ahead will also be yours, but the reward will be great.

Welcome to the first day of the rest of your life.

Michelle Hamburger
Lead Practitioner, Conners Clinic

PREFACE

Why I Do What I Do

I really had no intention of taking care of people with cancer when I started in practice. I did know that I was answering a *call* of sorts as I knew that I wanted to be a doctor by the time I was in high school. I graduated chiropractic school in 1986 and immediately started in solo practice; but as a chiropractor I was successful yet unfulfilled. I just felt, deep down, that I was supposed to serve at a deeper level. Not that there was anything wrong with helping people with back pain; for me, the gnawing urge to meet the spiritual needs of others was overwhelming.

I left practice in 1992 not knowing what I was to do next and we eventually ended up in Mexico as full-time missionaries. My wife and four children (at the time, now we have five as well as 17 grandchildren) served the poorest of the poor in the shanty towns surrounding Monterrey. I also taught at a seminary south of Monterrey, preached every chance I could get, we all ministered to students, built buildings, poured concrete, and did just about everything else a missionary would do.

Coming back to Minnesota was bittersweet. We went into the mission field completely self-supported and quickly ended up broke as we gave our money away every time we experienced need. Our heart ached for every little church we visited, every hungry baby, ministers who had no windows on their concrete block *home* and no blankets for their beds. Bringing a truckload of provisions to the thousands living in cardboard boxes seemed completely useless. Could anyone understand my broken Spanish messages? How much were we really helping these people? When we ran out of money to continue the work and it was obvious that God was indicating that we were finished, we scheduled our move to Minnesota.

Back in practice, I found the familiar hollowness of chiropractic that then drove me to deeper study in Nutrition, Neurology, and Functional Medicine. God soon saw fit to send me a patient with cancer, then another, and another. Over the years, success brought more people and I soon feared that I might be missing something. This led me to go back to school and obtain Fellowships in Integrative Cancer and Functional Medicine. Of course, this is a summary of many years, but I thought it best to spare you the boring details.

I don't *treat cancer*; that would be illegal, and I've always thought that treating a disease was just plain silly. *Figure out the reason WHY!* was the drive that God had placed in me. This has been my passion from the beginning: sickness (including cancer) is just a symptom, an expression of a deeper *cause*. If I could help identify the cause, the *symptom* would take care of itself!

God continued to send us patients with cancer. My thought was/is that since He sent me the patient, He would have to tell me how to fix them. And so, He usually does. However, I've been doing this too long to be ignorant of the fact that God doesn't always send me someone that is going to get *fixed* in the way that they or I desire. He is sovereign and His plan is bigger than our small, temporal wants. My passion must always be solely for God and I have to trust that He has placed me right where I am for whatever reason that He sees fit. I believe *obedience* is the operative word.

People now come to me with all sorts of diagnoses from autoimmune disease to cancer. My job is to lead members into an understanding of how their body can heal through the tools that God has provided, wisdom that can only come from above, and foods that were created to heal. Years ago, I retired my chiropractic license in Minnesota as I believed that God was leading me to a deeper, spiritual journey: caring for critically ill people; many with little hope. (Let's just say that neither the chiropractic nor the medical boards appreciate what I do, as they both tried to shut me down on numerous occasions.)

My prayer is that this book becomes more than just information. I pray that God will use it to touch someone, somewhere, who needs His hope. I remember back in 1998 when my family and I packed everything we owned into a small U-Haul trailer and drove back home from Mexico. Everyone else was sleeping at one point and I quietly reflected on our mission. I felt like we did nothing, that all the visits to the shanty-towns where we handed out necessities and shared the Gospel, all the preaching in the one-room churches, the teaching at the mission school, building dormitories, and learning a new language; it all seemed so fruitless. I cried to God asking Him, (or really whined at Him) complaining that I was now financially broke and that He could have at least shown us that our *sacrifice* produced something, for in Mexico we often felt we were simply placing drops of water in a bucket with no bottom.

God is gracious, even when we whine. It isn't often that I claim, *God spoke to me*, but in that old Chevy Suburban chugging north on Interstate 35, I know He clearly stated, "If I had you do all you did for just **one** person, would you have still done it?" My humble answer was obvious and my lesson complete: just shut up and be obedient and leave the results to the One who is sovereign over **all**!

Obedience is often a difficult lesson to learn. Jesus learned it through suffering (see Hebrews 5:8) so why do we assume anything less dramatic in our walk? I pray that I may say, as did the Apostle Paul as he recalled all his personal glories, "But what things were gain to me, these I have counted loss for Christ. Yet indeed I also count all things loss for the excellence of the knowledge of Christ Jesus my Lord, for whom I have suffered the loss of all things, and count them as rubbish, that I may gain Christ and be found in Him, not having my own righteousness, which *is* from the law, but that which *is* through faith in Christ, the righteousness which is from God by faith; that I may know Him and the power of His resurrection, and the fellowship of His sufferings, being conformed to His death, if, by any means, I may attain to the resurrection from the dead." – Philippians 3:7-11

INTRODUCTION

The Cancer Doctor's Cancer

I originally penned this book in 2010, and then updated it in 2016 with a second edition. As I type these letters, it is October 2019 and God has allowed some major events in my life that have shaped my care for others. Several years ago, I began experiencing abdominal symptoms that continued to persist and increase in intensity regardless of my efforts.

There was a time that I needed to imagine the feelings felt by my cancer patients. I'm empathic by nature, which I think makes me a better doctor, and I've had my share of physical injuries, broken bones, and sprained ankles...but cancer? I'd imagine their fear; I'd imagine their pain. I'd imagine their dread of an unknown future and console them with verses that assured that God would never leave them and that He desires to walk with them through their suffering, wherever it may lead. *There was a time.*

Flashback to December 2017. Alex sat in the chair adjacent to mine in my consult room. I shuffled through his CT report as he shared his desire to forgo any more chemotherapy treatments when he was told that the previous round was not effective, and the cancer has now progressed to his liver. I asked him the same question I ask all my cancer patients, "Tell me your story, I want to know you and how you got to this point."

I have to be honest. This consultation was a little different. It was just recently that I confirmed my own diagnosis and my selfish thoughts wandered to my own pain as he recalled that, "it all started in September of this year." Oh great. September was just three months ago and his first symptoms of any possible ill-health progressed from stomach aches to stage 4 in three months? I don't know why I was surprised; it was nothing that I haven't heard before, but this time it seemed more real. I guess I didn't have to imagine anymore.

There is nothing better than experiential knowledge in most things. I could read every book written about Abraham Lincoln and become the world's best authority on his life, yet I still don't know him. I've dedicated the last half of my career trying to understand cancer and I must say that I think I'm more committed than most doctors. My wife would say that I really have no life other than studying. Each patient has been my textbook; their disease, my obsession. I guess God's providential plan has an ironic twist in that I've now become my own textbook.

Alex continued. His timeline of events that shaped the last few months were clear. Scared by the sudden diagnosis, he started with surgery, resecting part of the large bowel followed by chemotherapy. The most recent scan shattered all his hopes, revealing that the chemotherapy *failed*. He was told he had months to live and here he sat, looking for comfort, grasping for a future. I understood; experientially.

Will this make me a better doctor or keep me from being one? Will my story be one that encourages many or will I be an example to the *real* doctors that standard oncology is the only way to go? The final chapter has yet to be written so I won't ponder the details with which God cannot yet trust me, but I do hope that the process may become a blessing to someone, somewhere, who is searching for hope that has been stolen away.

At this writing, Alex is still with us. His hope has been renewed, if only a little. I'll never understand why someone, calling themselves a doctor, would tell someone they had X amount of time to live. How arrogant have we become to think we know God's timeline? I wonder if the bit of success I've seen over the years has more to do with renewing hope than all the therapies and diets and nutrients. I wonder if more cancer patients die of a broken spirit than a broken body; I wonder what outcomes would be like if our medical system weren't so broken, if oncologists could work hand-in-hand with doctors like myself and if the patient's well-being was placed ahead of insurance documents. Most of all I wonder what God will do with this beautiful irony of the cancer doctor's cancer and I look forward, cautiously, to the ride.

I'm In the Boat With You

My diagnosis proved to be an extremely rare cancer called Metastatic Extra Mammary Paget's disease (EMPD.) Mine is stage 4, spread to the colo-rectal area, abdomen, and possibly bladder and bone (at this writing as of June, 2020.) According to a study at Mayo Clinic a few years ago, I should be dead by now. Actually, I should have been dead a while ago. Go figure; God's got different plans for the time being.

That being said, I wanted to update this book with both new findings as well as more information to help those who could never come see me and/or may read this book after I've been blessed to join the heavenly parade.

Some might ask, "Why would I take advice from someone with cancer let alone someone who may not survive cancer?" Good question. It seems fair to me. But, then I recall the grim 5-year survival rate of someone with metastasized EMPD (it's about the same as Pancreatic Cancer) and look at that recent Mayo study on Stage 4 EMPD to see that I, through the grace of God, am still kicking and even if my Father takes me home from this disease, I am fairing exceedingly better than the best Mayo offered the *best case scenario* in their study, and I without choosing to do **any** chemo. Besides, this book is about offering suggestions as opposed to giving recommendations.

You can find more information on everything that I am doing by going to our website ConnersClinic.com and look under the tab *My Personal Journey*. But, enough about me, let's get on with the book.

* * * * * * * *

I cannot take credit for what's in this book. The book of Ecclesiastes states, "What has been will be again, what has been done will be done again; there is nothing new under the sun." – Ecclesiastes 1:9

Information contained here is simply a small piece of nearly 30 years of practice experience learning from other doctors who've paved my way, scientists dedicated to finding answers, and patients who share their stories. I am also attempting to introduce what may be a new topic to some: Integrative Cancer Therapy. Years have passed since I completed my Fellowship on this subject and I desire to share a smidgen of information. This is in no way a complete work, it is a start; I am not an Oncologist, I am a doctor with advanced training in neurology, integrative cancer, anti-aging and functional medicine, nutrition, etc.

I am simply attempting to convey information and opinion; this is not a substitute for standard medical care. Any and all information in this book is NOT a substitute for standard medical care. Please consult your physician before considering any information in this book. This book is an opinion, not a protocol; it is the reader's responsibility to seek appropriate medical care and to understand that this book does not suggest or imply that treating cancer is anything but reserved for appropriate medical establishments. Please see the full disclaimer at the end of this book.

CHAPTER 1

Our Current State of Affairs

"Miracles are a retelling in small letters of the very same story which is written across the whole world in letters too large for some of us to see."

– C. S. Lewis

What is Cancer?

The American Cancer Society States:

"Cancer starts when cells in a part of the body start to grow out of control. There are many kinds of cancer, but they all start because of out-of-control growth of abnormal cells.

Cancer cell growth is different from normal cell growth. Instead of dying, cancer cells continue to grow and form new, abnormal cells. Cancer cells can also invade (grow into) other tissues, something that normal cells cannot do. Growing out of control and invading other tissues are what makes a cell a cancer cell.

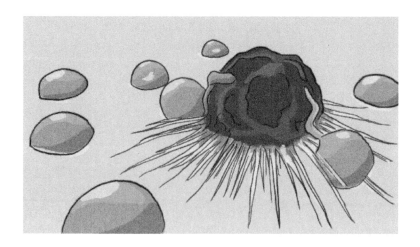

Cells become cancer cells because of damage to DNA. DNA is in every cell and directs all its actions. In a normal cell, when DNA gets damaged the cell either repairs the damage or the cell dies. In cancer cells, the damaged DNA is not repaired, but the cell doesn't die like it should. Instead, this cell goes on making new cells that the body does not need. These new cells will all have the same damaged DNA as the first cell does.

People can inherit damaged DNA, but most DNA damage is caused by mistakes that happen while the normal cell is reproducing or by something in our environment. Sometimes the cause of the DNA damage is something obvious, like cigarette smoking."

In short, cancer is defined as *uncontrolled cell replication*. There is *always* a reason, a cause! Something, at one time in the history of a particular cell, disrupts the replication cycle and/or it's *stop* mechanism, which caused the cell to begin to replicate. Also, at one time, the normal apoptotic (programmed cell death) mechanism failed. Remember, there is always a *cause*.

In truth, this happens often. Fortunately, most of the time progression of cell replication is thwarted by a healthy immune response recognizing the abnormal clump of cells and destroying it. Hence, most people don't end up with a diagnosis of cancer. It is when our fail-safe cellular protection programs, like a healthy immune response and our tumor suppressor system (we'll discuss this later) fail, cancer growth continues.

What Could You Do?

For the past several decades, the freedom of choice has not existed when it comes to treatment of cancer. Patients have been herded into the medical machine of surgery, chemotherapy, and radiation. Patients were shamed if they even thought about alternative care. The Marcus Welby generation idolized medicine and the demi-gods in white coats. Anyone daring to attempt a natural alternative was quickly labeled crazy and the practitioners quacks and money-mongers. Thank goodness for the information age; people can seek out answers once reserved for those with multiple letters behind their names. A new movement is beginning to take hold; it's a new horizon for those desiring to take a greater degree of responsibility for their health, and it couldn't have come too soon.

As public awareness of alternative cancer treatment increases, doctors have had to improve their skills on talking patients *out* of the safer, more reasonable alternative treatments. *Losing* the cancer patient to an alternative doctor could cost the hospital $300,000 to well over a million dollars according to Oncology Today as it listed out the average cost of conventional cancer treatment.

Remember, when a conventional doctor talks about alternative cancer treatments, they are usually repeating the lies that they have been told. For example, read the NCI Test Summary for Cancell (sold as Protocel in the US, a powerful, alternative cancer therapy.) NCI said Cancell showed "no biological activity" in the test, even when the study reported that, "Cancell performed amazingly well" against all cancers tested. It should have been front page news, but since they couldn't isolate the activity of its success, it was disregarded! It was another, "it works great but since we can't make any money with it, we'll slam it."

Desperate Doctors Avoid Losing Their License

Even if conventional doctors learn the truth about cancer or any other disease, clinic policies, hospital protocols, and pharmaceutical companies must be placated. There are rules from state medical boards and even laws passed (thanks to pharmaceutical lobbyists) to prevent doctors from even talking about alternative cancer treatments. Yes, believe it or not, it may be a felony for a medical doctor to even talk about something as safe and well-tested as Paw Paw, Essiac, Hoxsey, Herbal Therapy, vitamins, or Gerson Therapies.

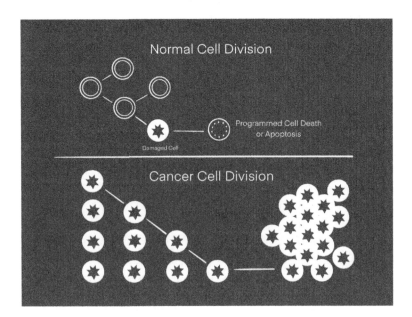

FDA Treatment Blockade

It takes $800 million (not a typo) and six to twenty years to get FDA approval of a cancer drug; it begins with submittal of an application (usually about 100,000 pages.) The median cost of doing so is around $19 million (according to Johns Hopkins, 2018.)

The best alternative cancer treatments cost a few hundred dollars a month and cannot be patented. That's the problem. If a natural substance cannot be patented, then it must be squashed. Natural treatments are nutritional in origin and since they are considered *plant-based*, they don't need FDA approval to the same degree as a drug would.

There is a misunderstanding out there that the vitamin industry isn't regulated; they are. The problem (if you owned a drug company) is that *plant-based* nutritional products cannot be patented. If you can't patent it, you can't make a ton of money with it. There is a systematic, carefully executed propaganda campaign against natural care of all disease. This is not a *conspiracy theory*, it's just plain economics; if you owned a drug company, you might make the same decisions. It's easy to justify actions to benefit stockholders and employees, after all, companies exist to make a profit.

But It's for Our Own Good? Really?

Let's be honest, conventional medicine is not *winning the war* on cancer. Despite the yearly fanfare regarding new cancer drugs, the percentage of Americans dying from cancer in 2019 was about the same as it was in 1970. But still, conventional doctors can't prescribe alternatives cancer treatments.

According to the Washington Post, there were 13,700 registered lobbyists in Washington, D.C. in 2009; many were paid by pharmaceutical companies doing their best to make sure that conventional doctors can never prescribe alternative cancer treatments.

According to Investopedia, the pharmaceutical industry has spent $3.9 **BILLION** over the past 20 years on lobbyists. CNN reported that the pharmaceutical industry spent about 27.5 million dollars lobbying our politicians in 2018 alone! Holy cow! It's no wonder a politician can have a net worth of 50 million after 20 years in congress making $150,000/year. It doesn't take an accountant to figure out they are receiving money from *other sources*.

In 1971, when President Richard Nixon proclaimed the official "War on Cancer" 1 out of every 21 Americans got cancer. Now we have a 1 out of 2.5 chance of developing cancer! Hello!!

All you need to do is go to this website:

https://surveillance.cancer.gov/statistics/types/survival.html

The above is a government website containing gobs of information on the 5-year survival rates of nearly every cancer. It is **not** improving! The way statistics are manipulated is through the whole idea of *early detection*. Since cancer treatment *success* is measured on surviving five years after the first date of diagnosis, all we need to do in order to give the perception of greater success is to diagnose the patient earlier. It's kind of like a company selling mutual funds including the *boom years* of 20% growth in their statistics to show that their fund averages 10% growth when really, it's 4% and more like 2% after all the hidden fees.

It gets worse. After 2003, the number of new cancer cases became artificially reduced which allowed agencies like the American Cancer Society to claim that progress is being made. In 2004 the Centers for Disease Control (CDC) reported that VA hospitals in at least 13 states are no longer reporting cancer cases and that reporting has been inconsistent in 14 additional states. Therefore, as many as 70,000 new cancer cases (about 5% of the national total) were not even reported. Any improvement in the number of cancer cases is therefore in doubt. This is called "manipulation of statistics."

Conventional Tactics

Conventional doctors may try and get you to immediately move forward and schedule their recommended treatment (chemotherapy, radiation…) Understand, taking their conventional treatments first may **not** be your best decision for a few reasons:

- Alternative cancer treatments may have a higher success rate than conventional treatments in your case. It may instead be the best thing for you to first address the environment of cancer growth and your overall health before you seek conventional care. Even for those who **will** choose standards of care at some point, beginning a course of therapy that supports immune health may greatly contribute to better outcomes.

- Conventional treatments ravage your body so severely, that it will be more difficult for alternative treatments to work if alternatives are taken after the conventional treatments. Alternative treatments do not necessarily *kill* cancer like a toxic chemotherapy. They require and promote a healthy body (cellular environment) since it is necessary for your immune system to do the *fighting*.

- Chemotherapy and radiation may cause cancer to spread, and even if it does *knock down* the original cancer, it leaves stronger stem cells and drug-resistant cells behind. Surgery may also spread cancer. Regardless of the decision-making process, cleaning up the body with detoxification and building up the immune system is essential.

Note: I recorded a video recently on the use of Hydrogen Peroxide for cancer citing an interesting article proving that, while hydrogen peroxide may help kill some cancers, it may also cause others to ***grow***! Understand, hydrogen peroxide is an oxidizing agent, like chemotherapy. Oxidizing agents ***can*** kill cells, even cancer cells, so this is how they work. However, as I reveal in my video, citing this recent study, oxidizing agents can also ***cause cancer growth*** through a process they termed, the *reverse Warburg Effect*. We'll talk more on this later, but you can watch my video here:

ConnersClinic.com/H2O2

The smart patient says, "I want to know all the side effects of the different treatments that can be used in my case and I will call your office for an appointment when I decide which treatment I want." Those who simply turn their care over to their doctor because he "knows best" have poor outcomes under any doctor's care. You ***must*** take responsibility for your healing!

My best advice to someone with a recent cancer diagnosis: "***slow down***" and become a student."

Smart cancer patients ask *tough* questions. They want to know ***why*** the cancer started growing in their body. They want to know ***why*** the environment around the cancer cells *allowed* it to *take hold*. They want to know if there are ***underlining causes***. They want to ***fix*** the underlining causes so their body can cure itself. Alternative treatment does not necessarily kill cancer, only your body can do that.

From an integrative perspective, we want to correct the environment that allowed the disease. *Integrative* doesn't mean *anti-medical*; it means "to sanely work together for the betterment of the patient." Chemotherapy and radiation may be the best option! However, if not coupled with correction of the *cause*, naturally boosting one's immune system, and creating a healthy internal environment through diet, detoxing, etc., it doesn't take a rocket scientist to figure out that the cancer has a pretty good chance of re-appearing *with a vengeance*.

Is Anyone Really "Cancer-Free"?

I was recently giving an educational talk on cancer and overall health and mentioned that someone with cancer **must** change their milieu that precipitated the cancer growth or simply doing conventional chemo, radiation, and/or surgery may result in the cancer "coming back." Apparently that statement didn't sit well with one listener who was not happy with the insinuation that her oncologist was wrong when he told her she was "cancer-free." Let's make one thing very clear: **none** of us are **ever** "cancer free!" I would never, ever, if it were legal for me to do so, tell a patient that they are cancer free. Does that sound pessimistic? Too bad; my job is **not** to be a foolish optimist; it is to be a realist. There is **always** hope for survival, but don't kid yourself into thinking you have it licked. Turn cancer into a chronic condition that you will *deal with* and *keep at bay* by continuing to do the right things! A false sense of security breeds failure of proper action, which can lead to catastrophe.

After **any** treatment choice is attempted, medical re-assessment is necessary/useful. The reexamination will show one of three things:

- The cancer has diminished, and the patient will know that he/she is on the right course. Don't stop and slip back to your previous lifestyle thinking that a medical miracle will bail you out of the consequences of your irresponsibility. Stay the course!

- The cancer has remained the same and the patient will know that they still have time to try other approaches. Sometimes "no change" is exactly what you want to hear as often it means that your body has *walled-off* the tumor and no further growth has happened! Stay the course!

- The cancer has advanced, and the patient will know that the treatment they chose didn't completely work or needs assistance. Remember, it is very possible that without your chosen plan of care you may not have even made it to the re-exam. If your cancer has progressed, re-assess your treatment plan and consider adding new ideas and new approaches. At this point the patient can either abandon the current course or add other alternatives.

Simple rule of thumb: if something *is* working, ***don't stop***. If it is ***not*** working, try something else! One needs no advanced degrees to understand this logic. I particularly don't care to know, nor am I intelligent enough to understand, all the mechanisms of ***how*** every, specific treatment works; I just care that it ***does***!

A few years ago, a patient entered my office with a diagnosis of B-cell chronic lymphocytic leukemia (B-CLL), also known as chronic lymphoid leukemia (CLL), scheduled at Mayo for treatment postponed for 30 days at the patient's request to *try* an alternative therapy. We had 30 days to make a difference; sadly, I had little hope given the short time we had to make a difference. We were all elated when conservative care proved miraculous for when she went back to her oncologist to hear, "whatever you've been doing, don't stop." The cancer was undetectable! Remember, we didn't *treat her cancer*; we aided her own nervous and immune response to help her body do the work; but it ***did*** work, and her oncologist cared enough to "not care how" and tell her to "not stop."

These types of stories are claimed antidotal, unbelievable, false, or simply the result of the placebo effect. I don't care! If my patients get better from the placebo effect, at least they got better! Heck, most my patients would let me throw angel dust on them if they thought it would help. Call me crazy but I think people just want to get better at a fair price and are not looking to over-analyze everything and remain sick. "I just want to get better." "I've been given **no** hope." "My oncologist won't even talk to me." These are all comments I hear too often.

People often ask me how the Rife (a light frequency generator we highly recommend) works. Though I share my theories, I tell them honestly, "I have no idea." Does that discount its validity? Everyone has a liver, but few could explain its functions, yet their liver still works. They don't care, as long as it's working. I don't (nor does anyone else) know exactly how every vitamin, mineral or enzyme works. No one yet has figured out exactly how aspirin works! Disease treatment is no different; I am most interested in *what* works and *that it works*; it is only my inquisitive mind that desires to know *how*.

The Foundation of Conventional Medicine is Sand

One of the most important theories of conventional medicine is known as monomorphism. It is based on the work of Louis Pasteur. On his deathbed he admitted that he was wrong and Bechamp (Pierre Antione) who promoted pleomorphism was right. The two (and their perspective camps) carried out on-going arguments on health/illness theories that greatly shaped society's approach to treatment. Conventional medicine has clung to monomorphism to the determent of patients everywhere.

Monomorphism vs. Pleomorphism

Under *pleomorphism*, bacteria and other microorganism are not seen as dangerous, invasive, pathogenic, nor infectious (in most instances.) They are seen as performing simple, necessary cleanup functions in response to cues from the local body tissues. Thus, it would make sense that you would treat an infectious illness by simply adjusting the inner terrain (the environment) of the body to allow it to become more healthful, thus eliminating the need for the presence of the *infectious* organisms. Any attempt to treat an infectious illness with antibiotics or other *aggressive* means (monomorphism) would be seen, in most cases, as short-sighted and would be attempting to treat a *symptom* of a deep imbalance, rather than addressing the deep imbalance. Further antibiotics and other aggressive antimicrobial means would actually further imbalance and disrupt the inner terrain, thus eventually leading to further degeneration.

While a more balanced approach to the debate between Monomorphism and Pleomorphism seems saner, throwing out one or another in a dogmatic overtone hurts the patient. There is a time and place for everything.

So, it is with cancer; though we want to destroy the growing cancer, we want to do so by improving the body's ability to heal; change the internal environment, and the cancer has no foothold.

Beware of the Hyperbole

A beautiful couple, madly in love, chase each other playfully on a sun-drenched beach as the waves caress their tanned legs. Cut to a middle-aged, smiling women clipping roses in what looks to be a garden outside an English cottage. Cut to an African American man in a driveway washing his Land Rover squiring water at his spouse as she runs, in slow-motion, towards the most beautiful sunset you could imagine. All this is done while a silver-tongued narrator declares the glories of a cancer drug as if those taking it will be transported into a utopian world. Cut to 30 seconds of a nearly inaudible, auctioneer-speed rambling of side effects one of which is death. End with blissful, romantic innuendos of the above characters clutching their partners with an indescribable devotion. One would think they are selling condoms.

Those *Great* New Cancer Drugs

In 2003 and 2004, there was a lot of publicity about the "great new cancer drugs." In March 2004, the Executive Editor of Fortune Magazine wrote an extensive article about these new drugs. The title of the article was all revealing, "Why We're Losing the War on Cancer."

Leaf reported that the two new blockbuster drugs, Avastin and Erbitux, aren't as effective as once reported. He states that Avastin (bevacizumab), "managed to extend the lives of some 400 patients with terminal colorectal cancer by 4.7 months" considering the possible side effects, that is not really worth the risk when there are safe effective alternative treatments available. Leaf further reported that Erbitux (cetuximab), used to treat cancers of the head and neck, did even worse. It "has not been shown to prolong patients' lives at all," Leaf states. Avastin profited 6.8 billion in 2018 alone.

There are many other reports on this out there.[1]

I know that it is typical for the Cancer industry and mainstream media to pump up any of the new therapies trying to sound like there has been a *new breakthrough*. Leaf even admits that Fortune magazine ran a cover article on Interleukin-2 with a "Cancer Breakthrough" headline that any honest oncologist would tell you, it wasn't.

This is not just an *American-capitalistic problem*. The article goes on to report that Europe seems to struggle with similar less-than-true advertising. The twelve new anticancer drugs approved in Europe between 1995 and 2000 did not improve survival or quality of life nor were they safer than the older

---

[1] https://www.curetoday.com/articles/avastin-falls-short-in-early-stage-colon-cancer

drugs. However, they were several times more expensive and provided the stockholders in drug companies a profit on false hope dished out to the suffering patients.

In 2005 Herceptin (over 7 billion in 2018, used to treat breast cancer) was hyped as "astonishingly effective, wonder drug." However, the truth is far different. *Ralph W. Moss, Ph.D.* has written a report on the Herceptin deception. Here is what Michael Janson, MD, past president of both the American College for Advancement in Medicine (ACAM) and the American Preventive Medical Association (APMA) has to say about this special report:

"Dr. Moss has once again cut through the hype of medical research and media reports with a keen, objective analysis that presents the true picture of scientific results regarding the latest "*miracle* in cancer therapy. He reveals the hollow core of the recent medical reports on Herceptin, showing that it is not what has been claimed, and that the statistics were manipulated to make it seem far better than it is, while underplaying the potential risks. The conflict of interest among the authors that he notes is a danger to honest researchers and to the public who might mistakenly take this drug (and many others) in inappropriate situations. Let's hope that his analysis gets wide attention."

In 2008 to 2009 a colon cancer trial was run to see if using Avastin soon after surgery would prevent reoccurrence. 2,700 colon cancer patients were involved:

- One group received six months of chemotherapy
- The other group received six months of the same chemotherapy and a year of Avastin

The results showed no significant difference between the survival rates of the groups. Still sales of Avastin remain in the top 6.8-billion-dollar range in 2018. It will be interesting to see if the manufacturer's marketing campaign (schmoozing doctors and giving lucrative charge backs) will be able to keep sales in the neighborhood. In July 2010 the New York Times reported that a drug advisory board voted 12 to 1 to revoke the previous approval of Avastin. This for a drug that, "has at times been hailed as a near miracle."[2]

Lung Cancer Drug Iressa?

From a Newsday article of December 18, 2004, "Shocking the medical and financial worlds, a highly touted lung cancer drug, Iressa (gefitinib), failed to help patients live longer in a major clinical trial." How can these hyped-up drugs get all the way to clinical trials? The promise of tremendous profits is the only explanation.

Ed Silverman, author of a 2015 article in the *Boston Globe*, pointed to lung cancer drug Iressa as a "cautionary tale" against using "surrogate endpoints" (signs that point to, but don't guarantee, a given clinical outcome) for FDA drug approvals. He stated that the FDA gave patients false hope, approving an expensive, ineffective drug, which manufacturer AstraZeneca would later have to pull from the market.

Well, Iressa is back on the market touting a more realistic success rate than originally promised. Though it has been shown to shrink tumors, Iressa-treated patients on average, however, did not fare any better than those who received the standard of care.

Understand, I have always supported whatever works. However, let's just be honest! **No** chemotherapy, targeted therapy drug, immunotherapy, radiation, or surgery is going to work on everyone. Alternative therapies also fail on numerous patients but why aren't pharmaceutical companies held to the same standards of honesty as everyone else?

---

[2] Pollack 2010

Immunotherapy

Over the past several years, immunotherapy has been the latest hope in medical intervention. Personally, I am a big supporter of immunotherapy, especially coupled with Rife; we've found it to be a great addition for many people. The problem is that it simply doesn't work for all cancers or all patients. There is a specific genetic test done to see if you qualify. Also, insurance companies may require that you *fail* traditional chemotherapy prior to trying immunotherapy.

Immunotherapy, also called by its *old name*, biologic therapy, is a type of cancer treatment that, according to their website, "boosts the body's natural defenses to fight cancer." It doesn't really do that. What it does is that it fools one's T-cells to interrupt a specific cell receptor responsible to keep immune cells from attacking one's own cells. This makes a lot of sense. Your own immune system is programmed so that it **won't** attack self-tissue. This is a good thing as it keeps us from literally destroying ourselves. However, cancer is self-tissue, and this is one of the reasons our immune system has in recognizing it (the growing cancer) as an enemy.

Immunotherapy is a group of drugs that, in simplest terms, block that *turn off* switch so our immune cells (specifically our T-cells) will attack the cancer. Again, the problem is that it simply doesn't work on all types of cancer our on all people. However, it is an extremely promising approach.

Immunotherapy isn't chemotherapy so it isn't a *toxic* treatment. It isn't without side effects though. Since it is turning off self-tissue recognition of immune cells, you can exhibit symptoms/disorders of just about any disease that ends in an *itis*. Colitis is probably the most common issue, but any autoimmune disorder is possible. The good thing is that a few months following discontinuation, usually these symptoms abate.

Coupling the immunotherapy drug with Rife therapy, in my opinion, is the **best**. I believe that the Rife helps both chemotherapy **and/or** immunotherapy **target** the cancer **much** better!

One other problem with immunotherapy (as well as CAR T-Cell Therapy discussed next) is that it requires a healthy and strong patient immune system. If you have been already revenged by chemotherapy and radiation, success may be limited.

Currently, an independent researcher is self-funding a project at Mayo Clinic in Rochester, MN to couple immunotherapy with **our product** Evolv Immune (a polysaccharide immune stimulant, see Chapter 5) and Evolv Entourage (a water soluble, nano CBD oil.) This is **super** exciting. Note: both these products are products that I personally take daily and are available in our store: shop.ConnersClinic.com

Some current immunotherapy drugs:

- Ipilimumab (Yervoy)
- Nivolumab (Opdivo)
- Pembrolizumab (Keytruda)
- Atezolizumab (Tecentriq)
- Avelumab (Bavencio)
- Durvalumab (Imfinzi)

CAR T-Cell Therapy

A novel, emerging, type of immunotherapy approach is called adoptive cell transfer (ACT): collecting and using patients' own immune cells to treat their cancer. There are several types of ACT, but the one that has advanced the furthest in clinical development is called CAR T-cell therapy.

In 2017, two CAR T-cell therapies were approved by the Food and Drug Administration, one for the treatment of children with acute lymphoblastic leukemia (ALL) and the other for adults with advanced lymphomas.

CAR T cells are the equivalent of "giving patients a living drug," explained Renier J. Brentjens, M.D., Ph.D., of Memorial Sloan Kettering Cancer Center in New York, an early leader in the CAR T-cell field.

As its name implies, the backbone of CAR T-cell therapy is our immune T-cells, which are a key killer cell of the immune system because of their critical role in orchestrating the immune response and destroying cells infected by pathogens. The therapy requires drawing blood from patients and separating out the T-cells. Next, using a disarmed virus, the T-cells are genetically engineered to produce receptors on their surface called chimeric antigen receptors, or CARs.

These new receptors are "synthetic molecules, they don't exist naturally," explained Carl June, M.D., of the University of Pennsylvania Abramson Cancer Center, during a recent presentation on CAR T-cells at the National Institutes of Health campus.

These new receptors allow the T-cells to recognize and attach to a specific protein, or antigen, on tumor cells, thereby helping one's own immune system attack the cancer. This is also a very promising therapy, but it also has some drawbacks that mainly involve cost. Currently, insurance is not paying for this therapy and costs range from 1.5 to 2.5 million per attempt. I created a video outlining this that you can view here:

ConnersClinic.com/car-t-cell

Why Doctors Prescribe the *Newest Drugs*

Doctors may not be prescribing the newest drugs because they are better for you because in truth, there is no way to know. Everyone's body chemistry is different; a treatment that worked for some people in a study on some university campus may not work *for you*. Conventional doctors do nothing to determine which of the available treatments for your cancer will work for you besides trial and error. They just prescribe the latest pharmaceutical drug. Pharmaceutical companies love this because the latest drug is usually the most expensive. Doctors may do this because:

- They do not want to appear to be behind the times. Should the patient have watched any TV program in the last few weeks, they were inundated with a host of promises with beautiful graphics of butterflies and sunset afternoons emotionally connected to the new version of medication. Patients ask for it!

- The doctors themselves are swept up by the hype. The "new cancer drugs" appear to be better because of the planned psychological manipulation that accompanies their release and patients demand them. We are all looking for a miracle drug to believe in!

- The side effects of new drugs are not well-known in the beginning and the doctors who care truly hope they may work better with less injury.

- New drugs *may* offer hope where previous drugs failed. We want to believe this is the main reason most doctors make recommendation; they really care about the patient and are willing to try new drugs because they've experienced the fragility of past recommendations.

The Wrong Approach?

Most cancer cells obtain their energy from fermentation. Normal cells obtain their energy from oxygenation (except muscle cells when they are completely exhausted) through the Kreb's cycle. This is a tremendous difference and one we must understand. Alternative cancer treatments such as Protocel and Herbal therapies target this difference. Conventional cancer research ignores this tremendous difference (as far as treatment goes) and continues to seek methods to destroy fast growing cells (which cancer cells are.) Our immune system contains mostly fast-growing cells and is also destroyed in the chemotherapy process. The worst thing you could do when you're sick is attack your own immune system. Again, is also destroyed with chemotherapy.

So understand: Cancer cells fall into the category of "rapidly reproducing cells." Some *normal* cells also fall into that same category, namely, immune cells, hair follicle cells, skin cells, intestinal cells, etc. Drugs aimed at killing rapidly reproducing cells (chemotherapy) cannot distinguish between cancer cells and normal cells. Chemotherapy kills immune cells, that's the *catch-22*.

Conventional "Truth"

In an Independent (UK) news article of December 8, 2003, Allen Rosesl, a vice-president of GlaxoSmithKline (a large international pharmaceutical company) was quoted as saying, "most (cancer) drugs work in 30 to 50 per cent of people" (who take them.) This is in stark contrast to a 2007 study published by the *Clinical Oncology*. The study was based on an analysis of the results of all the randomized, controlled clinical trials (RCTs) performed in Australia and the US that reported a statistically significant increase in 5-year survival due to the use of chemotherapy in adult malignancies (so the study was on the "good" drugs.)

Survival data were drawn from the Australian cancer registries and the US National Cancer Institute's Surveillance Epidemiology and End Results (SEER) registry spanning the period January 1990 until January 2004 (I gave you this website already so search it as well.) The authors found that the contribution of chemotherapy to 5-year survival in adults was:

- 2.3% in Australia
- 2.1% in the USA

They emphasize that, for reasons explained in detail in the study, these figures "should be regarded as the upper limit of effectiveness" (e.g., they are an optimistic rather than a pessimistic estimate.) So, where did Mr. Rosesl get the figure that his company's chemotherapy "works on 30-50%" of patients? I have no idea! It is amazing how the human mind can justify actions that benefit the flesh!

A study of over 10,000 patients shows clearly that chemo's supposedly strong track record with Hodgkin's disease (lymphoma) is actually a lie. Patients who underwent chemo were 14 times more likely to develop leukemia and 6 times more likely to develop cancers of the bones, joints, and soft tissues than those patients who did not undergo chemotherapy.[3]

As I previously stated, safe and effective plant-based treatments (nutrition, herbs) cannot produce large profits because they cannot be patented. Pharmaceutical companies need large profits to pay for the expensive FDA approved clinical trials, so plant-based treatments never get FDA approval to treat a disease. Nutritional companies simply cannot afford them!

As such, nutritional therapies go un-noticed and poo-poo-ed by doctors while chemotherapies get pushed by oncologists as

---

[3] NCI Journal 87:10

the standard of care regardless of the lack of evidence. From the December 12, 2002 issue of *Journal of the American Medical Association*, in a review with James Spencer Malpas, M.D., D.Phil. St. Bartholomew's Hospital London, United Kingdom:

"A recent randomized trial of treatment for stage one Multiple Myeloma by Riccardi and colleagues (*British Journal of Cancer* 2000; 82:1254-60) showed no advantage of conventional chemotherapy over no (no chemo at all) treatment."

The above statement is in direct contrast to popular belief that chemo is likely to help you. The reason for this belief is statements like this:

"1998 was truly one of the most exciting years for cancer research," said Harmon Eyre, MD, executive vice president for research and medical affairs for the American Cancer Society (ACS.) "While we are closer than ever to finding answers..." he continued, followed by a pitch for more donations.

Another popular belief that is repeated in movies and TV shows is that *not* taking chemotherapy is dumb, cowardice, and completely irresponsible. Nothing could be further from the truth. It is the smart cancer patient who does enough research to learn the fraud of conventional cancer theories and only the brave who stand up against the pressures of oncologists bent on forcing people into what is not in their best interest.

That being said, let's be perfectly clear: I believe there is a time and place for everything; and I am **not** against responsible use of chemotherapy, if needed. I have often begged a patient to consider using some chemotherapy. It **can** save lives, knock down a rapidly growing tumor, and give a person another chance to get on top of a downwardly spiraling situation. What I **am** against is standard protocols that disregard personal preference and individual need.

Understand, I do **not** get involved with the decision-making process of whether a patient should take chemo, radiation, surgery, or alternative care. However, I am sick and tired of hearing that people who choose to do the latter are crazy and ill-informed. Look at the real statistics and make a well-informed decision! *You* are the one who has the diagnosis, so *you* better do some of your own research. One need only do a search for chemotherapy effectiveness and you will read as many articles as you desire on the fallacies of their success.

I'm not even saying that chemo may not be necessary at times; just be wise, **not** dogmatic. Perhaps use these harsh approaches to squelch an aggressive tumor to allow more time to do what's right and necessary to change the milieu.

The Emperor Has No Clothes

"Once upon a time there lived a vain Emperor whose only worry in life was to dress in elegant clothes. He changed clothes almost every hour and loved to show them off to his people.

Word of the Emperor's refined habits spread over his kingdom and beyond. Two scoundrels who had heard of the Emperor's vanity decided to take advantage of it. They introduced themselves at the gates of the palace with a scheme in mind.

"We are two very good tailors and after many years of research we have invented an extraordinary method to weave a cloth so light and fine that it looks invisible. As a matter of fact, it is invisible to anyone who is too stupid and incompetent to appreciate its quality."

The chief of the guards heard the scoundrel's strange story and sent for the court chamberlain. The chamberlain notified the prime minister, who ran to the Emperor and disclosed the incredible news. The Emperor's curiosity got the better of him and he decided to see the two scoundrels.

"Besides being invisible, your Highness, this cloth will be woven in colors and patterns created especially for you." The emperor gave the two men a bag of gold coins in exchange for their promise to begin working on the fabric immediately.

"Just tell us what you need to get started and we'll give it to you." The two scoundrels asked for a loom, silk, gold thread and then pretended to begin working. The Emperor thought he had spent his money quite well: in addition to getting a new extraordinary suit, he would discover which of his subjects were ignorant and incompetent. A few days later, he called the old and wise prime minister, who was considered by everyone as a man with common sense.

"Go and see how the work is proceeding," the Emperor told him, "and come back to let me know."

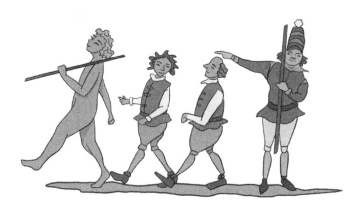

The prime minister was welcomed by the two scoundrels.

"We're almost finished, but we need a lot more gold thread. Here, Excellency! Admire the colors, feel the softness!" The old man bent over the loom and tried to see the fabric that was not there. He felt cold sweat on his forehead.

"I can't see anything," he thought. "If I see nothing, that means I'm stupid! Or, worse, incompetent!" If the prime minister admitted that he didn't see anything, he would be discharged from his office.

"What a marvelous fabric," he said then. "I'll certainly tell the Emperor." The two scoundrels rubbed their hands gleefully. They had almost made it. More thread was requested to finish the work.

Finally, the Emperor received the announcement that the two tailors had come to take all the measurements needed to sew his new suit.

"Come in," the Emperor ordered. Even as they bowed, the two scoundrels pretended to be holding large roll of fabric.

"Here it is your Highness, the result of our labour," the scoundrels said. "We have worked night and day but, at last, the most beautiful fabric in the world is ready for you. Look at the colors and feel how fine it is." Of course, the Emperor did not see any colors and could not feel any cloth between his fingers. He panicked and felt like fainting. But luckily the throne was right behind him and he sat down. But when he realized that no one could know that he did not see the fabric, he felt better. Nobody could find out he was stupid and incompetent. And the Emperor didn't know that everybody else around him thought and did the very same thing.

The farce continued as the two scoundrels had foreseen it. Once they had taken the measurements, the two began cutting the air with scissors while sewing with their needles an invisible cloth.

"Your Highness, you'll have to take off your clothes to try on your new ones." The two scoundrels draped the new clothes on him and then held up a mirror. The Emperor was embarrassed but since none of his bystanders were, he felt relieved.

"Yes, this is a beautiful suit and it looks very good on me," the Emperor said trying to look comfortable. "You've done a fine job."

"Your Majesty," the prime minister said, "we have a request for you. The people have found out about this extraordinary fabric and they are anxious to see you in your new suit." The Emperor was doubtful showing himself naked to the people, but then he abandoned his fears. After all, no one would know about it except the ignorant and the incompetent.

"All right," he said. "I will grant the people this privilege." He summoned his carriage and the ceremonial parade was formed. A group of dignitaries walked at the very front of the procession and anxiously scrutinized the faces of the people in the street. All the people had gathered in the main square, pushing and shoving to get a better look. An applause welcomed the regal procession. Everyone wanted to know how stupid or incompetent his or her neighbor was but, as the Emperor passed, a strange murmur rose from the crowd.

Everyone said, loud enough for the others to hear: "Look at the Emperor's new clothes. They're beautiful!"

"What a marvelous train!"

"And the colors! The colors of that beautiful fabric! I have never seen anything like it in my life!" They all tried to conceal their disappointment at not being able to see the clothes, and since nobody was willing to admit his own stupidity and incompetence, they all behaved as the two scoundrels had predicted.

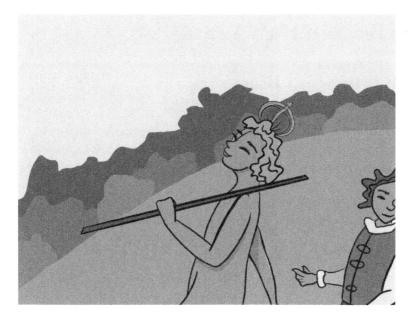

A child, however, who had no important job and could only see things as his eyes showed them to him, went up to the carriage.

"The Emperor is naked," he said.

"Fool!" his father reprimanded, running after him. "Don't talk nonsense!" He grabbed his child and took him away. But the boy's remark, which had been heard by the bystanders, was repeated over and over again until everyone cried:

"The boy is right! The Emperor is naked! It's true!"

The Emperor realized that the people were right but could not admit to that. He though it better to continue the procession under the illusion that anyone who couldn't see his clothes was either stupid or incompetent. And he stood stiffly on his carriage, while behind him a page held his imaginary mantle."

  –   Hans Christian Anderson

Lies and Half Truths

Publication Bias

How do you know who and what to trust? Research is supposed to give us hard evidence on what works, and medical research is supposed to be the basis of what we call *evidence-based medicine*. But what happens when the research is biased? Peer-reviewed randomized trials are to provide guidance for how medicine is practiced. Doctors trust in their published results and form protocols based upon proven success. However, trust has been eroded in recent years due to the exposure in several high-profile cases of alleged data suppression, misrepresentation, and manipulation.[4][5][6][7][8][9]

While most publicized cases have involved pharmaceutical drug trials, it is scary to reveal that Grandma's medicine received FDA's approval due to a positive outcome in 22 trials yet the 37 that showed negative results were *never published*.[10]

---

[4] McHenry LB, Jureidini JN (2008) Industry-sponsored ghostwriting in clinical trial reporting: A case study. Account Res 15: 152–167

[5] Jureidini JN, McHenry LB, Mansfield PR (2008) Clinical trials and drug promotion: Selective reporting of study 329. Int J Risk Safety Med 20: 73–81

[6] Psaty BM, Kronmal RA (2008) Reporting mortality findings in trials of rofecoxib for Alzheimer disease or cognitive impairment: A case study based on documents from rofecoxib litigation. JAMA 299: 1813–1817

[7] Curfman GD, Morrissey S, Drazen JM (2006) Expression of concern reaffirmed. N Engl J Med 354: 1193

[8] Whittington CJ, Kendall T, Fonagy P, Cottrell D, Cotgrove A, et al. (2004) Selective serotonin reuptake inhibitors in childhood depression: Systematic review of published versus unpublished data. Lancet 363: 1341–1345

[9] Mitka M (2008) Controversies surround heart drug study: Questions about Vytorin and trial sponsors' conduct. JAMA 299: 885–887

[10] Dwan K, Altman DG, Arnaiz JA, Bloom J, Chan A-W, et al. (2008) Systematic review of the empirical evidence of study publication bias and outcome reporting bias. PLoS ONE 3: e3081. doi:10.1371/journal.pone.0003081

This is like a basketball coach with a record of 3-8 declaring success for a 3-0 winning season because the losses were never recorded. If we only publish the results of studies that *prove* our bias, is it really research? These examples highlight the harmful potential impact of biased reporting on patient care, and the violation of ethical responsibilities of researchers and those who fund it.

Biased reporting arises when two main decisions are made based on the significance of the data: whether to publish the trial at all, and if so, what data to report in the publication. Strong evidence for the selective publication of research trials has been available for decades but more recent cohort studies identified major discrepancies: favorable results were often highlighted while unfavorable data were suppressed; definitions of primary outcomes were changed; and methods of statistical analysis were modified without explanation in the journal article.[11] [12] [13] [14] [15] [16] [17] [18] [19] [20] [21] [22] [23] [24]

---

[11] Song F, Eastwood AJ, Gilbody S, Duley L, Sutton AJ (2000) Publication and related biases. Health Technol Assess 4: 1–115

[12] Dickersin K (1997) How important is publication bias? A synthesis of available data. AIDS Educ Prev 9: 15–21

[13] Rising K, Bacchetti P, Bero L (2008) Reporting bias in drug trials submitted to the Food and Drug Administration: A review of publication and presentation. PLoS Med 5: e217. doi:10.1371/journal.pmed.0050217

[14] Turner EH, Matthews AM, Linardatos E, Tell RA, Rosenthal R (2008) Selective publication of antidepressant trials and its influence on apparent efficacy. N Engl J Med 358: 252–260

[15] Melander H, Ahlqvist-Rastad J, Meijer G, Beermann B (2003) Evidence b(i)ased medicine—Selective reporting from studies sponsored by pharmaceutical industry: Review of studies in new drug applications. BMJ 326: 1171–1173

[16] Hemminki E (1980) Study of information submitted by drug companies to licensing authorities. BMJ 280: 833–836

[17] Chan A-W, Hróbjartsson A, Jørgensen KJ, Gøtzsche PC, Altman DG (2008) Discrepancies in sample size calculations and data analyses reported in randomized trials: Comparison of publications with protocols. BMJ. In press

[18] Chan A-W, Hróbjartsson A, Haahr MT, Gøtzsche PC, Altman DG (2004) Empirical evidence for selective reporting of outcomes in randomized trials: Comparison of protocols to published articles. JAMA 291: 2457–2465

[19] Hahn S, Williamson PR, Hutton JL (2002) Investigation of within-study selective reporting in clinical research: Follow-up of applications submitted to a local research ethics committee. J Eval Clin Pract 8: 353–359

[20] Pildal J, Chan A-W, Hróbjartsson A, Forfang E, Altman DG, et al. (2005) Does unclear allocation concealment in trial publications reflect poor methods or poor reporting of adequate methods? Cohort study of trial protocols and corresponding published reports. BMJ 330: 1049–1052

[21] Chan A-W, Krleža-Jeric K, Schmid I, Altman DG (2004) Outcome reporting bias in randomized trials funded by the Canadian Institutes of Health Research. CMAJ 171: 735–740

[22] Scharf O, Colevas AD (2006) Adverse event reporting in publications compared with sponsor database for cancer clinical trials. J Clin Oncol 24: 3933–3938

In a study published in *PLoS Medicine*, Lisa Bero and colleagues revealed that, "a substantial amount of primary outcome data submitted to the FDA was found to be missing from the literature (of new drug trials.) One quarter of trials in their sample were unpublished—predominantly those with unfavorable results. Not only were data suppressed for the unpublished trials, but an additional quarter of primary outcomes were omitted from journal articles of published trials. These findings are consistent with two recent reviews of FDA documents and journal articles, one of which was published in *PLoS Medicine* in September 2008."

It's not that anyone is saying that research is falsified; it's just that research that doesn't reveal what the drug company wanted may never get published. How is a doctor to know that the drug prescribed with an attached positive research data really had six other studies that failed? Since the interests of patients are the only thing of importance, it is difficult to justify why healthcare providers have access to *only* a biased subset of information.

---

[23] Soares HP, Daniels S, Kumar A, Clarke M, Scott C, et al. (2004) Bad reporting does not mean bad methods for randomised trials: Observational study of randomised controlled trials performed by the Radiation Therapy Oncology Group. BMJ 328: 22–24
[24] Al-Marzouki S, Roberts I, Evans S, Marshall T (2008) Selective reporting in clinical trials: Analysis of trial protocols accepted by The Lancet. Lancet 372: 201

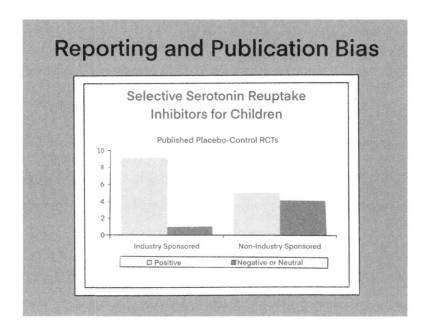

Always look at the bias! What financial interest is there in that prescription drug? The doctor wants you to get better, but the drug company wants a consumer for life! Could there be a bias in the pharmaceutical information supplied to the clinic? You decide.

A 2008 study stated that a substantial amount of primary outcome data submitted to the FDA was found to be missing from the literature; this is information that the FDA used to accept a drug yet wouldn't release to clinicians. 25% of trials (in their sample studied) were unpublished; predominantly those with unfavorable results. Other recent reviews of FDA documents and journal articles[14][25] reveal similar results, one of which was published in *PLoS Medicine* in September 2008.[25]

---

[25] Lee K, Bacchetti P, Sim I (2008) Publication of clinical trials supporting successful new drug applications: A literature analysis. PLoS Med 5: e191. doi:10.1371/journal.pmed.0050191

One study just openly stated its results as, "Studies with significant or positive results were more likely to be published than those with non-significant or negative results, thereby confirming findings from a previous HTA report. There was convincing evidence that outcome reporting bias exists and has an impact on the pooled summary in systematic reviews. Studies with significant results tended to be published earlier than studies with non-significant results, and empirical evidence suggests that published studies tended to report a greater treatment effect than those from the grey literature."[11] It's difficult to expound upon their statements.

Another study wanted to determine whether, "The reporting of outcomes within published randomized trials has previously been shown to be incomplete, biased and inconsistent with study protocols. We sought to determine whether outcome reporting bias would be present in a cohort of government-funded trials subjected to rigorous peer review." Their conclusion stated, "Selective reporting of outcomes frequently occurs in publications of high-quality government-funded trials."

Biased reporting of results of new drug trials is particularly concerning because these journal articles are often the only peer-reviewed source of information on recently approved drugs for healthcare providers (though I'm sure they receive plenty of literature from drug reps.) There are also substantial cost implications if the efficacy is overestimated and the drugs overused, as new molecular entities are among the most expensive pharmaceuticals on the market[26] and profit is necessary.

The FDA and other regulatory agency submissions represent the final description of how the trial was conducted and

---

[26] Morgan SG, Bassett KL, Wright JM, Evans RG, Barer ML, et al. (2005) "Breakthrough" drugs and growth in expenditure on prescription drugs in Canada. BMJ 331: 815–816

analyzed prior to journal publication. However, details from these submissions are not publicly available in most countries and rarely viewed by doctors. Although the FDA website posts summaries of reviews, their content and availability are variable, and sections are often redacted.[13 26 27] Furthermore, regulatory agency submissions are prepared by companies *after* data analysis and do not represent the full data; these may also be subject to biased reporting. Study protocols (how it was conducted) constitute the most comprehensive description of study design; access to these are particularly difficult to obtain.[28 29] The SPIRIT initiative (Standard Protocol Items for Randomized Trials) aims to address these deficiencies by producing evidence-based recommendations for key information to include in a trial protocol.[30]

Someone once said that you can make statistics say anything you want. I believe that careful consideration must be taken prior to undertaking any medical care, and that goes for alternative care as well. Unfortunately, the trial literature *is* biased, and much remains to be done to establish reliable, comprehensive data/results disclosure processes worldwide,

---

[27] Turner EH (2004) A taxpayer-funded clinical trials registry and results database. PLoS Med 1: e60. doi:10.1371/journal.pmed.0010060
[28] Chan A-W, Upshur R, Singh JA, Ghersi D, Chapuis F, et al. (2006) Research protocols: Waiving confidentiality for the greater good. BMJ 332: 1086–1089
[29] Lurie P, Zieve A (2008) Sometimes the silence can be like the thunder: Access to pharmaceutical data at the FDA. Law Contemporary Problems 69: 85–97
[30] Chan A-W, Tetzlaff J, Altman DG, Gøtzsche PC, Hróbjartsson A, et al. (2008) The SPIRIT initiative: Defining Standard Protocol Items for Randomized Trials [conference abstract]. German J Evid Quality Health Care (suppl) 102: S27

but also to start heeding the calls for increased access to full protocols and regulatory agency submissions.[18 27 31 32 33]

I always tell patients that are Christians, "pray about your care and make sure you have complete peace in your heart about the path you are going to follow." It is wise to listen to other trusted friends in whom you value their counsel. Try to keep from making decisions from fear, and *do not* let anyone pressure you into anything. Even with a cancer diagnosis, you always have more time than you may be pressured into believing to make a conscious and sane decision.

Here is even more *damning data* exposing the problems of publication bias:

"Dealing with the positive publication bias: Why you should really publish your negative results"
https://www.ncbi.nlm.nih.gov/pmc/articles/PMC5696751

"Is positive publication bias really a bias, or an intentionally created discrimination toward negative results?"
https://www.ncbi.nlm.nih.gov/pmc/articles/PMC6753760

"Open laboratory notebooks: good for science, good for society, good for scientists"
https://www.ncbi.nlm.nih.gov/pmc/articles/PMC6694453

---

[31] Krleža-Jeric K, Chan A-W, Dickersin K, Sim I, Grimshaw J, et al. (2005) Principles for international registration of protocol information and results from human trials of health related interventions: Ottawa statement (part 1). BMJ 330: 956–958
[32] Lassere M, Johnson K (2002) The power of the protocol. Lancet 360: 1620–1622
[33] Hawkey CJ (2001) Journals should see original protocols for clinical trials. BMJ 323: 1309

"But This is the Way We've Always Done it."

Medulloblastoma: A Childhood Brain Cancer

Medulloblastomas are the most common brain tumors in children. They usually form deep in the brain between the brainstem and the cerebellum. Although it is thought that medulloblastomas originate from immature or embryonic cells at their earliest stage of development, the exact cell of origin, or *medulloblast* has yet to be identified.

Symptoms are mainly due to secondary increased intracranial pressure due to swelling and a subsequent blockage in the brain and the cerebral spinal fluid. The child develops neurological symptoms, can become listless, nauseous, having episodes of vomiting, and headaches. Soon after, the child may develop a stumbling gait, frequent falls, and diplopia. Other neurological findings are also frequent and facial sensory loss or motor weakness may be present. The tumor is distinctive and usually diagnosed on an MRI.

Treatment nearly always begins with surgery; maximal resection of the tumor. The *standard protocol* includes the addition of radiation, but here's where treatment differences begin to emerge. Some studies reveal radiation alone to be as effective as a combination of radiation with chemotherapy.[34] Other studies attempt to prove better outcomes with chemotherapy added but fail to prove their point as they

---

[34] Medulloblastoma: Progress over time Robert I Smee1, Janet R Williams1, Katie J De-loyde1,*, Nicola S Meagher2, Richard Cohn3 Article first published online: 13 APR 2012 DOI: 10.1111/j.1754-9485.2012.02349.x

compare one chemotherapy regimen to another and then conclude that chemotherapy is a wise addition.[35] [36]

Increased intracranial pressure may be controlled with a ventriculoperitoneal shunt that is surgically placed to drain the inflammation.

Their Proof

Here's a study published in the *Journal of Oncology*, VOLUME 24, NUMBER 2, SEPTEMBER 1 2006 that was ***given to me by an Oncologist to prove the need for continued maintenance chemotherapy*** on an 8-year-old girl with Medulloblastoma who has already had chemotherapy and radiation:

Phase III Study of Craniospinal Radiation Therapy Followed by Adjuvant Chemotherapy for Newly Diagnosed Average-Risk Medulloblastoma

Roger J. Packer, Amar Gajjar, Gilbert Vezina, Lucy Rorke-Adams, Peter C. Burger, Patricia L. Robertson, Lisa Bayer, Deborah LaFond, Bernadine R. Donahue, MaryAnne H. Marymont, Karin Muraszko, James Langston, and Richard Sposto

ABSTRACT

Purpose: To determine the event-free survival (EFS) and overall survival of children with average-risk medulloblastoma

---

[35] Packer RJ, Cogen P, Vezina G, et al: Medulloblastoma: Clinical and biologic aspects. Neuro Oncol 1:232-250, 1999

[36] Packer RJ, Sutton LN, Elterman R, et al: Outcome for children with medulloblastoma treated with radiation and cisplatin, CCNU, and vincristine chemotherapy. J Neurosurg 81:690-698, 1994 Outcome for children with medulloblastoma treated with radiation and cisplatin, CCNU, and vincristine chemotherapy. Packer RJ, Sutton LN, Elterman R, Lange B, Goldwein J, Nicholson HS, Mulne L, Boyett J, D'Angio G, Wechsler-Jentzsch K, et al. Source Division of Neurology, Children's National Medical Center, George Washington University, Washington, DC

and treated with reduced-dose craniospinal radiotherapy (CSRT) and one of two postradiotherapy chemotherapies.

Methods: Four hundred twenty-one patients between 3 years and 21 years of age with nondisseminated medulloblastoma (MB) were prospectively randomly assigned to treatment with 23.4 Gy of CSRT, 55.8 Gy of posterior fossa RT, **plus one of two adjuvant chemotherapy regimens**: lomustine (CCNU), cisplatin, and vincristine; or cyclophosphamide, cisplatin, and vincristine.

Results: Forty-two of 421 patients enrolled were excluded from analysis. Sixty-six of the remaining 379 patients had incompletely assessable postoperative studies. Five-year EFS and survival for the cohort of 379 patients was 81% +/- 2.1% and 86% +/- 9%, respectively (median follow-up over 5 years.) EFS was unaffected by sex, race, age, treatment regimen, brainstem involvement, or excessive anaplasia. EFS was detrimentally affected by neuroradiographic unassessability. Patients with areas of frank dissemination had a 5-year EFS of 36% +/- 15%. Sixty-seven percent of progressions had some component of dissemination. There were seven second malignancies. Infections occurred more frequently on the cyclophosphamide arm and electrolyte abnormalities were more common on the CCNU regimen.

Conclusion: *This study discloses an encouraging EFS rate for children with nondisseminated MB treated with reduced-dose craniospinal radiation and chemotherapy*. Additional, careful, step-wise reductions in CSRT in adequately staged patients may be possible.

Let's break this down:

1. Starting with the purpose of the study, it states, "Purpose: To determine the event-free survival (EFS) and overall survival (OS) of children with average-risk medulloblastoma and treated with reduced-dose

craniospinal radiotherapy (CSRT) and one of two postradiotherapy chemotherapies."

a. EFS (event-free survival) in research study terms are usually measured in percentage and denote those in the study that survived (as opposed to those that died) that didn't experience a specific event. As stated in page 2 of the study under "Statistical Considerations," "The primary end point for analysis was time to a treatment failure event (EFS) measured from the time of study enrollment." Therefore, data was measured for each patient until an event occurred. An event was defined in the same paragraph as, "the first occurrence of death from any cause, relapse, progressive disease, or development of a second malignancy."

b. OS (overall survival) simply denotes those in the study group that remain alive at the end of the study as defined, "The secondary end point was time to death from any cause, from which actuarial survival probability was computed."

c. "Average risk medulloblastoma" refers to the fact that medulloblastoma can be classified into several risk groups and candidates for this study were considered average risk.

d. "Treated with reduced-dose craniospinal radiotherapy (CSRT) and one of two postradiotherapy chemotherapies." This sets the parameters of the study as to what is actually being measured and is my greatest concern. Why?

i. This study is comparing efficacy between two chemotherapy regimens: lomustine (CCNU), cisplatin, and vincristine; or cyclophosphamide, cisplatin, and vincristine.

ii. It is **not** comparing efficacy between chemotherapy and doing nothing.

iii. It is **not** comparing efficacy between chemotherapy and doing a natural approach.

iv. It is **not** comparing efficacy between chemotherapy and doing a specific alternative therapy. The study states exactly what is being compared: two chemotherapy regimens. Therefore, **one** regimen will probably show better success than the other regimen. What does this prove? It proves that one regimen showed better success than another in this study.

e. What you **cannot** extrapolate from this study:

i. You **cannot** extrapolate that chemotherapy is necessary for this type of cancer.

ii. You **cannot** extrapolate that chemotherapy is better then doing nothing, doing something else, or even requiring the patient to chant and throw dried rattlesnake venom over their left shoulder.

f. There is **only** one piece of information that can be gathered from the data from this study: Comparing chemotherapy regimens, which one worked better? Remember this because when the authors write their opinion at the conclusion, they extrapolate far more than possible from their own data.

2. Next let's move on to the study's method: "Four hundred twenty-one patients between 3 years and 21 years of age with nondisseminated medulloblastoma (MB) were prospectively randomly assigned to treatment with 23.4 Gy of CSRT, 55.8 Gy of posterior fossa RT, plus one of two adjuvant chemotherapy regimens: lomustine (CCNU), cisplatin, and vincristine; or cyclophosphamide, cisplatin, and vincristine."

   a. First, we see that four hundred twenty-one patients were included in this study.

   b. Then we see the inclusions:

      i. Patients were between 3 years and 21 years of age.

      ii. Patients had a nondisseminated (not dispersed, localized) medulloblastoma

      iii. All patients had radiation therapy to their brain

      iv. Patients were randomly divided into two groups that received the two separate chemotherapy cocktails.

   c. What **can** we understand from the method?

      i. This was a fairly large study (as studies go) and all received radiation therapy

      ii. All patients received chemotherapy of one of two types

   d. What we **cannot** extrapolate from understanding the method:

      i. We have no idea the health of any individuals in this study

      ii. We have no idea of the diets, other therapies explored by the parents, family habits, or lifestyle changes made by any individuals in either group.

      iii. We cannot compare anything other than that which is measured. In this case, all that is measured is EFS and OS, by percentage, of those in these two groups.

3. Now is where it gets exciting; let's see the results: "Forty-two of 421 patients enrolled were excluded from analysis. Sixty-six of the remaining 379 patients had incompletely assessable postoperative studies. Five-year EFS and survival for the cohort of 379 patients was 81% plus/minus 2.1% and 86% plus/minus 9%, respectively (median follow-up over 5 years.) EFS was unaffected by sex, race, age, treatment regimen, brainstem involvement, or excessive anaplasia. EFS was detrimentally affected by neuroradiographic inaccessibility. Patients with areas of frank dissemination had a 5-year EFS of 36% plus/minus 15%. Sixty-seven percent of progressions had some component of dissemination. There were seven second malignancies. Infections occurred more frequently on the cyclophosphamide arm and electrolyte abnormalities were more common on the CCNU regimen."

    a. Forty-two patients were excluded for reasons disclosed later in the writing which leaves 379 remaining for the study.

    b. The five-year EFS of the two groups was 81% +/- 2.1%, and 86% +/- 9%. From this data you can conclude:

        i. Group number two appears to have had a better EFS rate than group number one.

        ii. Given the +/- 2.1%, and +/- 9% error rate pretty much negates the above statement that group number two's success rate was better.

  c. From the above data, you ***cannot*** conclude:

        i. You ***cannot*** conclude that success or lack thereof in either group compares to any other treatment.

        ii. It is both illogical and impossible to compare success rates of these two groups to any other group utilizing any other therapy or, for that matter, doing nothing. There is ***no*** data in this study that allows such extrapolation.

  d. "EFS was unaffected by sex, race, age, treatment regimen, brainstem involvement, or excessive anaplasia. EFS was detrimentally affected by neuroradiographic inaccessibility." This tells us other factors affecting/not affecting the results.

  e. "Patients with areas of frank dissemination had a 5-year EFS of 36% plus/minus 15%. Sixty-seven percent of progressions had some component of dissemination." This tells us that patients with dissemination (widely dispersed in the tissue or other tissues) had a markedly lower 5-year EFS rate. It does ***not*** tell us if this EFS rate was worse/better in group one or group two.

  f. "Sixty-seven percent of progressions had some component of dissemination. There were seven second malignancies. Infections occurred more frequently on the cyclophosphamide arm and electrolyte abnormalities were more common on the CCNU regimen." From this we find:

57

  i. Sixty-seven percent of progressions (those whose cancer progressed) had some component of dissemination.

   1. This does **not** tell us how many patients in the study had *progressions* only that some did

   2. This tells us that 67% of those that did had dissemination

  ii. There were seven second malignancies though the study does not define if these were diagnosed as new, distinct tumors or metastatic lesions

  iii. The data also states that other complications were present such as infections and electrolyte abnormalities yet does not fully define this or the numbers that experienced them.

4. Conclusions: "This study discloses an encouraging EFS rate for children with nondisseminated MB treated with reduced-dose craniospinal radiation and chemotherapy. Additional, careful, step-wise reductions in CSRT in adequately staged patients may be possible."

  a. "This study discloses an encouraging EFS rate for children with nondisseminated MB treated with reduced-dose craniospinal radiation and chemotherapy." Really? As stated previously by the data itself, this study compares **two** groups of patients receiving two different chemotherapy cocktails. The only conclusion that can possibly be drawn directly from this study is that one chemotherapy cocktail fared better than another. Nothing more can be concluded from data collected!

b. "Additional, careful, step-wise reductions in CSRT in adequately staged patients may be possible." This speaks to the fact that this study utilized a reduced (from common) dose of radiation on all subjects. The only way to conclude that, "Additional, careful, step-wise reductions in CSRT in adequately staged patients may be possible," is to compare the success (EFS) of patients on this study to patients on other identical studies utilizing a higher dose of radiation which the authors state in the study proper.

  i. Authors state in study proper that, "The EFS rate compares favorably with results obtained after treatment with radiotherapy alone, including a contemporary prospective trial which found a 64.8% EFS rate for nondisseminated patients treated with 36 Gy of CSRT and supports the use of chemotherapy for all children with medulloblastoma." However, to compare one study result to another, you must compare apples to apples, identical parameters except the variable being studied. The authors cite this study (an un-identical comparable) in the above quote: "Low-stage medulloblastoma: final analysis of trial comparing standard-dose with reduced-dose neuroaxis irradiation."[37] The problems with this comparison:

    1. The above study's purpose was comparing doses of radiation usage, "To evaluate prospectively the effects on

---

[37] Journal of Clinical Oncology. 2000 Aug;18(16):3004-11

survival, relapse-free survival, and patterns of relapse of reduced-dose (23.4 Gy in 13 fractions) compared with standard-dose (36 Gy in 20 fractions) neuroaxis irradiation in patients 3 to 21 years of age with low-stage medulloblastoma, minimal postoperative residual disease, and no evidence of neuroaxis disease."

2. In comparing dosage use of radiation, this study revealed, "At 8 years, the respective EFS proportions were also 67% (SE = 8.8%) and 52% (SE = 11%) (P =.141)."

ii. The above statement from the study proper in quoted point i. also cites this (another un-identical comparable) study: "Results of a randomized study of preradiation chemotherapy versus radiotherapy alone for nonmetastatic medulloblastoma: The International Society of Paediatric Oncology/United Kingdom Children's Cancer study group PNET-3" Published in the *Journal of Clinical Oncology* 21:1581-1591, 2003. The problem with this comparison:

1. Its methods were distinct and different, as stated in its purpose, "to determine whether preradiotherapy (RT) chemotherapy would improve outcome for Chang stage M0–1

medulloblastoma when compared with RT (radiation) alone."

2. The results of this study revealed that long-term survival of those receiving chemotherapy prior to radiation fared no better than those who did radiation alone, "There was no statistically significant difference in 3-year and 5-year OS between the two arms."

iii. To extrapolate any further data from this study other than that which the study compares (one chemotherapy regimen to another) you must compare studies that utilize identical methods with a variable of comparison.

iv. To extrapolate that this study *proves* the validity of the use of chemotherapy over anything other than the chemotherapy that was used in comparison is overreaching. It is as if you formulated an experiment where you would juice two varieties of oranges; let's say Mandarin and Valencia. The results of the experiment revealed that our population group preferred the juice from the Valencia oranges. What could we conclude?

1. Could we conclude that our study proves that everyone should drink Valencia juice?

2. Could we conclude that nothing other than Valencia juice is affective in satisfying the population because 81% of those in our study prefer it?

3. Could we conclude that the population does not prefer apple juice?

4. Could we even conclude that Valencia is the superior orange for juicing?

We obviously could **not** conclude any of the above yet that is exactly the logic used in taking a study comparing two types of the same therapy, rating one superior than another, and then stating that it is superior to **all** therapy, even those it has not been compared to.

The logic is fuzzy at best.

More Studies Cast Doubt in Standard Protocols

I know this all seems complicated, so let's look at a few more studies. Here's one published in the *Journal of Clinical Oncology* in 1999 Mar;17(3):832-45:

Metastasis stage, adjuvant treatment, and residual tumor are prognostic factors for medulloblastoma in children: conclusions from the Children's Cancer Group 921 randomized phase III study

Zeltzer PM, Boyett JM, Finlay JL, Albright AL, Rorke LB, Milstein JM, Allen JC, Stevens KR, Stanley P, Li H, Wisoff JH, Geyer JR, McGuire-Cullen P, Stehbens JA, Shurin SB, Packer RJ

University of California at Irvine Medical Center, Orange, USA

ABSTRACT

Purpose: From 1986 to 1992, 'eight-drugs-in-one-day' (8-in-1) chemotherapy both before and after radiation therapy (XRT) (54 Gy tumor/36 Gy neuraxis) was compared with vincristine, lomustine (CCNU), and prednisone (VCP) after XRT in children with untreated, high-stage medulloblastoma (MB).

This means that this study compares two groups of patients: those receiving an 8-in-1 chemotherapy cocktail and another group receiving a cocktail of vincristine, lomustine (CCNU), and prednisone (VCP.) Both groups received XRT, that is, radiation therapy.

Immediately, from the purpose, you can discern data that can and cannot be gathered from this study regardless of results.

- It is logical to expect that one of the two groups may have a better outcome then the other.

- It is logical to then state that patients in similar scenarios as the patients in this study may do better on one protocol than the other based on outcome of this study.

- It is completely illogical to imply in any way that results of this study can be used to determine the efficacy of any other therapy other than the comparison of the two in the study.

A medulloblastoma study published in Nature, July 2012, states, "Despite recent treatment advances, approximately 40% of children experience tumor recurrence, and 30% will die from their disease. Those who survive often have a significantly reduced quality of life."[38] This paints a different picture then the 2006 study (six years previous) that an oncologist used to *prove* that her recommended therapy would result in an 81% cure rate. So how can one study give data that 81% are cured and another state that 40% have tumor recurrence, and 30% will die from their disease? It's easy, just look at what is compared to achieve the numbers. If you want to prove something, simply compare two products that you wish your audience to use and run a study. One will win and you can now convince the masses that it is superior to all; even those it was never compared to.

An article published in the April 2012 issue of *Journal of Medical Imaging and Radiation Oncology*, stated when measuring Medulloblastoma treatment outcomes at the Prince of Wales Hospital Cancer Centre, "The 5-year PFS (progression-free survival) was 69.7%. The 5-year PFS for patients treated pre and post 1990 was 66.1% and 71.8%, respectively. The 5-year CSS (cancer-specific free survival) for high- and low-risk patients was 61.1% and 78.4%, respectively."[34] And this was for surgical resection and radiation ***only***!

A study published in March of 2012 on the commonly used chemotherapy agent cisplatin attempted to see why, "cancer cells often develop resistance to cisplatin, which limits therapeutic effectiveness of this otherwise effective genotoxic drug." They found that what is a common problem in many other cancers, an inhibited estrogen-beta receptor (which is actually an apoptotic receptor), "interfere(s) with cisplatin-induced cytotoxicity in human medulloblastoma cell lines."[39]

---

[38] Nat Rev Neurol. 2012 May 8;8(6):340-51. doi: 10.1038/nrneurol.2012.78 - The clinical implications of medulloblastoma subgroups. Northcott PA, Korshunov A, Pfister SM, Taylor MD. Division Molecular Genetics, German Cancer Research Center (DKFZ), 69120 Heidelberg, Germany

[39] PLoS One. 2012;7(3):e33867. Epub 2012 Mar 16. Inhibition of ERβ induces resistance to cisplatin by enhancing Rad51-mediated DNA repair

This just means that there is a percentage of medulloblastoma patients (and other cancer patients with ERbeta inhibition) that will not respond as desired to cisplatin usage.

There are other studies that have shown remarkably favorable outcomes for medulloblastoma patients *not* utilizing chemotherapy. Published in the *International Journal of Radiation Oncology and Biological Physiology* in February, 2012, twenty-five children with medulloblastoma receiving radiation alone showed a "3-year relapse-free survival and overall survival of 83.5% and 83.2%, respectively."[40]

Oncologists seemingly ignore studies that call for a novel approach to treating childhood cancers. Published in February, 2012, "Brain Tumors in Children- Current Therapies and Newer Directions" points out the need to discover new therapies given cell biologists discoveries in "major targets like the Epidermal Growth factor Receptor (EGFR), Platelet Derived Growth Factor Receptor (PDGFR), Vascular Endothelial Growth factor (VEGF) and key signaling pathways like the MAPK and PI3K/Akt/mTOR."[41]

---

in human medulloblastoma cell lines. Wilk A, Waligorska A, Waligorski P, Ochoa A, Reiss K. Source Neurological Cancer Research, Department of Medicine, LSU Health Sciences Center, New Orleans, Louisiana, United States of America

[40] Int J Radiat Oncol Biol Phys. 2012 Aug 1;83(5):1534-40. Epub 2012 Feb 16. Early clinical outcomes demonstrate preserved cognitive function in children with average-risk medulloblastoma when treated with hyperfractionated radiation therapy. Gupta T, Jalali R, Goswami S, Nair V, Moiyadi A, Epari S, Sarin R. Source Department of Radiation Oncology, Advanced Centre for Treatment Research and Education in Cancer and Tata Memorial Hospital, Mumbai, India

[41] Indian J Pediatr. 2012 Feb 1. [Epub ahead of print] Brain Tumors in Children- Current Therapies and Newer Directions. Khatua S, Sadighi ZS, Pearlman ML, Bochare S, Vats TS. Source Division of Pediatric Neurooncology, Department of Pediatrics, Children's Cancer Hospital, MD Anderson Cancer Center, 1515 Holcombe Boulevard, Unit 87, Houston, TX, 77030, USA

One study published in January 2012 revealed the pathway that Curcumin (the Indian spice AKA turmeric) utilizes blocks inflammation and induces apoptosis (programmed cell death, necessary to stop cancer.)[42] I'm willing to bet that your oncologist didn't refer to this study when he recommended this nutrient.

Even studies that reveal possible causes of cancers seem ignored. An October, 2011 study revealed the astonishing fact repeated by alternative practitioners for decades, "that a large proportion of primary medulloblastomas and medulloblastoma cell lines are infected with HCMV and that COX-2 expression, along with PGE2 levels, in tumors is directly modulated by the virus."[43]

That's crazy! Why hasn't the oncological community jumped on this and begun recommending anti-viral nutritional protocol? Is it possible that this study was overlooked because there are no anti-viral drugs worth using? Is it in the least bit contraindicative to bombard an immune system with destructive chemotherapy if you know you will be creating an enormous opportunity for the virus to replicate uninhibited?

Not to get too technical in this book, but there are many other studies that reveal information that make excessive use of chemotherapy contraindicative:

---

[42] BMC Cancer. 2012 Jan 26;12:44. Anaphase-promoting complex/cyclosome protein dc27 is a target for curcumin-induced cell cycle arrest and apoptosis. Lee SJ, Langhans SA. Source Nemours/Alfred I, duPont Hospital for Children, Wilmington, DE 19803, USA
[43] J Clin Invest. 2011 Oct;121(10):4043-55. doi: 10.1172/JCI57147. Epub 2011 Sep 26. Detection of human cytomegalovirus in medulloblastomas reveals a potential therapeutic target. Baryawno N, Rahbar A, Wolmer-Solberg N, Taher C, Odeberg J, Darabi A, Khan Z, Sveinbjörnsson B, FuskevÅg OM, Segerström L, Nordenskjöld M, Siesjö P, Kogner P, Johnsen JI, Söderberg-Nauclér C. Source Karolinska Institutet, Department of Women's and Children's Health, Childhood Cancer Research Unit, Stockholm, Sweden

- A 2011 study[44] proves that a Th2 chemokine (a chemical produced in a hyper Th2 response which is the response the immune system is *stuck* in if suppressed.)

- An upregulation of chemicals that increase cell replication necessary in growth and healing but **not** desired in cancer are stimulated by a suppressed immune system. Transcription factor Forkhead box M1 (FoxM1) is one of these "stimulators of cell division" that a healthy immune system keeps at bay. If your immune system is suppressed (like in aggressive chemotherapy usage) transcription (cell growth and replication) is less uninhibited! This is just one reason that chemo, though it can kill a growth tumor, also causes cancer growth![45]

- MicroRNA-21, an oncogene that is up regulated in a variety of cancers increases cancer growth, which is stimulated by a high sugar diet and a suppressed

---

[44] Mol Cancer. 2011 Sep 24;10:121. A MCP1 fusokine with CCR2-specific tumoricidal activity. Rafei M, Deng J, Boivin MN, Williams P, Matulis SM, Yuan S, Birman E, Forner K, Yuan L, Castellino C, Boise LH, MacDonald TJ, Galipeau J. Source The Montreal Center for Experimental Therapeutics in Cancer, McGill University, Montreal, Canada

[45] J Biol Chem. 2011 Jul 22;286(29):25586-603. Epub 2011 May 25. MicroRNA-21 orchestrates high glucose-induced signals to TOR complex 1, resulting in renal cell pathology in diabetes. Dey N, Das F, Mariappan MM, Mandal CC, Ghosh-Choudhury N, Kasinath BS, Choudhury GG. Source Veterans Affairs Research, South Texas Veterans Health Care System, San Antonio, Texas, USA

immune response.[45 46 47]

- Other oncogenes (genes that, when upregulated, increase cancer growth) and apoptotic pathways are

---

[46] Eur J Cancer. 2011 Nov;47(16):2479-90. doi: 10.1016/j.ejca.2011.06.041. Epub 2011 Jul 19. MicroRNA-21 suppression impedes medulloblastoma cell migration. Grunder E, D'Ambrosio R, Fiaschetti G, Abela L, Arcaro A, Zuzak T, Ohgaki H, Lv SQ, Shalaby T, Grotzer M. Source Oncology Department, University Children's Hospital of Zurich, Switzerland

[47] Brain Pathol. 2012 Mar;22(2):230-9. doi: 10.1111/j.1750-3639.2011.00523.x. Epub 2011 Sep 15. Genetic alterations in microRNAs in medulloblastomas. Lv SQ, Kim YH, Giulio F, Shalaby T, Nobusawa S, Yang H, Zhou Z, Grotzer M, Ohgaki H. Source - International Agency for Research on Cancer (IARC), Lyon, France Neuro-Oncology Program, University Children's Hospital of Zurich, Switzerland

possibly affected by excessive chemotherapy use[48] [49] [50]
[51] [52] [53] [54] [55] [56] [57] [58] [59] [60]

---

[48] Grotzer MA, Janss AJ, Fung K, et al: Trkc expression predicts good clinical outcome in primitive neuroectodermal brain tumors. J Clin Oncol 18:1027-1035, 2000

[49] Pomeroy SL, Tamayo P, Gaasenbeek M, et al: Prediction of central nervous system embryonal tumor outcome based on gene expression. Nature 415:436-442, 2002

[50] Segal RA, Goumnerova LC, Kwon YK, et al: Expression of the neurotrophin receptor trkc is linked to a favorable outcome in medulloblastoma. Proc Natl Acad Sci U S A 91:12867-12871, 1994

[51] MacDonald TJ, Rood BR, Santi MR, et al: Advances in the diagnosis, molecular genetics, and treatment of pediatric embryonal CNS tumors. On- cologist 8:174-186, 2003

[52] Gilbertson RJ, Pearson AD, Perry RH, et al: Prognostic significance of the c-erbb-2 oncogene product in childhood medulloblastoma. Br J Cancer 71:473-477, 1995

[53] MacDonald TJ, Brown KM, LaFleur B, et al: Expression profiling of medulloblastoma: PDGFRA and the RAS/MAPK pathway as therapeutic targets for metastatic disease. Nat Genet 29:143-152, 2001

[54] Grotzer MA, Hogarty MD, Janss AJ, et al: Myc messenger RNA expression predicts survival outcome in childhood primitive neuroectodermal tumor/medulloblastoma. Clin Cancer Res 7:2425-2433, 2001

[55] Rood BR, Zhang H, Weitman DM, et al: Hypermethylation of Hic-1 and 17p allelic loss in medulloblastoma. Cancer Res 62:3794-3797, 2002

[56] Gajjar A, Hernan R, Kocak M, et al: Clinical, histopathologic, and molecular markers of prognosis: Toward a new disease risk stratification system for medulloblastoma. J Clin Oncol 22:984-993, 2004

[57] Lamont JM, McManamy CS, Pearson AD, et al: Combined histopathological and molecular cytogenetic stratification of medulloblastoma patients. Clin Cancer Res 10:5482-5493, 2004

[58] Herms J, Neidt I, Luscher B, et al: C-MYC expression in medulloblastoma and its prognostic value. Int J Cancer (Pred Oncol) 89:395-402, 2000

[59] Ray AM, Ho M, Ma J, et al: A clinicobiological model predicting survival in medulloblastoma. Clin Cancer Res 10:7613-7620, 2004

[60] Eberhart CG, Kratz J, Wang Y, et al: Histopathological and molecular prognostic markers in medulloblastoma: C-myc, N-myc, TrkC, and Anaplasia. J Neuropathol Exp Neurol 63:441-449, 2004

- Other studies showing that novel, natural alternatives to chemotherapy exist.[61] [62] [63] [64] Unfortunately, unless pharmaceutical companies can create patented medications from them, don't expect to hear about them soon.

Many studies openly reveal the inadequacies of current treatment protocols:

- *"The 5-year EFS for patients receiving standard-dose irradiation is suboptimal,* and improved techniques and/or therapies are needed to improve ultimate outcome. Chemotherapy may contribute to this

---

[61] Mol Neurobiol. 2011 Dec;44(3):223-34. Epub 2011 Jul 8. MicroRNAs in brain tumors : a new diagnostic and therapeutic perspective? Hummel R, Maurer J, Haier J. Source Department of General and Visceral Surgery, University of Muenster, Waldeyerstrasse 1, Muenster, Germany
[62] J Neurooncol. 2012 Jan;106(1):59-70. Epub 2011 Jul 7. Norcantharidin impairs medulloblastoma growth by inhibition of Wnt/β-catenin signaling. Cimmino F, Scoppettuolo MN, Carotenuto M, De Antonellis P, Dato VD, De Vita G, Zollo M. Source - CEINGE, Centro di Ingegneria Genetica, Biotecnologie Avanzate, Via Gaetano Salvatore 486, 80145 Naples, Italy
[63] Evidence-Based Complementary and Alternative MedicineVolume 2012 (2012), Article ID 154271, 4 pagesdoi:10.1155/2012/154271 Research Article Norcantharidin Induces HL-60 Cells Apoptosis In Vitro You-Ming Jiang,1 Zhen-Zhi Meng,1 Guang-Xin Yue,2 and Jia-Xu Chen1,3 1School of Pre-Clinical Medicine, Beijing University of Chinese Medicine, Beijing 100029, China2Institute of Basic Theory of TCM, China Academy of Chinese Medical Sciences, P.O. Box 83, Beijing 100700, China3Department of Basic Theory in Chinese Medicine, Henan University of Traditional Chinese Medicine, Zhengzhou 450008, China Received 29 February 2012; Revised 3 May 2012; Accepted 3 May 2012
[64] J Ethnopharmacol. 1989 Sep;26(2):147-62. Medical uses of mylabris in ancient China and recent studies. Wang GS. Source Institute of Pharmacy, Beijing Fourth Pharmaceutical Works, China

improvement."[65]

- "The addition of chemotherapy to standard radiotherapy improves the rate and length of disease-free survival for those children with MB/PNET *who have the most extensive tumors at diagnosis. It remains to be determined which drug or drug combinations are the most effective in MB/PNET, and which patients are most likely to benefit from chemotherapy.*"[66]

- "After 3600 cGy of radiation therapy, children <7 years of age at the time of diagnosis have declines in *overall intelligence of between 20 and 30 points within three years of the completion of radiation therapy.*"[67]

- Later the same study admits, *"It is also increasingly clear that long- term survivors of medulloblastoma may have difficulties in organization and attention, and such "executive" function disabilities will greatly impair learning. Most children <7 years of age with medulloblastoma who are treated with surgery and radiation will require special education placement, and a significant number of older children will also need some type of classroom help."*

- Oncologists readily use studies done on patients included under specific criteria and use them to *prove* the benefits for everyone. In one patient's case the

---

[65] Thomas PR, Deutsch M, Kepner JL, et al: Low-stage medulloblastoma: Final analysis of trial Comparing standard-dose with reduced-dose neuroaxis irradiation. J Clin Oncol 18:3004-3011, 2000www.jco.org 4207 Information downloaded from jco.ascopubs.org and provided by at UNIV MINNESOTA on February 1, 2012 from Copyright © 2006 American So1c6ie0t.y94o.f4C5l.i1n5ic6al Oncology. J Clin Oncol. 2000 Aug;18(16):3004-11

[66] Packer RJ: Chemotherapy for medulloblastoma/primitive neuroectodermal tumors of the posterior fossa. Ann Neurol 28:823-828, 1990

[67] Packer RJ, Cogen P, Vezina G, et al: Medulloblastoma: Clinical and biologic aspects. Neuro Oncol 1:232-250, 1999

study that the oncologist handed me to *prove* her position on continued chemotherapy stated, *"To be eligible for study entry, patients had to be older than 18 months of age at diagnosis and have a subtotal resection, evidence of metastatic disease, and/or brainstem involvement."*[68] Our patient **would not have been eligible for the study**! She had **no** evidence of metastatic disease, was considered to have had a total resection (not subtotal), and **no** brainstem involvement. Yet, she is being recommended for the same care **based** on this study!

- I later checked the citings of the "proof study" to find that it referenced studies clearly stating that chemo should be recommended in high risk MB (which our patient was **not**), "In the past two decades, chemotherapy has proven to be an increasingly more effective modality in the treatment of medulloblastoma. Current evidence suggests that chemotherapy be included as part of standard treatment for all patients *with high-risk medulloblastoma."*[69]

- It even referenced a study that proved, *"There was no statistically significant difference in 3-year and 5-year OS between the two arms"* (OS = Overall Survival and the two arms being two groups in the study, one with radiation

---

[68] Packer RJ, Sutton LN, Elterman R, et al: Outcome for children with medulloblastoma treated with radiation and cisplatin, CCNU, and vincristine chemotherapy. J Neurosurg 81:690-698, 1994 Outcome for children with medulloblastoma treated with radiation and cisplatin, CCNU, and vincristine chemotherapy. Packer RJ, Sutton LN, Elterman R, Lange B, Goldwein J, Nicholson HS, Mulne L, Boyett J, D'Angio G, Wechsler-Jentzsch K, et al. Source Division of Neurology, Children's National Medical Center, George Washington University, Washington, DC

[69] Friedman HS, Schold SC: Rational approaches to the chemotherapy of medulloblastoma. Neurol Clin 3:843-854, 1985

alone and one with chemotherapy plus radiation)[70]

- *"The 2-year results of this study suggest that children with brain tumors treated with CRT are cognitively impaired and that these deficits worsen over time. The younger the child is at the time of treatment, the greater is the likelihood and severity of damage. These children, although not retarded, have a multitude of neurocognitive deficits which detrimentally affects school performance. New treatment strategies are needed for children with malignant brain tumors."*[71]

- *"This study represents the largest series of patients with average-risk MB/PNETs treated with a combination of reduced-dose RT and adjuvant chemotherapy whose intellectual development has been followed prospectively. Intellectual loss was substantial but suggestive of some degree of intellectual preservation compared with effects associated with conventional RT doses.* However, this conclusion remains provisional, pending further research."[72]

- "In the past two decades, chemotherapy has proven to be an increasingly more effective modality in the treatment of medulloblastoma. Current evidence suggests that chemotherapy be included as part of standard treatment for all patients *with high-risk medulloblastoma.*"

---

[70] Taylor RE, Bailey CC, Robinson K, et al: Results of a randomized study of preradiation chemotherapy versus radiotherapy alone for nonmetastatic medulloblastoma: The International Society of Paediatric Oncology/United Kingdom Children's Cancer study group PNET-3 study. J Clin Oncol 21:1581- 1591, 2003

[71] Packer RJ, Sutton LN, Atkins TE, et al: A prospective study of cognitive function in children receiving whole-brain radiotherapy and chemotherapy: 2-year results. J Neurosurg 70:707-713, 1989

[72] Ris MD, Packer R, Goldwein J, et al: Intellectual outcome after reduced-dose radiation therapy plus adjuvant chemotherapy for medulloblastoma: A Children's Cancer Group study. J Clin Oncol 19: 3470-3476, 2001

- The German Society of Pediatric Hematology and Oncology (GPOH) conducted a randomized, prospective, multicenter trial (HIT '91) *"in order to improve the survival of children with medulloblastoma by using postoperative neoadjuvant chemotherapy before radiation therapy as opposed to maintenance chemotherapy after immediate postoperative radiotherapy."*[73]

- *"Reduced-dose craniospinal radiation therapy can be proposed in standard-risk medulloblastoma provided staging and radiation therapy are performed under optimal conditions."*[74]

What *Is* Clear

One thing we *do* know as we investigate all the existing data on Medulloblastoma is this: we have a long way to go before we know everything! This is exactly the point. You cannot argue that continued excellence in surgical procedures is a major contributor to greater treatment success and that some chemotherapy and radiation may be necessary in this aggressive cancer. You also cannot rule out both the need for and the efficacy of an alternative, natural approach. For an oncologist to force the parents of a child into their protocol because, "the research supports it," is ludicrous. There is *no* research that supports the traditional approach of chemo and radiation and then maintenance chemotherapy to be *any* more effective than a natural protocol following radiation. Why? Because it simply doesn't exist!

---

[73] Kortmann RD, Kuhl J, Timmermann B, et al: Postoperative neoadjuvant chemotherapy before radiotherapy as compared to immediate radiotherapy followed by maintenance chemotherapy in the treatment of medulloblastoma in childhood: Results of the German prospective randomized trial HIT '91. Int J Radiat Oncol Biol Phys 46:269-279, 2000

[74] Oyharcabal-Bourden V, Kalifa C, Gentet JC, et al: Standard-risk medulloblastoma treated by adjuvant chemotherapy followed by reduced-dose craniopsinal radiation therapy: A French Society of Pediatric Oncology study. J Clin Oncol 22:4726- 4734, 2005

What **can** we say? Is it wrong to recommend maintenance chemo? No. Is it wrong to make it illegal to try something else? Yes. Chemotherapy can kill as easily as it can save, so let's stop pretending anything else!

Again, I'm **not** trying to be negative to standards of care, chemotherapy, radiation, or surgery. I am pointing out the Orwellian system that already exists in the heavily egocentric profession we call medicine.

More Studies

In the previous version of this book I listed numerous studies that supported an alternative approach to cancer. To conserve space so I could add new content, I've omitted this and simply point you to our website where many of these are listed:

> ConnersClinic.com/alternative-cancer-treatment-case-studies

Are We Really Getting the Truth?

In 1986 McGill Cancer Center scientists surveyed 118 oncologists who specialized in lung cancer. They were asked if they would take chemo if they developed lung cancer. Three-quarters replied that they **would not take chemo**.[75] Although 1986 seems like a long time ago, chemo drugs have changed very little since then, if at all.

In 1984 an unusual convention of doctors was held in Chicago. Nine eminent physicians from across the United States spoke to an auditorium packed with colleagues. The conference, entitled "Dissent in Medicine" was to discuss the

---

[75] "Reclaiming Our Health" by John Robbins, 1996. Published by HJ Kramer, Box 1082, Tiburon, CA 94920

propensity of the nation's medical hierarchy to propagate half-truths. Among the speakers was Alan S. Levin, M.D., professor of immunology at the University of California, San Francisco, Medical School, who stated that "Practicing physicians are intimidated into using regimes which they know do not work. One of the most glaring examples is chemotherapy, which does not work for the majority of cancers."

Ulrich Abel was a German epidemiologist and biostatistician. In the eighties, he contacted over 350 medical centers around the world requesting them to furnish him with anything they had published on the subject of cancer. By the time he published his report and subsequent book[76] he may well have known more about chemotherapy than any other person.

His report, later reviewed by the German Magazine *Der Spiegel* in 1990 and summarized by Ralph Moss in an article entitled "Chemo's *Berlin Wall* Crumbles,"[77] described chemotherapy as a "scientific wasteland" and that neither physician nor patient were willing to give it up even though there was no scientific evidence that it worked:

"Success of most chemotherapies is appalling...There is no scientific evidence for its ability to extend in any appreciable way the lives of patients suffering from the most common organic cancer... Chemotherapy for malignancies too advanced for surgery, which accounts for 80% of all cancers, is a scientific wasteland." – Dr. Uhlrich Abel

Let's hear from a couple of physicians and doctors who have not yet succumbed to the heavy hand of the cancer industry:

"...as a chemist trained to interpret data, it is incomprehensible to me that physicians can ignore the clear evidence that chemotherapy does much, much more harm than good." – Alan C Nixon, PhD, former president of the American Chemical Society.

---

[76] "Chemotherapy of Advanced Epithelial Cancer", Stuttgart: Hippokrates Verlag GmbH, 1990
[77] Cancer Chronicles, Dec 1990, p.4

Walter Last, writing in The Ecologist, reported recently: *"After analyzing cancer survival statistics for several decades, Dr. Hardin Jones, Professor at the University of California, concluded '...patients are as well or better off untreated.' Jones' disturbing assessment has never been refuted."*

Professor Charles Mathe declared: *"If I contracted cancer, I would never go to a standard cancer treatment center. Cancer victims who live far from such centers have a chance."*

"Many medical oncologists recommend chemotherapy for virtually any tumor, with a hopefulness undiscouraged by almost invariable failure," – Albert Braverman MD.[78]

"Most cancer patients in this country die of chemotherapy. Chemotherapy does not eliminate breast, colon, or lung cancers. This fact has been documented for over a decade, yet doctors still use chemotherapy for these tumors," – Dr. Allen Levin, MD UCSF, *The Healing of Cancer.*

"Despite widespread use of chemotherapies, breast cancer mortality has not changed in the last 70 years," – Thomas Dao, MD[79]

Alternative Therapies science journal recently published two articles showing that since the 1970's, 280 peer-reviewed studies, 50 of which were human studies involving 8,521 patients, have consistently shown that natural treatments containing antioxidants and other nutrients do not interfere with other therapeutic treatments, such as traditional chemo and radiation.[80] [81] In fact, not only do they not interfere, the research has shown that these natural treatments can actually

---

[78] 1991 Lancet 1991 337 p901 Medical Oncology in the 90s

[79] NEJM Mar 1975 292 p 707

[80] Simone, C.B., et al. Antioxidants and Other Nutrients Do Not Interfere with Chemotherapy or Radiation Therapy and Can Increase Kill and Increase Survival, Part I. Alternative Therapies. 2007 Jan/Feb; 13(1): 22-28

[81] Simone, C.B., et al. Antioxidants and Other Nutrients Do Not Interfere with Chemotherapy or Radiation Therapy and Can Increase Kill and Increase Survival, Part II. Alternative Therapies. 2007 Mar/Apr; 13(2): 40-47

enhance the therapeutic effects of other treatments, while decreasing side effects and protecting normal tissue.[80] [81] Furthermore, in 15 human studies, 3,738 patients who took natural treatments actually had increased survival times.[80] [81]

The joke, of course, is that the same oncologists who pontificate on the dangers of natural treatments also prescribe amifostine and dexrazoxane, two prescription antioxidants generally used during chemo and radiation treatments. Amifostine is owned by MedImmune and dexrazoxane (Zinecard) is owned by Pfizer; both put a particular spin on natural antioxidants so they can be labeled and sold as prescriptions. Both these pharmaceutical companies rank in the list of some of the largest: MedImmune reported $1.5 billion in revenue in 2005, it was bought by AstraZeneca for $15.6 billion in 2007; Pfizer reported $48 billion in revenue in 2007 and $68 billion in 2010, and is consistently ranked in the top 7 biggest pharmaceutical companies in the world. Traditional oncology has to get its story straight. Either natural treatments are bad, or, they are a huge support and provide major benefits for patients undergoing traditional chemo and radiation.

Tamoxifen and Breast Cancer

Another example of distortion is an Oxford University study published in The Lancet which touts the effectiveness of today's conventional cancer treatments. It supports the use of chemotherapy and states that women who used tamoxifen for five years reduced the breast cancer death rate by one-third. *Really??* This story was picked up by many newspapers and got wide distribution. However, if you look closely at the statistics, you find that your odds of getting breast cancer without using tamoxifen is 1.3%, and with tamoxifen it drops to .68%. That represents a 49% difference between the two numbers (as cited), but just a little over one-half of one-percent difference (.62%) in real terms. This is a prime example of how drug companies manipulate statistics! One half percent in real world terms is vastly different from the 49% improvement stated in the studies, and hardly worth this risk:

- Tamoxifen can cause cancer of the uterus, ovaries, and gastrointestinal tract while it reduces the risk by .62% (that's **point** 62%, **not** 62%, .62%!!) Talk about quackery! These are the same criminals that control the FDA and shut-down natural health clinics for false advertising! Is this really a whole lot different than Nazi Germany's propaganda campaign of the 1930's and 1940's?

- A study at Johns Hopkins found that tamoxifen promotes liver cancer, and other studies have shown it produces a risk of other cancers including endometrial. Though the risk is small, it still exists.[82]

- In 1996, a division of the World Health Organization, the International Agency for Research on Cancer, declared tamoxifen a Group I carcinogen.

- In an abruptly curtailed NCI study, 33 women that took tamoxifen developed endometrial cancer, 17 suffered blood clots in the lungs, 130 developed deep vein thrombosis (blood clots in major blood vessels) and many experienced confusion, depression, and memory loss.

- In 2014, the American College of Obstetricians and Gynecologists released an opinion letter that recommended **not** using Tamoxifen in patients with various stipulations, including those with atypical endometrial hyperplasia, noting the risk of endometrial cancer.[83]

---

[82] https://www.ncbi.nlm.nih.gov/pubmed/9469370
[83] https://www.acog.org/clinical/clinical-guidance/committee-opinion/articles/2014/06/tamoxifen-and-uterine-cancer

The point isn't that Tamoxifen should never be used, nor is it that Tamoxifen is a bad drug. The point is that we don't always receive the *full story* behind these "miracle drugs."

Again, choose wisely.

Taxol Spreads Breast Cancer?

Taxol (paclitaxel) is often called the "gold standard of chemo." The following report gives you a good idea of the dangers of even the best chemo.

As reported at the 27th Annual San Antonio Breast Cancer Symposium, Dec 2004, (abstract 6014), using a technique that quantifies circulating tumor cells, German investigators from Friedrich-Schiller University in Jena, have shown that neoadjuvant chemotherapy with paclitaxel (Taxol) causes a massive release of tumor cells into the circulation (measured as *circulating tumor cells* or CTC's), while at the same time reducing the size of the tumor. The finding could help explain the fact that complete pathologic responses do not correlate well with improvements in survival. Let me think, should we shrink the original tumor but spew millions of CTC's all over the body at the same time? You decide.

In one study, according to Katharina Pachmann, M.D., professor of experimental oncology and hematology, breast cancer patients undergoing neoadjuvant chemotherapy gave blood samples in which epithelial, antigen-positive cells were isolated. Such cells are detected in most breast cancer patients but are rarely found in normal subjects. The investigators measured the levels of circulating tumor cells (CTC's) before and during primary chemotherapy with several different cytotoxic agents.

Paclitaxel (Taxol) produced the greatest degree of tumor shrinkage but also the greatest release of circulating tumor cells. In three different paclitaxel-containing regimens, circulating cell numbers massively increased, whereas tumor size decreased. These cells remained in the circulation for at least five months after surgery.

The tumor shrinks, but more cells are found in the circulation. This corresponds with a high pathologic complete response during paclitaxel treatment, but in the end, this is not reflected in improved survival. These cells are alive in the circulation and can easily *settle* somewhere else; called metastasis, the deadliest of all cancers.

A 2018 study confirmed the pro-metastatic effects of chemotherapy. An international team of scientists led by Michele De Palma at EPFL has shed new light into this process. Working with experimental tumor models, the researchers found that two chemotherapy drugs frequently used for patients, paclitaxel and doxorubicin, induce mammary tumors to release small vesicles called exosomes. Under chemotherapy, the exosomes contain the protein annexin-A6, which is not present in the exosomes released from untreated tumors. "It seems that loading of annexin-A6 into exosomes is significantly enhanced in response to chemotherapy," explains Ioanna Keklikoglou, first author of the study.

After being released from a chemotherapy-treated tumor, like breast cancer, the exosomes circulate in the blood. Upon reaching the lung, the exosomes release their content, including annexin-A6. This stimulates the lung cells to release another protein, CCL2, which attracts immune cells called monocytes.

This immune reaction (the spike in monocytes) can be dangerous, as previous studies have shown that monocytes can facilitate the survival and growth of cancerous cells in the lung, which is one of the initial steps in metastasis. "In short, our study has identified a new link between chemotherapy and breast cancer metastasis," says De Palma.

Again, is Taxol always a bad idea? I don't think so. But, let's stop talking about it (as well as other chemotherapy drugs) as the gold standard and the **only** way to treat cancer. It comes with risks! Not only is there a good chance that it won't work, there's a good chance that it will make you **worse**. There's also more than a good chance that it will make you really sick and leave you with an extremely suppressed immune system.

I'm just asking for the **whole truth**!

5-FU (a common chemo drug) and Colon Cancer

The conclusion of a long-term research project by the National Surgical Adjuvant Breast and Bowel Project (NSABP) was published in the August 4, 2004 edition of the *Journal of the National Cancer Institute*. The new study throws doubt on the value of the MOF regimen which uses 5-FU, the most common anti-colon cancer agent used by conventional medicine. 5-FU is "moderately effective at shrinking existing tumors, but the effect is almost always temporary."

A 2010 study revealed that 5-FU has serious detrimental effects on healthy brain cells stating, "Thus, 5-FU appears to have a lasting negative impact on cognition and to affect cellular and biochemical markers in various brain regions."[84]

Sonia Amin Thomas has written an excellent article on the adverse effects of 5-FU published in Cancer Cell & Microenvironment, 2016.[85]

If these facts are known, then why do doctors turn so quickly to these harsh drugs?

---

[84] https://www.ncbi.nlm.nih.gov/pubmed/20738018
[85] Sonia Amin Thomas, et al. Adverse effects of 5-fluorouracil: focus on rare side effects. Can Cell Microenviron 2016; 3: e1266. doi: 10.14800/ccm.1266

Here's an article I wrote for my *Doctor's Only* newsletter:

The Aging Effects of Chemotherapy

Does chemotherapy have long-term side effects beyond the known immediate toxicity? Though most patients never get a chance to consider, let alone voice a concern over long-term side-effects of chemo as they get herded through the traditional oncological procedures, new studies suggest they exist. Depending on the regimen of chemotherapy chosen, potential long-term adverse effects include premature menopause, cognitive impairment, cardiovascular and neuromuscular toxicity, and secondary malignancies as the chemo may kill rapidly replicating cells but then leaves circulating tumors cells to thrive. Recently, two groups of investigators have studied whether premature aging is also a possible effect.

Sanoff and colleagues[86] cite evidence that "adjuvant chemotherapy may confer effects consistent with molecular aging of 10 to 15 years in breast cancer patients." The observed cellular senescence is due to the drugs activation of INK4/ARF locus on chromosome 9p21.3, which codes for the tumor-suppressor proteins p16INK41 and ARF in peripheral blood T cells. Studies have also shown that other markers of aging, including decreased leukocyte telomere length (LTL) and expression of senescence-associated cytokines such as interleukin 6 are present in a much higher degree post-chemo.[87]

Post-chemo expression of p16INK4a and ARF corresponds to an almost 15-year chronological aging in the hematologic compartment, specifically CD3+ lymphocytes. The

---

[86] Sanoff HK et al. J Natl Cancer Inst 2014 Mar 28. Duggan C. J Natl Cancer Inst 2014 Mar 13

[87] THE FRANZ BUSCHKE LECTURE: LATE EFFECTS OF CHEMOTHERAPY AND RADIATION THERAPY: A NEW HYPOTHESIS PHILIP RUBIN, M.D. Chairman, Division of Radiation Oncology, University of Rochester Cancer Center, Rochester, NY 14642

senescence-associated cytokines VEGFA (vascular endothelial growth factor A) and monocyte chemotactic protein-1 were also persistently elevated with adjuvant chemotherapy.

Understand, chemotherapy has three main applications. It is thought to be curative for only a small number of malignancies including childhood leukemia, Hodgkin's and non-Hodgkin's lymphoma. It has a palliative role for most metastatic epithelial malignancies. Finally, it is used in an adjuvant role in several types of epithelial malignancies particularly breast cancer. First employed in the mid 1970s, adjuvant chemotherapy has been associated with up to a 30% relative improvement in long-term overall survival in high risk breast cancer but demonstrates significantly less absolute improvement.

Now that adjuvant chemotherapy is being recommended in nearly every cancer case, both the relative and absolute improvement in overall survival is even less impressive. With a growing number of long-term cancer survivors, we are only now able to define the delayed implications of adjuvant chemotherapy. These long-term side effects include acceleration of neurocognitive decline, musculoskeletal complications such as early onset osteoporosis, premature skin and ocular changes and the most common long-term complaint; mild to profound fatigue. This complex of problems is suggestive of early onset frailty.[88]

If I may offer some suggestions, those exposed to chemotherapy might consider:

- Green Tea Extract (EGCg) at a daily dose of 1500-2500mg. This can help promote osteoblastic activity and decrease overall IL-6 levels.

---

[88] Possible acceleration of aging by adjuvant chemotherapy: A cause of early onset frailty? Ronald Eric Maccormick, Medical Hypotheses, Volume 67, Issue 2, 2006, Pages 212–215

- Resveratrol at a dose of 10-20mg TID. Don't be fooled into believing that drinking a glass or two of red wine supplies your resveratrol needs. A fluid ounce of red wine averages around 90 micrograms of resveratrol. The studies on resveratrol supplementation suggest 20mg (20,000mcg) of resveratrol is needed to positively affect aging. Therefore, 20mg resveratrol provides approximately 220 times the amount of resveratrol found in one fluid ounce of red wine. Since a glass of wine is approximately 5 and 1/3 ounces, a person taking one 20mg resveratrol supplement may ingest the equivalent amount of resveratrol found in 41 glasses of red wine. Needless to say, that is a lot of red wine and no one needs the alcohol. When reversing the telomere decay from the effects of chemotherapy, I suggest a higher dose of resveratrol and throughout the day. Since resveratrol has a very short half-life in the body, it is very necessary to spread out the dosage over time.

- Liver pathway support. It is essential to support methylation and other detoxification pathways. There are numerous good products on the market available to do so and I suggest you keep patients on something for this for life.

- Decrease brain inflammation. We use a product we've developed that we call BAM (Brain Anti-inflammatory Mix) but generally you want to use herbs such as Ginkgo, Turmeric, Boswelia, White Willow Bark, Ginger Root, Nettle Root Extract, Arnica Extract, and Celery seed. You can add Bacopa to this list as well as ALA, NAC, etc.

- Heal the barriers (gut and brain) with appropriate nutrition and diet.

- Decrease any other inflammatory causes.

Well, once again, I hope this helps!

Does Our Medicare System Encourage Fraud?

From *Cure Your Cancer* by Bill Henderson (another book I highly recommend):

"Our government's Medicare system encourages the fraud and abuse that is rampant among oncologists. For example, the chemotherapy drug Etoposide is sold wholesale to oncologists for $7.50 for a 100mg dose. The allowable Medicare reimbursement, however, is $129.34 per dose. The consumer (you and I) pay a co-payment of $25.87; almost three and a half times the doctor's cost! Medicare pays the rest from our tax dollars.

See the 2013 "monthly cost sheet" from Sloan Kettering.[89]

According to the *Journal of the American Medical Association* (*JAMA*), the average oncologist makes $253,000 a year ($259,000 according to the website Payscale.) Of this, 75% is profit on chemotherapy drugs administered in his or her office. All of these drugs, like Tamoxifen and Etoposide, treat the symptoms of cancer, not its causes.

A recent survey of the 64 oncologists working at the McGill Cancer Therapy Center in Montreal, Canada found that 58 of them (91%) said they would not take chemotherapy or allow their family members to take it for cancer treatment. Why? Too toxic and not effective."

---

[89]

https://www.mskcc.org/sites/default/files/node/25097/documents/chemo-prices-table-bach-center-health-policy-and-outcomes-6-13-14.pdf

People are Waking Up

In the Seattle Post-Intelligencer article of September 5, 2002, entitled, "Many cancer patients getting relief from alternative treatments, study shows," Carol Smith reported that, "Seven out of 10 adult cancer patients in Western Washington are using alternative therapies…" The survey, done in conjunction with Bastyr University in Kenmore and the Oregon Health & Science University in Portland, was based on interviews with 356 patients who had breast, prostate, or colon cancer.

A 2018 article published in Current Oncology stated, "Cancer patients are increasingly seeking out complementary and alternative medicine (cam) and might be reluctant to disclose its use to their oncology treatment team."

Data from the Centers for Disease Control and Prevention's National Health Interview survey of more than 3,100 cancer patients revealed that one-third of people with a cancer diagnosis use complementary and alternative medicines (CAM) such as herbal supplements, meditation, yoga, and acupuncture. Though standard medicine sees this as a "dangerous trend," it suggests that people are beginning to wake up to the facts.

From Physician and Author Dr. Cynthia Foster MD:

"Cytotoxic chemotherapy kills cancer cells by way of a certain mechanism called 'First Order Kinetics.' This simply means that the drug does not kill a constant number of cells, but a constant proportion of cells. So, for example, a certain drug will kill 1/2 of all the cancer cells, then 1/2 of what is left, and then 1/2 of that, and so on. So, we can see that not every cancer cell necessarily is going to be killed. This is important because chemotherapy is not going to kill every cancer cell in the body. The body has to kill the cancer cells that are left over after the chemotherapy is finished. This fact is well known by oncologists. Now, how can cancer patients possibly fight even a few cancer cells when their immune systems have been disabled and this is yet another stress on the body, and they're bleeding because they have hardly any platelets left from the toxic effects of the chemotherapy? This is usually why, when chemotherapy is stopped, the cancer grows again and gets out of control. We have now created a vicious cycle, where doctors are trying to kill the cancer cells, and the patient is not able to fight the rest, so the doctors have to give the chemotherapy again, and then the patient can't fight the rest of the cancer cell, and then the doctors give the chemotherapy again, and so on."

A patient using *Protocel*, one of our alternative cancer therapies, wrote, "The radiologist who read my recent breast ultrasound says 'it' (my original grape-size tumor) is shrinking, seeing only a 'distal acoustic shadowing' as opposed to the original 'organized mass.' The technician commented to me, 'How do they expect us to get images of something we can't see (anymore)?'

Cancer is scary, make no bones about it. Hearing the "C" word can send chills down your spine. But take heart! There is **always** *time to make rational (not emotional) decisions about your care. There are* **always** *choices other than chemo or radiation for those willing to search and do a little study.*

Integrative Cancer Therapy is what we are all about; this means a collaborative approach where we work alongside your oncologist to give the cancer patient the greatest hope. Check out our website on cancer/detoxification and the testimonials of cancer patients. You'll find that we care for people, we don't treat cancer; we search for causes, we don't treat symptoms; we don't kill cancer, we help your body heal itself. My AMA Fellowship in Integrative Cancer Therapy gives me connections with the country's best minds in alternative solutions.

"There are no studies that prove alternative therapies..." Or, Are There?

For those that claim alternative approaches lack objective data to support them, this just is **not** true. Anyone with a computer can Google, "_____ and cancer" while filling in the blank with whatever approach they are looking at (Curcumin, Artemesinin, Astragalus, would be some examples) and they could wade through the sites that *slam* such an approach to find peer-reviewed, published studies on most of the herbal *cures*.

Below are just a ***few*** of these examples:

Triptolide Inhibits Lung Cancer Cell Migration, Invasion, and Metastasis.
https://www.ncbi.nlm.nih.gov/pubmed/26298168

Triptolide Inhibits the Proliferation of Prostate Cancer Cells and Down ...
journals.plos.org/plosone/article?id=10.1371/journal.pone.0037693

Triptolide inhibits the migration and invasion of human prostate cancer ...
www.sciencedirect.com/science/article/pii/S0753332216312008

Targeted treatment of cancer with artemisinin and artemisinin-tagged ...
https://www.ncbi.nlm.nih.gov/pubmed/16185154

Antitumor Activity of Artemisinin and Its Derivatives: From a Well ...
https://www.hindawi.com/journals/bmri/2012/247597/

Oridonin inhibits breast cancer growth and metastasis through ...
www.sciencedirect.com/science/article/pii/S1319016417301019

Proteus mirabilis inhibits cancer growth and pulmonary metastasis in a ...
journals.plos.org/plosone/article?id=10.1371/journal.pone.
0188960

Clove extract inhibits tumor growth and promotes cell cycle arrest and ...
https://www.ncbi.nlm.nih.gov/pubmed/24854101

Astragalus extract inhibits proliferation but enhances apoptosis in ...
https://www.ncbi.nlm.nih.gov/pubmed/27731799

Livistona extract inhibits angiogenesis and cancer growth. - NCBI – NIH
https://www.ncbi.nlm.nih.gov/pubmed/11605065

Green tea (Camellia sinensis) extract inhibits both the metastasis and ...
www.arthroplastyjournal.org/article/S0955-2863(13)00260-
X/fulltext

Should I Do Chemo?

The only person that can answer this question is you! Since I am schooled in an integrative approach to cancer, I do not believe that all chemotherapy is bad. Low-dose chemo and insulin potentiated chemotherapy have shown to be tremendous aides in slowing fast-growing tumors, but remember, chemo does not kill cancer stem cells and can create drug resistant circulating tumor cells. Former White House press secretary Tony Snow died in July 2008 at the age of 53, following a series of chemotherapy treatments for colon cancer. Three years prior to his death, Snow had his colon removed and underwent six months of initial chemotherapy after being diagnosed with colon cancer (remember, chemo does **not** kill cancer stem cells, it only *knocks-down* the current cancer.)

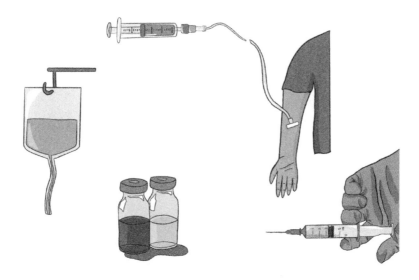

Two years later (2007), Snow's cancer returned (because it was never really gone, the stem cells remained) and he underwent surgery to remove a growth in his abdominal area, near the site of the original cancer. "This is a very treatable condition," said Dr. Allyson Ocean, a gastrointestinal oncologist at Weill Cornell Medical College. "Many patients, because of the therapies we have, are able to work and live full lives with quality while they're being treated. Anyone who looks at this as a death sentence is wrong." But of course, we now know, Dr. Ocean was dead wrong because he *only* looked at traditional methods (chemo, radiation, and surgery) to treat Snow and his other patients.

The media headlines proclaimed that Snow died from colon cancer, although they knew he didn't even have a colon (it was surgically removed in 2005) anymore. As is all too common when the *cause* is not addressed, the malignant cancer had "returned" (from the drug-resistant circulating tumor cells and stem cells) and "spread" to the liver and elsewhere in his body. Now unable to heal the *causes* of the original cancer (in addition to the newly created ones), Snow's body developed new cancers in the liver and other parts of the body, and he was finished.

The mainstream media, of course, still insist Snow died from colon cancer while they ignore the fact that it was really the treatment that killed him. Maybe I should say that it was the *lack of treatment* that killed him. As we (in the cancer world) continue to ignore the truth that cancer is a symptom of a body's inability to manage its environment and think that we are *treating* the patient by *killing the cancer*, bodies will continue to pile up at the door of the morgue.

Is Chemo Right for You?

While making that decision, remember, it is extremely difficult for even the healthiest patient to heal from this condition while being subjected to the systemic poisons of chemotherapy and deadly radiation. If you are bitten by a poisonous snake and don't get an antidote for it, isn't it likely that your body becomes overwhelmed by the poison and, therefore, cannot function anymore?

Before Tony Snow began his chemo treatments for his *second bout* with colon cancer, he still looked healthy and strong. But after a few weeks into his treatment, he started to develop a coarse voice, looked frail, turned gray, and lost his hair. Does this sound familiar? Did the cancer do all this to him? Certainly not! It wasn't the cancer that destroyed Snow's immune system, eroded epithelial tissue, non-selectively destroyed all reproducing tissue, and poisoned his body. It was the chemical toxins we call "therapy" because it's the "best we have to work with." I have no doubt that his doctors were caring individuals trying to make the best decision in an attempt to save Snow's life. If they are heroes, they are fighting the wrong battle.

Do the mainstream media ever report about the overwhelming scientific evidence that shows chemotherapy has zero benefits in the five-year survival rate of colon cancer patients? Or how many oncologists stand up for their cancer patients and protect them against chemotherapy treatment which they very well know can cause them to die far more quickly than if they received no treatment at all? Can you trustingly place your life into their hands when you know that most of them would not even consider chemotherapy for themselves if they were diagnosed with cancer? What do they know that you don't? The news is spreading fast that in the United States physician-caused fatalities now exceed 750,000 each year. Perhaps, many doctors no longer trust in what they practice, for good reasons.

You **must** define the battle you are fighting! There can be a time and place for chemotherapy. If your purpose is to slow down an aggressive cancer so you have time to clean-up the environment that allowed it to flourish, then go for it. If you are seriously taking steps to change your life, your diet, your emotions, your health, then explore low-dose chemo or a less aggressive chemotherapy regimen. If you are putting yourself in the hands of your oncologist and rolling the dice on traditional medicine alone without taking responsibility for the reason the cancer is growing in your body…well I hope you are feeling lucky!

Put it this way: traditional approaches to cancer are optional (and may be the best choice in your case), but the "alternative" approaches like lifestyle changes, dietary changes, Rife, detoxification, and many others are just **not optional**!

Just think about it: how messed up are we in our thinking? Eating right, exercising, proper nutrition, stress management, getting normal nerve flow to the tissues through chiropractic care, massage therapy, colon therapy, physical therapy, herbal therapy, etc., are considered "alternative." For goodness sake, these things are not alternative, secondary choices; they are primary, necessary steps to health. These are the Biblical approaches that should be considered *first*.

Traditional drugging, cutting, and burning should be considered "alternative;" they are un-natural, invasive, and oftentimes inappropriate. Granted, traditional medicine has a large place in our healthcare needs and saves lives in emergency situations every day, but don't go there first.

In adults, a cancer diagnosis means the cells have been multiplying for years to reach the numbers (well over a million cells) to be diagnosed by any means. There is a reason they are not being killed by their immune system, and our first order of events should be attempting to find that reason and change the milieu of the body that has allowed it to grow. Whatever your decision is regarding surgery, chemotherapy, and radiation, make it balanced with doing everything possible to heal your body.

Biblically, we are called to ask for wisdom: "If any of you lacks **wisdom**, let him ask God, who gives generously to all without reproach, and it will be given him." – James 1:5. We **must** take a balanced, unbiased approach to living. I am **not** here to bash traditional care, I'm here to bring balance and encourage you to seek God and His wisdom **first**. Surrendering your will to anyone, whether it's a doctor or a preacher, is wrong. James writes, "But the wisdom from above is first pure, then peaceable, gentle, open to reason, full of mercy and good fruits, impartial and sincere." – James 3:17.

Be open, gentle, pure, impartial, and sincere in the way you seek truth and in the way you make decisions. Don't let anyone **rush** you down a path you are not perfectly clear you should take. **Slow down** and become a student of truth.

I'll be praying for you!

CHAPTER 2

Uncovering Causes

"Truth is generally the best vindication against slander."

– Abraham Lincoln

How Cancer Spreads

When cancer spreads to other areas in the body it is called metastasis and can be the deadliest. But remember, the original cancer cells are growing in an anaerobic (without oxygen) environment. In order to spread, a cancer cell must first detach from the primary cancer and move through the wall of a blood vessel to get into the bloodstream.

These mobile cancer cells are called circulating tumor cells (CTC's) or cancer stem cells and look a little like speculated burrs not unlike the burrs you may find on you pant legs after a walk through the meadow, only microscopic.

When CTC's enter the bloodstream, the circulating blood sweeps them along until they stick somewhere, usually in another opportunistic position that enables it to lodge and multiply.

This can be a complicated journey but as long as the host (the patient) has done little to strengthen their immune system's ability to defend against secondary attacks like this, it is common. Most CTC's do not survive this journey and there is a simple, yet profound nutritional approach that can help assure they do not. Besides everything the patient should be doing to strengthen their immune response, oxygenate their tissue, alkalize their body, and feed their cells good nutrition, every cancer patient *must* be taking one simple nutrient to help prevent metastasis: Modified Citrus Pectin (MCP.)

MCP isn't even an expensive product and does a wonderful job grabbing these little CTC's in their claws to escort them out of the body. Like any approach to cancer, MCP is just one addition to the arsenal that every patient should consider, but like always, correct the cause!

Again, to help prevent metastasis, take 1-3 scoops of MCP per day along with everything you are doing to upregulate your immune system to help kill these cells.

Here's another recent article I wrote for my *Doctor's Only* newsletter:

Chronic Biotoxin Load a Precursor for Cancer and...

Several recent studies confirm that patients with chronic biotoxins are more susceptible to cancer.[90] [91] Certain gram-negative bacteria have the ability to alter intracellular

---

[90] Achenbach CH et al. HIV viremia and incidence of non-Hodgkin lymphoma in patients successfully treated with antiretroviral therapy. Clin Infect Dis 2014 Feb 12

[91] Indian J Med Paediatr Oncol. 2013 Oct;34(4):323-6. doi: 10.4103/0971-5851.125259. Human immunodeficiency virus Infection in a patient of chronic myelogenous leukemia. Tuljapurkar VB, Phatak UA

communication pathways that disrupts normal function.[92] H. pylori, a chronic biotoxin most notably associated with gastric ulcers, gastric, duodenal, and esophageal cancers have been shown to initially increase gastric epithelial apoptosis through a specific pathway (called the TRAIL apoptotic system) increasing stomach cell premature death leading to symptoms associated with ulcers. Later in its progressive cycle it blocks other apoptotic pathways leading to an inability of normal, programmed cell death as well as a disruption of cellular replication phase, hence, cancer.

Another example is Chlamydophila pneumonia, a common etiological agent of respiratory tract infections that can linger for decades as a sub-clinical pathogen linked to lung cancer, arthritis, Alzheimer's disease, multiple sclerosis, sarcoidosis and erythema nodosum.[93]

During chronic, systemic Helicobacter pylori infection, bone marrow-derived-mesenchymal stem cells (BMD-MSCs) have been found to migrate to distant tissue sites causing various carcinomas.[94] [95] Other reports on Propionibacterium acnes (P. acnes, a gram-positive skin infection) suggest that this bacterium is also prevalent in the prostate, is associated with acute and chronic prostatic inflammation, and might have a role in prostate carcinogenesis.[96]

---

[92] Clin Me. 2002 Mar-Apr;2(2):147-52. Helicobacter pylori: 20 years on. Marshall B

[93] Adv Clin Exp Med. 2014 January-February;23(1):123-126. Infections Caused by Chlamydophila pneumoniae

[94] Adv Biomed Res. 2014 Jan 9;3:19. doi: 10.4103/2277-9175.124650. Effect of Helicobacter pylori infection on stromal-derived factor-1/CXCR4 axis in bone marrow-derived mesenchymal stem cells

[95] World J Gastroenterol. 2014 Feb 14;20(6):1485-1492. Helicobacter pylori-related chronic gastritis as a risk factor for colonic neoplasms

[96] LoS One. 2014 Feb 28;9(2):e90324. doi: 10.1371/journal.pone.0090324. Intracellular Propionibacterium acnes Infection in Glandular Epithelium and Stromal Macrophages of the Prostate with or without Cancer

Clinically we recently saw a 4-year old female previously diagnosed with Ollier disease and left with no hope and a dismal future. Ollier disease is a grossly deforming bone disorder where multiple enchondromas form in epiphyseal plates and intraosseously near growth plate cartilage.

We concluded, after testing, that there existed a biotoxin source to her disease that sparked a TH2 dominant autoimmune attack on the epiphyseal growth plates. Modern medicine may scream *foul* based on the fact that their named disease was first classified as a genetic variant therefore the "once written into a textbook, never shalt thou alter" rule applies (as often is the case), but I really don't give a hoot!

A quick search of recent studies may support my theory of causation in this case. Schipani and Provot[97] discovered the relationship between parathyroid-hormone-related peptide (PTHrP), parathyroid hormone (PTH), and the PTH/PTHrP receptor in endochondral bone development in such proliferative diseases. These proteins act as a switch that regulates bone growth and cellular differentiation of chondrocytes, as well as their replacement by bone cells.

Disruption of this mechanism, in this case by a parasitic infiltration, *flips the switch* and creates problems.

In future newsletters I'll follow up with this and a plethora of other case studies to help convince you to at least consider biotoxin sources for chronic disorders, but for now…

What you need to consider:

1. Do not disregard the possibility of chronic infection as a causative agent in your patient's health picture regardless of revealed negative testing.

---

[97] Birth Defects Res C Embryo Today. 2003 Nov;69(4):352-62. PTHrP, PTH, and the PTH/PTHrP receptor in endochondral bone development. Schipani E, Provot S

2. Testing for chronic, subclinical infections is inaccurate at best. The doctor would do better to make an informed (through symptomatology) decision if they don't have access to someone who can test with other measures such as AK. No one reading this remembers, but there existed a time that doctors actually made decisions based on years of experience and wisdom gleaned more from pouring over case studies and consulting with elder peers as opposed to dependency on MRIs and Labs.

Inflammation and Oxidation

Inflammation is really a double-edged sword. It is a necessary component of healing for in it contains the chemicals of your immune response that kill invaders and promote healing. While it is beneficial at one level, it is also detrimental in chronic forms. Much like most things in life, balance is the key to success. In cancer, the chronic inflammation of a Th2 immune response suppresses the needed Th1 response, which is largely responsible for controlling cancer cell growth.

Reasoning

Alexander Fleming, the discoverer of penicillin, once said, "If the soil causes the disease; the cure to the disease also lies in it." We might say, "The cure for cancer lies in the cause of cancer, namely, the imbalanced immune system."

For instance, while TNFalpha, Natural Killer Cells (NKC), T-cells, and Macrophages, some of the pro-inflammatory chemicals of the Th1 (immediate, killer-cell side) immune response bring inflammation, it also brings the cure, the correction, the stimulus that leads to cancer suppression.

Also, it is noted that while pro-oxidants produced in the body mediate inflammation, antioxidants (such as glutathione) suppress this response. Inflammation is an important part of the body's response to both internal and external environmental stimuli. This response serves to counteract the insult incurred by these stimuli to the body; survival is always the body's goal. When acute inflammation, as seen in a fever, is manifested for a short period of time, it has a therapeutic consequence. However, when inflammation becomes chronic or lasts too long, it can prove harmful and may lead to disease. It's all about balance.

To summarize: If we are going to kill cancer cells, we **need** an immune upregulation. When we stimulate the immune system, we get an inflammatory response (increased inflammation.) This is a **good** thing. This is why some patients may experience an increase size of the cancer mass or even an increase in pain when starting treatment. That can be a **good** sign.

For more help with this, see my blog, *Cancer: Good Pain/Bad Pain*:

ConnersClinic.com/cancer-good-pain-bad-pain

Pro-Oxidants vs. Antioxidants

A similar relationship exists in pro- vs. antioxidants. It seems we are overwhelmed with information about the importance of increasing antioxidants in our diet; the truth be told: any cancer care without pro-oxidation would prove fruitless. To understand this, let's discuss the mechanisms.

A free radical is a reactive molecule that tends to damage cell parts, so we tend to think that this is always *bad*. *Not* true. However, when DNA is damaged, this can mean damaged genes, but this is precisely why our body replicates cells and the *old* cell dies. If the genes controlling cell multiplication are harmed, cell growth/replication can get stuck in the *on* position and cause cancer; this is an example of imbalance.

Cancer cells are very active, reproducing and growing, causing an increased load of free radicals within the cancer cell. Cancer cells are not good at handling more free radicals, since they already have more in them than normal cells and they tend to spew them out of the cells forming a *slime layer of waste* that makes it more difficult for immune killer cells to penetrate. At first thought, maybe it would be wise to flood the cancer with antioxidants until we understand that, at the root, the cancer is growing without oxygen, fermenting its energy, we then arrive at a different solution.

Normally the body makes energy through oxidation and is able to quench free radicals produced with substances called antioxidants. Antioxidants lessen the amount of free radical-induced injury and bring balance. This *tug-of-war* continues and may be illustrated in exercise.

We go to the gym and work our muscles, breaking tissue down in the presence of a depleting supply of oxygen (almost a semi-cancerous state) for muscles to *recover* stronger, bigger, thriftier in their use of oxygen, healthier in what we call *better shape*.

Cancer is similar in that the cells have created a survival mechanism to grow and thrive in a hypoxic environment. Since pro-oxidant strategies increase free radicals, it may better seem that the way to kill cancer cells is by bombarding them with pro-oxidants. This would lead to more free radicals within cancer cells, and injury and eventual death to the cancer cells.

The mechanism of many chemotherapy drugs, as well as radiation, in destroying cancer cells is by causing free radical increase within cancer cells. This is the same mechanism in many of the apoptogens (cancer killers) in a nutritional approach.

Many nutraceuticals that are normally considered to be antioxidants actually have a pro-oxidant, cancer-killing effect on cancer cells. Curcumin, for example, is just one antioxidant that acts as a pro-oxidant to a cancer cell. It also elicits anti-inflammatory benefits that aide in breaking down the barrier for an immune assault on the growing cancer mass. Selenium, EGCG (from Green Tea Extract), high dose Vitamin C, ALA, and others also act like this. Some so-called antioxidants at high levels have other ways of killing cancer cells, like inhibiting certain enzymes (for example, Curcumin inhibits topoisomerase II) that hinder normal apoptosis (normal, programmed cell death.)

Therefore, we have to be careful taking dogmatic stances in our nutritional approach. The "antioxidants are good for you so excess amounts of antioxidants must be better" ignores the very principles of health that regulate homeostasis: balance. Mixing different nutrition can be counterproductive as well; for instance, use of Curcumin along with Glutathione has shown to be a very wrong approach. Extensive research within the past half-century has indicated that Curcumin, the yellow pigment in curry powder, exhibits antioxidant, anti-inflammatory, and pro-apoptotic (aiding in normal cell death) activities.

Recent studies have investigated whether the anti-inflammatory and pro-apoptotic activities assigned to Curcumin are mediated through its pro-oxidant/antioxidant mechanism. Much data has revealed that TNF-mediated NF-κB (markers found to accelerate cancer) activation was inhibited by Curcumin; therefore, Curcumin acts to slow cancer growth. Glutathione, normally a great antioxidant (some would argue that it is the body's greatest,) reversed the inhibition: that means that Glutathione *negated* the cancer stopping benefits of Curcumin. This is just one example of what can go wrong with taking too many supplements!

Cellular pro-oxidants, called reactive oxygen species (ROS), are constantly produced in our body. As stated, excessive ROS can induce oxidative damage in the cell and promote a number of degenerative diseases including accelerated aging and even cancer. Cellular antioxidants protect against the damaging effects of ROS and have long been the sales-pitch of health practitioners. However, we cannot ignore *normal balance*; in moderate concentrations, ROS are necessary for a number of protective reactions. ROS are essential mediators of antimicrobial phagocytosis (killing bio-toxins), detoxification reactions carried out by the cytochrome P-450 complex (the main liver and cellular detox pathway), and apoptosis which eliminates cancerous and other life-threatening cells. Can you say *balance* again?

Excessive ingestion of antioxidants could dangerously interfere with these protective functions, while temporary depletion of antioxidants can enhance anti-cancer effects of apoptosis. This is just another lesson against *cookbook nutrition*. This is where practitioners educated in Kinesiology may have an advantage in determining the correct approach for the patient. Functional medicine testing measuring ROS baselines may also prove effective on determining a nutraceutical attack, as each patient is different.

Chronic Inflammation

Chronic inflammation is the real problem. It almost always lurks beneath the surface of nearly every chronic disease including diabetes, cancer and every autoimmune disorder. Most of the time you can't see or feel it, but this low-grade, constant type of inflammation increases the risk of every leading cause of death.

To understand and therefore control inflammation is a major key to conquering cancer. I have often said that cancer is a Th2 dominant disorder that imposes a Th1 immune suppression. What do I mean by this? Your Th1 system is the main *killer* portion of your immune response that also helps *kill* cells that are supposed to die and be cleaned out of the body like cancer cells. If the Th1 system is suppressed, cancer has a better chance to proliferate.

Both sides of the immune system fire inflammation. The Th1 system creates a more acute inflammation where the Th2 system enables a slower, more insidious inflammation that may go largely unnoticed by the patient. It is common for a person with a Th2 dominant autoimmune condition to be completely unaware of their problem and blame stiffness, arthritis, brain fog, and other chronic inflammatory symptoms on *old age* or worse, allowing a doctor to give them a medication that suppresses the symptoms and allows the problem continue.

Let's look at a common condition in America: high cholesterol. Millions are diagnosed with this every year and placed on some statin drug that readily lowers their numbers and gives the patient a false sense of victory. Was the reason *why* the liver was producing an excess amount of cholesterol ever addressed? What causes your body to make cholesterol?

Cholesterol is a necessary ingredient to life; it is the precursor to all your hormones including Vitamin D. Side note: Since Vitamin D is crucial in apoptosis (normal cell death that is **not** happening in cancer) and every cancer patient is arguably low in serum Vitamin D levels **and** since cholesterol is the precursor to Vitamin D production, do you think there is a correlation between the 80 billion dollar per year Lipitor industry and our rise in cancer rates? It doesn't really take a rocket scientist to figure some of this stuff out!

Excess cholesterol isn't good either, but why is the body making too much? I think that **this** is the type of question that must be asked! Your body makes cholesterol for numerous reasons, but one is in response to inflammation. See the connection? If a person has chronic inflammation, they can have elevated cholesterol. Find the source of inflammation!

Vicious Cycles

Illness is an outcome of vicious cycles. Here's just one possibility: A person is exposed to a high amount of toxins in their lifetime, some of which settle in their tissue. An immune response from a completely normal immune reaction, let's say, to an infection of some sort, causes a spike in the Th1 system to kill the infector. This Th1 immune response carries a slurry of different chemicals that are just looking for something to kill (because that is the only thing your immune system does.) If the infection is easily quenched, excess Th1 cytokines may *find* a toxin lodged in your tissue that the immune system was never supposed to *turn on* against.

If these chemicals initiate a response against such a toxin, we have a problem. Since the immune system only kills things, its attempt to *kill* a toxin will simply result in a constant, ramped-up response that destroys local tissue and leaves inflammatory cytokines that choke-off detoxification pathways and clog extracellular spaces. This is really the definition of how an autoimmune disease begins!

If the subsequent immune response is dominant in Th1 chemicals, it is called a Th1 dominant autoimmune condition and is marked by more acute destruction and often leads to a greater number of symptoms for the patient that may cause them to seek help and receive a diagnosis. A greater number of Th2 chemicals leads to a Th2 dominant autoimmune response that can be just as destructive but is often slower in process and more insidious, leaving the patient with diffuse, lower-grade symptoms that may go undiagnosed and undetected. The Th2 response still breeds chronic inflammation and chronic inflammation down-regulates cell receptors against things that aide in normal cell death (like Vitamin D receptors that are supposed to help old cells die and not become cancerous.)

We are left with a breeding ground for cancer!

I could give a hundred different examples of *vicious cycles* but the important thing to understand is that **every** disease is a product of one. Failure for you and your doctor to *dig back* and figure out the vicious cycle that has led you to your problem is just **wrong**. To give the patient a label of cancer or any disease for that matter, without finding the reason it is there is malpractice in my book. I thought that this is what a doctor was supposed to do. Any educated individual can *Google* their symptoms and compare their lab results to patterns to reach a reasonable diagnosis; it's **why** the problem exists that must be solved!

Other Possible Causes of Cancer

We'll be covering multiple dietary causes to cancer in Chapter 4, from sugar and glutamine to chemicals in our food supply, GMOs, BPAs and other hormone disruptors…the list is almost endless. You could literally write volumes on these subjects, but I want to cover what we believe to be a few of the most common causes we see.

We know a number of factors that increase the risk of many different kinds of cancer, from genetic BRCA, P53 gene suppression, smoking, obesity, diet, and even stress. The truth is that **only a sick person will get cancer**. When I say "get cancer" I mean actually be diagnosed with cancer. We all have cancer cells growing in us every day; our immune system is either winning the battle or it isn't.

When our immune system is overwhelmed, for a myriad of reasons, cancer cells (rapidly replicating cells) start to *take hold*. There is **not** one cause of any cancer; there are a multitude of risk factors.

Maybe it would be easier to picture it this way: If we had a scale and we placed "healthy, life-giving, and nurturing" things on one side and then placed "not-so-good-for-us" things on the other side, the scale would tip toward either health or sickness. You see, cancer isn't any different than any other disease as far as whether it develops in us or not. We really don't need a $5 billion government study to prove that a life consumed with overwhelming stress, coffee, donuts, cigarettes, and drugs isn't good for us.

Understanding the above helps us see that the first step in caring for a cancer patient is to fix the environment. We need to *clean up* the person's body, modulate any underlining autoimmune disorder, deal with toxins, molds, parasites, and even hidden emotional scars that may have paved the way for cancer cells to grow.

There is a reason for everything, a cause for every effect. Find someone who will search for these.

Genetics

I think about 5% of cancers are caused genetically. That being said, most with cancer have defects in genetic pathways that might contribute to their diagnosis. Defects in tumor suppressor genes would be one example. BRCA gene defects (the gene that is the tumor suppressor gene for breast cancer and ovarian cancer) can increase a person's cancer risk.

God gave us a *fail-safe* method to deal with cells that go into rapid replication: tumor suppressor genes. These are genes within the cell that *turn on* in the presence of rapid replication to stimulate cell death. When a cell goes into rapid replication, it's an abnormal process, but it happens on a regular basis to all of us.

However, should the cell begin replicating every day or multiple times a day, our tumor suppressor genes kick on a pathway to stimulate apoptosis or cell death. It's a protective measure to keep us from getting a cancer diagnosis. So, you could say that we all have cancer, which is true. By this we mean that we all have cells in rapid replication. These tumor suppressor genes kick on and cause cell death and kill the cell and protect us from ever having a diagnosis. People with defects on their tumor suppressor genes, and we'll use the BRCA genes as an example, have an increased risk of cancer because they're not turning on that important, protective pathway as well as they should.

Another class of genes, called *oncogenes*, can contribute to cancer. An oncogene is a mutated gene whose protein product (that which it makes) is produced in higher quantities or whose altered product has increased activity and thereby acts in a dominant manner stimulating growth. Oncogenes (when defected) can hinder necessary cell death and/or stimulate replication. More than 100 oncogenes have been identified.

Defects in other pathways, such as detoxification pathways, can also contribute to a cancer diagnosis. There is so much to this subject that I've written a separate book on it: *Cancer Genes*. It's really a video-book and it's available for ***free*** on our website at ConnersClinic.com/cancer-genes

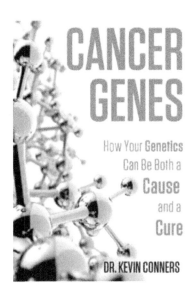

Genetically Modified Foods

Genetically modified organism (GMO) food has been around for decades. Most corn and soy purchased in the United States is GMO food. Proponents argue that there are no ill-effects on humans, but I completely disagree. I'm not in the minority with my belief that changing the genetic structure of a food product is playing with disaster. Recent studies reveal that GMO corn destroys the intestinal lining of mice causing absorption problems and leaky gut syndrome. What is it doing to our gut?

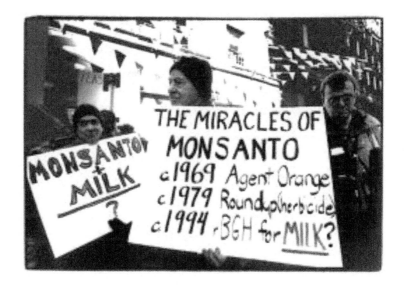

Today's GMOs are based on adding new genes to crops like corn, soy, and cotton in order to alter the way the plants function, make them more tolerant to disease and bugs, and (maybe the number one reason) enable companies to patent the seed and create an endless need for farmers to repurchase year after year. Gone are the days of saving seeds; it's against the law; Monsanto owns the patent.

To say that our food supply (laced with toxins, filled with additives, colorings and chemicals, and now genetically altered) doesn't negatively affect our bodies is ludicrous. This book does not contain enough space to discuss these things in detail and I have recommended various books for your personal research but suffice it to say that removing these poisons from your diet is of the utmost importance.

Bottom line: Eat only organically grown foods. Do your own research into the foods you put into your mouth and make sure they are not genetically modified. If we all create a greater demand for good food, the supply will follow.

For more information on this subject, search "GMO" on our blog at ConnersClinic.com/blog

Pesticides and Herbicides

Just recently Monsanto was slapped with another giant lawsuit. This is actually their third lawsuit (as of 2019) of people who are making claims that their cancer is caused by *RoundUp*. *RoundUp* is their major weed killer that's now in just about everything in our food supply. This couple both had Hodgkin's lymphoma, and brought a $2 billion lawsuit. If these lawsuits keep coming, it could be bankruptcy for Monsanto/Bayer (Bayer bought Monsanto out.) If you're still using *RoundUp* you guys, you have to stop.

Pesticides are so widely used in agriculture that you can just about guarantee we all have an increased the risk of cancer. Some studies have suggested that pesticides could increase the risk of leukemia, lymphoma, brain tumors, breast cancer, and prostate cancer, but they are so widespread that they can affect everyone and every cell. For now, researchers are afraid, so they say that the evidence is not strong enough to show a definite link, possibly because of pressures *from above*.

Obviously, due to the consequences, human studies are difficult to obtain so we must rely on animal research. However, it needn't take more than a childlike understanding to draw the correlations.

Agricultural Workers and Farmers

People exposed to higher levels of pesticides as part of their job (for example in industry or farming) may be at higher risk of certain cancers, particularly leukemias and lymphomas.

The International Agency for Research into Cancer (IARC) have looked at the evidence and said that regularly spraying pesticides as part of your job *probably* increases the risk of cancer. But for most individual pesticides, the evidence was either too weak to come to a conclusion, or only strong enough to suggest a *possible* effect.

However, in animal studies, many pesticides are proven carcinogenic, (e.g. organochlorines, creosote, and sulfallate) while others (notably, the organochlorines DDT, chlordane, and lindane) are tumor promoters. Some contaminants in commercial pesticide formulations also may pose a carcinogenic risk. In humans, arsenic compounds and insecticides used occupationally have been classified as carcinogens by the IARC. Human data, however, are limited by the small number of studies that evaluate individual pesticides. Epidemiologic studies, although some-times contradictory, have linked phenoxy acid herbicides or contaminants in them with soft tissue sarcoma (STS) and malignant lymphoma; organochlorine insecticides are linked with STS, non-Hodgkin's lymphoma (NHL), leukemia, and, less consistently, with cancers of the lung and breast; organophosphorous compounds are linked with NHL and leukemia; and triazine herbicides with ovarian cancer.

Information is disseminating though. A 2013 study posted on the American Cancer Society's site states, "A growing number of well-designed epidemiological and molecular studies provide substantial evidence that the pesticides used in agricultural, commercial, and home and garden applications are associated with excess cancer risk. This risk is associated both with those applying the pesticide and, under some conditions, those who are simply bystanders to the application."

A 2009 study revealed, "Our observation is consistent with a previous literature reporting suggestive associations between parental exposure to pesticides and risk of astrocytoma (in the child of the parent.)" What? Parents who use or are exposed to pesticides and herbicides and the **children** have an increased risk of **brain cancer**? Crazy!

A 2015 study concluded, "We found that childhood exposure to indoor residential insecticides was associated with a significant increase in risk of childhood leukemia." This stuff is **bad**; **please** stop using it!

We have found that pesticides and herbicides are one of the most common causes of cancer. Knowing this, I feel we need to touch on how to help rid oneself of these things.

These compounds (and there are dozens) take thousands of years to breakdown. Once we ingest them, breathe them in, or absorb them through the skin, our body **needs** to get rid of them. Unfortunately, the way our body does so is through our cellular and liver detoxification pathways.

I talk a lot about these detoxification pathways in my book *Cancer Genes* because these pathways can be hindered (slowed) by defects on specific genetic pathways. The PON1 and Cytochrome P450 pathways, for example, are essential for getting rid of these large chemicals. Defects on these, which are common, can cause slower rates of detoxification and a greater chance of you depositing these potentially cancer-causing chemicals inside the cells which can, at some later date, interrupt the replication cycle causing cancer.

See more on detoxification at the end of this chapter.

Other Toxic Food Additives

Since the mandate of the FDA includes protecting public health by assuring the safety of the food supply, why is this government organization allowing a staggering number of additives to adulterate our food? Many of these "allowable" additives have dire consequences to the health this very agency is supposed to protect.

Drug and chemical companies have secretly flourished since the advent of commercially processed foods in the 1950's. Many of these chemicals, added as "non-food substances", have come into common usage to preserve and enhance the taste and appearance of products made with cheap ingredients.

Increasingly, these additives, such as indigestible gums, have been used to replace real food ingredients. The use of food additives has allowed food producers to make higher profits at the expense of public health.

Currently, the FDA allows thousands of different food additives, although a 2013 study found that *almost 80% of them lack the relevant information needed to estimate the amount that consumers can safely eat.*

Nearly None Have Any Safety Testing

In the FDA's own database, 93% of food additives lack reproductive or developmental toxicity data. Of the totality of FDA-regulated additives, both directly and indirectly allowed in food, almost two-thirds don't have publicly available feeding data. The report concluded that in the absence of toxicology data on the majority of chemicals added to food, their safety in humans may be questioned.

To explain the FDA's negligence, some cite a decades-old loophole that allows companies to confer GRAS (generally recognized as safe) status to the additives they plan to use, without any FDA oversight. But if the FDA were genuinely interested in protecting the public, it would have moved long ago to close that loophole; leading you to conclude that maybe, just maybe, there's a bit of sneakiness going on to have these overlooked.

The same apologists say companies regularly introduce new additives without ever informing the FDA, so this regulatory body just doesn't know about them. Yet, the FDA has been able to track down small raw milk producers halfway across the country to put them out of business, send the FBI to raid a cancer center using natural treatments in Tulsa, and put a small company out of business for making elderberry juice concentrate. Clearly the FDA has its ear to the ground. Can somebody say *payoff*?

How to Protect Yourself

Since the drug and chemical companies can literally do anything that brings them profit regardless of harm produced, and the government agency created to protect the public will wink at anything as long as you can line someone's pocket, you need to protect yourself. The best way to start is by scrutinizing the label of every food item before buying. If there is a listing that is not food, chances are good it is referring to a food additive. Do some research and decide whether you want the substance in your body.

Here are a few of the most commonly used dangerous food additives:

- **BHT and BHA**: These are preservatives for fats and oils. They are found in cereals, vegetable oil, potato chips, popcorn, and other packaged foods. Both can be found in Harry and David's popular Moose Munch bars. Studies have concluded that **BHT** and **BHA** may cause cancer in rats.

- **Azodicarbonamide**: A chemical used in the rubber and plastics industries to produce shoe soles and yoga mats. It's also used as a dough conditioner in low quality breads, other baked goods, and in the buns and breads used in several fast food chains. Subway has agreed to discontinue its use but didn't set a time frame. Azodicarbonamide has also been found to cause cancer in rodents.

- **MSG**: MSG is an excitotoxin that makes below average food taste good. It's in many salad dressings, potato chips, hot dogs, canned soup and tuna, frozen dinners, prepared gravies, and much more. It kills sensitive neurons in the brain. According to natural health authority Russell Blaylock MD, there is a link between sudden cardiac death and excitotoxic damage caused by MSG and artificial sweeteners.

- **Acesulfame-K**: This additive is replacing toxic aspartame in products such as candy, drinks, chewing gum and anything else that's sweet. And as is usually the case, it is as deadly as what it replaces. Acesulfame-K is a potassium salt containing methylene chloride, a known carcinogen. It may also cause liver and kidney impairment, and problems with eyesight.

- **Sodium Nitrate**: Sodium nitrate is a preservative used in conventionally produced bacon, ham, hot dogs, lunchmeats, and other processed meats. Nitrates can be converted to cancer-causing chemicals known as nitrosamines.

- **Blue 1 and Blue 2**: These are food dyes used in beverages, candy, and baked goods. Blue 2 is also used in pet food. Both have been found to hyperactivity and potentially cause brain tumors in mice.

- **Red 3**: Another food coloring used in bottled cherries, fruit cocktail, candies, and baked goods. Causes thyroid tumors in rats and potentially in humans.

- **Yellow 6**: Yet another food dye which is found in pickles, pepperoncini, and sausages, as well as gelatin, baked goods, and candy, yellow 6 may cause adrenal gland and kidney tumors.

We can only guess the agenda of the FDA. But once you start reading labels, don't be surprised if it becomes an empowering habit!

Heavy Metals and Other Toxins

In the late phase of the Roman Empire, it was considered a privilege of the reigning aristocracy to drink out of lead cups and many of the water lines in the city of Rome were made out of lead. It took several hundred years before the physicians of the time established the link between mental illness — affecting mostly the aristocracy — and the contamination of the drinking water with lead. In the 1700s, the use of mercury for the treatment of both acute and chronic infections gained favor and again, it took decades before the toxic effects of mercury were recognized within the medical community. In the time of Mozart, who died of mercury toxicity during a course of treatment for syphilis, any pathologist in Vienna was familiar with the severe grayish discoloration of organs in those who died from mercury toxicity and other organ-related destructive changes caused by mercury.

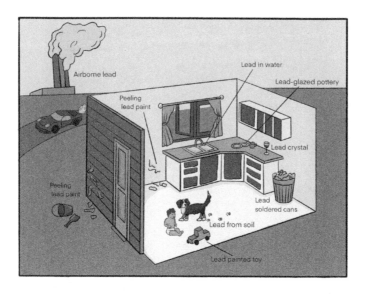

In the case of mercury, the therapeutic dilemma is most clear. Mercury can be used to treat infections, but (not unlike modern chemotherapy) also causes a different type of illness and may kill the patient. The same is true for most metals: small doses may have a therapeutic effect for a short term, lifesaving direction, but then cause their own illness. Most metals have a very narrow therapeutic margin before their neurotoxic (and in some cases carcinogenic effect) outweigh the benefits. Toxic metals can be used to kill fungi, bacteria, and maybe even viruses. However, many of these microbial invaders adapt to a toxic metal environment.

It is important to note that we are not speaking solely of metals on the periodic table, but other elements as well. We have a distorted view of nutrients in this country, thinking that since a little Iron will help my anemia, a lot would be better. If a little iodine is necessary for my thyroid, a lot is even more optimal. *Wrong*! Iron toxicity may be the most common of all *secret killers* along with Iodine (the major causative agent for Hashimoto's disease.)

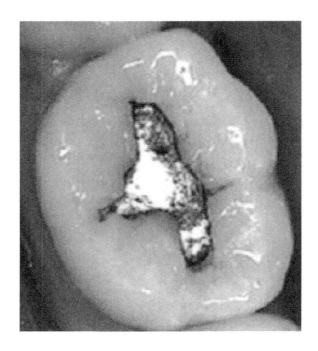

It is difficult for our bodies to adapt to high doses of anything; toxic metals harm the cells of the body, whereas the invading microorganisms can often thrive in a heavy metal environment. Research shows that microorganisms tend to congregate in those body compartments that have the most toxic metals. This is in part because the body's own immune cells are incapacitated in those areas where the microorganisms multiply and thrive in an undisturbed way. The teeth, jawbone, Peyer's lymphoid patches in the gastrointestinal wall, the ground-system (connective tissue) and the autonomic ganglia are common sites of metal storage and the place where microorganisms thrive. Fat cells are the easiest place for your body to shunt excess toxin exposure since they are the cells with the spiritual gift of accommodation; they just invite everyone in. Tissue that is most densely vasculated will receive the greatest concentration of toxins. Furthermore, virus, bacteria, molds and fungi settle in those bodily areas are least vasculated, vasoconstricted (the blood vessels are in spasm) and hypoperfused (reduced blood flow) by blood, nutrients and oxygen, which foster the growth of anaerobic germs, fungi and viruses.

The list of symptoms of mercury toxicity alone, published by DAMS (Dental Amalgam Support Group) includes virtually all illnesses known to mankind. Chronic fatigue, depression and joint pains are the most common on the list. Mercury alone can mimic or cause any illness currently known, or at least contribute to it.

Through the use of the PCR test (polymerase chain reaction, a type of genetic testing) virtually any illness seems to have a chronic infection (autoimmune) response either at its core or *because of* another cause. A study performed by the VA Administration (published in JADA, April 1998) on 10,000 US veterans, showed that most coronary heart disease really starts as an infection (an autoimmune response and subsequent inflammation) of endothelial cells (cells lining of the blood vessel, the intimal layer) and, in most cases was caused by microorganisms from the mouth. Another study showed that close to 70% of all TMJ syndromes in women are caused or contributed to by Chlamydia trachomatis. Childhood diabetes is often caused by either a Cytomegalovirus or influenza virus infection. These all become autoimmune diseases though they are seldom diagnosed as such and therefore, they are treated symptomatically.

It is obviously a doctor's first-most importance to diagnosis and remove antigens (chronic, hidden infections, toxic metals, chemicals) or at the very least, combine this with treatment of the patient. As long as compartmentalized toxic metals or other antigens are present in the body, microorganisms have a fortress that cannot be conquered by antibiotics, nutrition, herbs, ozone therapy, UV light therapy, etc.

To diagnose metal deposits in the different body compartments on a living patient is not always easy. Most "scientific" tests are based on grinding up tissue and then examining it with a microscope, spectroscopy, or other laboratory-based procedures. This of course is impractical, so we have to rely on the next best option: analysis of hair, blood, and/or urine.

Among the detoxifying agents most commonly used are DMPS, DMSA, IV Vitamin C, Glutathione, sulfur compounds such as DL-Methionine and Cysteine, branched chain amino acids, Chlorella, Porphrazyme, Chitosan, activated charcoal, cilantro, and yellow dock. We also use specialized tools like the Rife, Ion Cleanse, LBG, etc. with great success.

Remember to follow the detoxification guidelines in this chapter and seek professional help!

Effective therapy thus must incorporate the following:

- Diagnosing the site of toxic metal compartmentalization

- Diagnosing the exact type of metal

- Determining the most appropriate and least toxic metal removal agent

- Determining other appropriate synergistic methods and agents (e.g. kidney drainage remedies, blood protective agents — garlic or Vitamin E, agents that increase fecal absorption and excretion of mobilized toxin, exercise, lymphatic drainage, etc.)

- Diagnosing any secondary infection

- Determining an appropriate antibiotic (actually termed anti-microbial to distinguish from antibacterial agents) regimen (medical antibiotics, antifungals, antivirals, ozone therapy, Rife, etc.)

- Monitoring the patient carefully from visit to visit to respond quickly to untoward effects most often caused by plugged up exit routes. With this approach, many patients that were chronically ill and did not respond to other approaches will improve or get well

However, the thoughts expressed thus far do not answer one important question: Why do patients deposit the mercury, lead, aluminum, and other heavy metals and toxins in a specific area of their body? Some deposit toxins in their hypothalamus (and develop multiple hormone problems), or in their limbic system (depression.) Others deposit it in the adrenal glands (fatigue), or in their bones (osteoporosis, leukemia.)

Some tend to accumulate toxins in the pelvis (interstitial cystitis), in the autonomic and sensory ganglia (chronic pain syndromes), fatty tissue like the breast (cancer); some in the connective tissue (scleroderma, lupus, rheumatism, fibromyalgia), or in the cranial nerves (tinnitus, cataracts, TMJ problems, loss of smell), or in the muscles (fibromyalgia.) There seems to be multiple causes:

- Past physical trauma (such as closed head injury) will make the brain susceptible to becoming a storage site for lead, aluminum and mercury

- Food allergies often cause low-grade inflammation in a susceptible site of the body, setting up those areas to become targets for toxic deposits

- Geopathic stress due to living or sleeping near underground water lines or electrical equipment and transformers. Metals apparently concentrate in the body regions most compromised

- Physical scars from surgery, trauma, or an infection can create abnormal electrical signals that can alter the function of the ANS (autonomic nervous system.) The abnormal impulses often cause areas of vasoconstriction and hypoperfusion, which again become metal storage sites

- Structural abnormalities: TMJ problems and cranial-sacral dysfunctions often are responsible for impairment of blood flow and lymphatic drainage in affected areas

- Biochemical deficiencies: For example, a chronic zinc deficiency makes the prostate susceptible since it has a large turnover of zinc. In lieu of zinc (Zn^{++}), the prostate incorporates other 2-valent metals (such as Hg^{++}, Pb^{++}.) Another example of this would be iodine deficiency and the thyroid

- Environmental toxicity (solvents, pesticides, wood preservatives, etc.) has a synergistic effect with most toxic metals. Metals will often accumulate in body parts that have been chemically injured.

Unresolved psycho-emotional trauma and unresolved problems in the family system can be another hidden issue. You can find more information on how to test for your toxic load at ConnersClinic.com/measuring-toxic-load

Vaccines

The **Polio Virus** has been around for centuries. Yet the virus seldom caused paralysis until the late 1800's. In fact, 95% of polio cases occur without symptoms, just a mild fever. But in less than 1% of the victims, the virus penetrates the blood-brain barrier to cause paralysis and death. As the fear of a polio epidemic in the US spread in the 1950's, polio vaccines were rushed to market and vaccination became compulsory.

Dr Maurice Hilleman, one of the most renowned vaccine developers in the world with over three dozen vaccines to his credit headed Merck's vaccine program. On examining the injectable Salk polio vaccine and the oral Sabine vaccine, he isolated the **SV40** Simian Live Virus from both and discovered that **most polio vaccines given to the public were contaminated with cancer causing viruses**.

As expected, the government kept these revelations secret, warning neither doctors nor the public while the vaccines continued to be administered for decades. **SV40** was so virulent that it became a popular tool for cancer researchers to rapidly transform healthy animal cells into tumor cells. In fact, from 1955 to 1963 up to 98 million children and adults in the United States were exposed to **SV40** Simian Live virus, a known carcinogen, due to contaminated polio vaccines.

In the March 1977 issue of Science, Jonas and Darrell Salk made the startling revelation that, **"Live virus vaccines against influenza or poliomyelitis may in each instance produce the disease it is intended to prevent..."** This should make every thinking person pause and consider whether vaccines do more harm than good.

On January 26, 1988, the Washington Post featured a story about polio from a national conference that concluded that all new cases of polio have come from the vaccine itself. None of the original *wild type* polio virus has caused a single case of polio in the United States since 1979. The program should have been discontinued long before, but it wasn't, due to collusion between Big Pharma and government regulators, known as the Medical Cartel, exposed in the book *Cancer Vortex*.

The CDC posted on its own website (which was taken down shortly after the post went viral.)

View an archived copy of the web page at:

ConnersClinic.com/polio

This report revealed that as many as 30 million Americans could be at risk for developing cancer due to polio vaccine tainted with Simian Virus 40 (SV40) found in some species of monkey.

This story is not new; many of us who thoroughly researched the vaccination issue before choosing whether or not to immunize were already aware of this fact years ago.

I became aware of the tainted polio vaccines from 1955-1963 in the late 1990's and it was one of the primary motivators for me to choose a "no shots, no way" approach for my children. What **is** new is that the CDC is finally admitting it.

What took you so long CDC? Many of the folks vaccinated with the tainted polio stock are already **dead** from cancer with many more getting diagnosed each and every day!

Here's the exact language from the **CDC Fact Sheet**. I am reprinting it here in its entirety because the CDC decided to take it down shortly after the post went viral.

- SV40 is a virus found in some species of monkey

- SV40 was discovered in 1960. Soon afterward, the virus was found in polio vaccine

- More than 98 million Americans received one or more doses of polio vaccine from 1955 to 1963 when a proportion of vaccine was contaminated with SV40; it has been estimated that 10-30 million Americans could have received an SV40 contaminated dose of vaccine

- SV40 virus has been found in certain types of cancer in humans, but it has not been determined that SV40 causes these cancers

- The majority of scientific evidence suggests that SV40-contaminated vaccine did not cause cancer; however, some research results are conflicting, and more studies are needed

- Polio vaccines being used today do not contain SV40. All of the current evidence indicates that polio vaccines have been free of SV40 since 1963. (**Note**: *This claim by the CDC is false. SV40-contaminated oral polio vaccines were produced from early 1960s to about 1978 and were used throughout the world.*)

- In the 1950s, rhesus monkey kidney cells, which contain SV40 if the animal is infected, were used in preparing polio vaccines. Because SV40 was not discovered until 1960, no one was aware in the 1950s that polio vaccine could be contaminated

- SV40 was found in the injected form of the polio vaccine (IPV), not the kind given by mouth (OPV.) (Editor's note: this claim by the CDC is patently false. SV40 was found in oral polio vaccines after 1961. A study determined that the procedure used by the manufacturer to inactivate SV40 in oral poliovirus vaccine seed stocks based on heat inactivation in the presence of $MgCl_2$ did not completely inactivate SV40)

- Not all doses of IPV were contaminated. It has been estimated that 10-30 million people actually received a vaccine that contained SV40

- Some evidence suggests that receipt of SV40-contaminated polio vaccine may increase risk of cancer. However, the majority of studies done in the U.S. and Europe which compare persons who received SV40-contaminated polio vaccine with those who did not have shown no causal relationship between receipt of SV40-contaminated polio vaccine and cancer. (*Editor's note: Oh really? SV40 has already been detected in some human tumors. That is far and beyond **some evidence**)

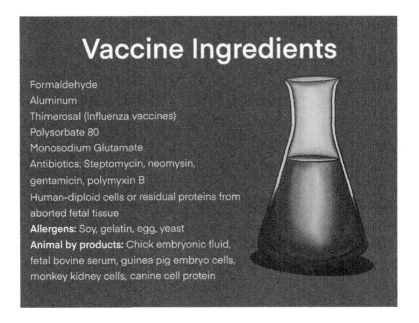

Vaccine Ingredients

Formaldehyde
Aluminum
Thimerosal (Influenza vaccines)
Polysorbate 80
Monosodium Glutamate
Antibiotics: Steptomycin, neomysin, gentamicin, polymyxin B
Human-diploid cells or residual proteins from aborted fetal tissue
Allergens: Soy, gelatin, egg, yeast
Animal by products: Chick embryonic fluid, fetal bovine serum, guinea pig embryo cells, monkey kidney cells, canine cell protein

Possibly more shocking than the fact that it took 50 years for the CDC to admit to this is that it took 3 years once SV40 was discovered in 1960 to finally recall the tainted stock and reformulate the vaccine. Over 100 million Americans were vaccinated with the contaminated polio vaccine before action was taken off the market but 30 million seems like a very lowball number of the true extent of the problem!

With baby boomers suffering from cancer, by some estimates,

at the mind-boggling rate of 1 in every 3 individuals (up from 1 in 8,000 only a few decades prior and the highest rate of any age group), it would seem that something is terribly amiss, don't you think?

The government has a penchant for doling out bad news a little at a time to minimize public outrage.

Even if the CDC does finally admit that SV40 is a cause for this enormous explosion in cancer of boomers in their late 40's, 50's, and 60's, can these folks or their grieving families do anything about it?

You can read more on vaccines and cancer here:

ConnersClinic.com/vaccines-and-cancer

ConnersClinic.com/are-vaccines-un-christian

Fluoride Toxicity

While fluoride deserves a book on its own, I will briefly mention it here and refer you to several web pages where I discuss this in detail. Fluoride, added to water supplies and dental hygiene, is perhaps the greatest medical lie next to vaccines. I simply cannot express my disgust enough to do it justice. It's a poison. Period. Stop drinking it and using it!

See more here:

ConnersClinic.com/fluoride-toxicity

ConnersClinic.com/environmental-toxins

More information on other environmental toxins can be found here:

ConnersClinic.com/environmental-toxins

ConnersClinic.com/autoimmune-casues

ConnersCinic.com/parent-kid-toxins

ConnersClinic.com/deodorant

ConnersClinic.com/are-we-all-poisoned

ConnersClinic.com/b-vitamins-help-detox-pesticides

Hormone Disruptors

We have long preached that you are not what you eat, but you are what you fail to detoxify. Toxins that can't pass out of the body, for whatever reason, are stored in the fat cells. Breast tissue is particularly vulnerable to environmental toxins since breasts are made up of fat cells. Breast tissue is also influenced by hormonal activity, with a large body of research linking environmental pollutants to unhealthy hormonal signaling throughout the body. Many environmental toxins are not water-soluble, making breast tissue even more susceptible.

In particular, many pesticides and heavy metals tend to gravitate toward fatty tissues. Numerous studies have found high levels of such toxins in breast tissue and breast milk. Many of these compounds, known as *POPs* (Persistent Organic Pollutants), remain in the environment for a long time and continue to bio accumulate up the food chain. There's another group of chemicals that pose an issue for breast health and other hormone related areas, such as prostate, ovarian, and uterine health.

Known as endocrine disruptors, environmental estrogens, or xenoestrogens, these chemicals mimic estrogen and other hormones and trick the body into using them.

Common examples include Bisphenol A (BPA) and phthalates

found in certain plastics and food packaging. Xenoestrogens can trigger excessive stimulation of hormone-sensitive tissues, with widespread impacts on human and environmental health. Foods and supplements that help remove pollutants from the body provide a multitude of long-term benefits, not just for breast health but overall longevity. Sulphur-containing foods such as broccoli, kale, cabbage, cauliflower, onions, and garlic all contain compounds that aid in detoxification.

For comprehensive breast health support, we recommend several products below that give a unique integrative formula designed to promote optimal hormone health:

Aromatase Inhibitors

Both conventional wisdom and clinical trials have supported blocking aromatase for breast cancer (or any hormone positive cancer) patients, but when oncologists speak of an aromatase inhibitor, they mean a drug.

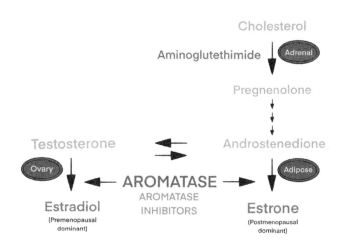

Aromatase inhibitors work by blocking the enzyme aromatase,

which turns the both hormones stored in fat cells into *bad estrogens* and androgens into estrogens thereby increasing the risk of cancer promotion. The idea is to reduce estrogens, especially in hormone-receptor-positive cancer patients.

There are three main aromatase inhibitor drugs:

- Arimidex (chemical name: anastrozole)
- Aromasin (chemical name: exemestane)
- Femara (chemical name: letrozole

Aromatase inhibitors don't stop the ovaries from making estrogen, so clinically they are mainly used to treat postmenopausal women. Tamoxifen, though not technically an aromatase inhibitor because its action is to shutdown estrogen production, is generally given to premenopausal women. Both classes of drugs do a good job in removing estrogen, but the cost is high.

Taking tamoxifen may increase your risk of uterine cancer, stroke, or a blood clot in the lung, which can be fatal.

The manufacturer warns to "tell your doctor" if you have:

- A history of stroke or blood clot
- Liver disease
- High cholesterol or triglycerides (a type of fat in the blood)
- A history of cataracts, or
- If you are receiving chemotherapy or radiation

It is not known whether tamoxifen passes into breast milk or if it could harm a nursing baby. This medicine may slow breast milk production. You should not breast-feed while taking tamoxifen.

In my experience, most women do **not** like the estrogen-draining effects of tamoxifen!

130

Aromatase inhibitor drugs tend to cause fewer serious side effects than tamoxifen, such as blood clots, stroke, and endometrial cancer. But aromatase inhibitors can cause more heart problems, more bone loss (osteoporosis), and more broken bones than tamoxifen, at least for the first few years of treatment.

Though it is standard practice to prescribe estrogen-blocking medications in ER+, PR+, and HER2+ cancer patients for at least 5 years post-diagnosis, a recent study revealed continued use may be beneficial: Women who had already completed 5 years of letrozole received either letrozole or placebo for 5 additional years. Five-year disease-free survival was slightly higher with letrozole than with placebo (95% vs. 91%), but overall 5-year survival was similar in the two groups. Because aromatase inhibitors do have adverse effects, discussions on whether to proceed with an additional 5 years of treatment (total, 10 years) should be informed by this trial: NEJM JW Gen Med Aug 1 2016 and *N Engl J Med* 2016; 375:209.

Is There a Natural Alternative?

When we attempt to support cancer patients naturally, we typically aren't trying to block estrogen production like the drugs do; we would rather support healthy, normal elimination of estrogens through proper metabolism. However, some women may over-express estrogen in a state of *hyper-aromatization* and do well on nutrients such as Chrysin, Quercetin, Naringenin, Resveratrol, Apigenin, Genistein, Grape Seed Extract, and Oleuropein, all *natural slowers* of aromatase.

Generally, our desire is to support healthy metabolism by supporting the cytochrome P-450 pathways (also look at these genes.) Compounds found in vegetables from the Brassica plant family, such as cabbage, brussels sprouts, and broccoli, are essential for this. I3C and DIM are found in these foods. Glutathione S transferase is also upregulated by the sulfur constituents in cruciferous vegetables, so make sure you look at and support genetic defects in the Transsulfuration genetic pathway.

Other nutrients that support healthy estrogen balance may include Norway spruce lignan extract and Hops extract. Plant lignans are phytonutrients commonly found in small amounts in unrefined whole grains, seeds, nuts, vegetables, berries, and beverages, such as tea (green tea) and coffee. The friendly bacteria in our intestines convert plant lignans into the *human* lignans called enterodiol and enterolactone. Aromatic-PN is a concentrated, naturally occurring plant lignan called 7-hydroxymatairesinol, which is derived from the Norway spruce (Picea abies.) In humans, 7-hydroxymatairesinol is a direct metabolic precursor of enterolactone.

Enterolactone is a phytoestrogen that binds to estrogen receptors and has both weak estrogenic and weak antiestrogenic effects. The latter accounts for much of its cell-protective capacity. Additionally, in vitro work has demonstrated that enterolactone affects aromatase and the biosynthesis of estrogen and has strong free radical scavenging and antioxidant properties.

The protective effect of lignans and enterolactone on tissues, including those of the prostate and breast, is encouraging. At the same time, the estrogenicity of HMR and enterolactone, although milder than estradiol, offers promising applications for women with menopausal concerns. For instance, in a randomized, single-blind, parallel group pilot study, 20 menopausal women taking 50mg/d of hydroxymatairesinol for eight weeks experienced half as many hot flashes as compared to pretreatment. Furthermore, high serum enterolactone has repeatedly been associated with cardiovascular health.

Fermented soy may also be a great addition to help balance estrogens. Note: fermented soy acts opposite that of unfermented soy!

Summary

Aromatase Inhibiting Medications

- Block the conversion of other hormones to estrogens
- Are widely prescribed in hormone positive cancer patients, especially those that are post-menopausal
- Carry the risk for numerous dangerous side-effects

Tamoxifen Medications

- Block the production of all estrogens
- Are widely prescribed to pre-menopausal breast cancer patients
- Carry the risk of numerous dangerous side-effects and unwanted changes and symptoms

Natural Alternatives That We Use

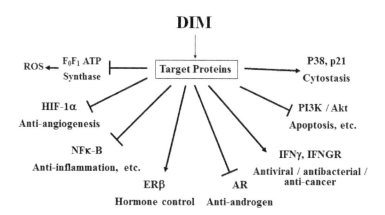

Cruciferous vegetables such as broccoli, cauliflower Brussel sprouts and cabbage

DIM

> shop.ConnersClinic.com/DIM

Quercetin

> shop.ConnersClinic.com/quercetin

Turmeric (Curcumin)

> shop.ConnersClinic.com/curcumin

Astragalus

> shop.ConnersClinic.com/astragalus

Scutellaria Barbata (adds to the effectiveness of DIM)

> shop.ConnersClinic.com/clear-inflam

Fermented Soy

> shop.ConnersClinic.com/soy

More information may be found here:

> ConnersClinic.com/aromatase-inhibitors

Electromagnetic Fields (EMFs)

Electromagnetic fields (EMFs) from cell phones, cell phone towers, power lines, high power lines, normal home electrical wiring, airport and military radar, all types of electrical substations, electrical transformers, computers, and other home appliances all have the potential to disturb human body cells. I believe that EMFs can contribute to the cause of brain tumors, other cancers including leukemia, a variety of birth defects, miscarriages, and all sorts of chronic illnesses.

Dr. David Carpenter, Dean at the School of Public Health, State University of New York believes it is likely that up to 30% of all childhood cancers come from exposure to EMFs. The Environmental Protection Agency (EPA) warns "There is reason for concern" and advises "prudent avoidance."

Martin Halper, the EPA's Director of Analysis and Support says, "I have never seen a set of epidemiological studies that remotely approached the weight of evidence that we're seeing with EMFs. Clearly there is something here."

The initial concern over possible problems with EMFs exploded after Paul Brodeur wrote a series of articles in the New Yorker Magazine in June 1989. His articles had a catalytic effect on scientists, reporters and concerned people throughout the world. In November 1989, the Department of Energy reported that "It has now become generally accepted that there are, indeed, biological effects due to field exposure."

The EMF issue gained more publicity in 1990 when alarming reports appeared in *Time*, the *Wall Street Journal*, *Business Week* and popular computer publications. ABC's Ted Koppel and CBS's Dan Rather both aired special segments on EMFs.

One prominent cardiovascular surgeon, Dr. Stephen Sinatra, MD, has written several books on the subject that I recommend you read. Search for his name on Amazon.

By 1990, over one hundred studies had been conducted worldwide and at least two dozen epidemiological studies on humans indicated a link between EMFs and serious health problems. In response to public pressure, the Environmental Protection Agency (EPA) began reviewing and evaluating the available literature and drafted several reports.

The EPA recommended in a 1990 report that EMFs be classified as a Class B carcinogen, stating that EMFs are a "probable human carcinogen and joined the ranks of

135

formaldehyde, DDT, dioxins and PCBs." After the 1990 EPA draft report was released, utility, military and computer lobbyists forced a final revision did ***not*** classify EMFs as a Class B carcinogen and the following explanation was added:

"At this time such a characterization regarding the link between cancer and exposure to EMFs is not appropriate because the basic nature of the interaction between EMFs and biological processes leading to cancer is not understood."

After the EPA placated to the various pressures (I never said they accepted bribes) the report also stated: "In conclusion, several studies showing Leukemia, Lymphoma and cancer of the nervous system in children exposed to supported by similar findings in adults in several occupational studies also involving electrical power frequency exposures, show a consistent pattern of response that suggest a causal link."

When questioned about the contradictory nature of these statements, the EPA responded that it was "not appropriate" to use the probable carcinogen label until it could demonstrate how EMFs caused cancer and exactly how much EMF is harmful.

Power Lines

Electrical generating stations both create and lose energy. The giant power lines that transmit the high-voltage electricity to be down-graded at local stations and transformers give off an enormous amount of stray electricity that disperses into the air and travels through our bodies. All power lines radiate electromagnetic fields into the environment; how much are the power lines near your home radiating? The amount of EMFs coming from a power line depends on its particular configuration, the age of the wires, other interferences in the conductivity, and even your home, work or environment that may contribute to the EMFs attraction. Power companies know which power line configurations are best for reducing

EMFs, but most don't feel the evidence supports costly changes in the way they deliver electricity.

An electrical substation is an assemblage of circuit breakers, disconnecting switches, and transformers designed to hold and transmit electricity to neighborhoods. Substations have been blamed for causing cancer clusters among nearby residents. Paul Brodeur wrote about several such cancer clusters in the July 9, 1990 issue of the New Yorker Magazine and I've personally seen areas of specific cities that have high incidences of brain cancers.

A key component of a utility's electrical distribution network depends upon numerous, small transformers mounted on power poles around town. A transformer looks like a small metal trash can, usually cylindrical, mounted at the top of the pole. Even when electrical service is placed underground, you will often see a metal box (usually square) located on the ground near the street. Many people don't realize that when they see a transformer, the power line feeding the transformer is 4000 to 13,800 volts and is transforming that voltage down to a usable (120v/240v) service for the nearby homes.

EMFs near a transformer can be quite high, but due to its small structure, the field strength diminishes rapidly with distance, as it does from any point source. For this reason, having a transformer located near your home is usually not a major source of concern, although just to make sure, everyone should measure the field strength around it. To di this you can use a meter called a gauss meter.

Your Home

With our patients that have a diagnosis of cancer, we sometimes make a point to go to their home and measure the extent of EMFs that may be a contributing factor in their recovery. We not only want to measure EMFs in their home but also sources of environmental toxins like chemicals gasifying off carpets or building materials, hidden fungus or mold, and chemicals used in the home. I just believe that we cannot leave any stone unturned!

If your home has high EMF readings, it is important to determine the sources of the EMF so that remedial action can be taken using *grounding*. Many times, a particular room will have higher EMF readings due to the configuration of the wiring, the appliances in the home, or something nearby.

Sometimes, the source of a high magnetic field is incorrect/faulty wiring/grounds. If you suspect that your home is wired improperly, obtain the services of a licensed electrician. Warning: Do not touch electric wires, even if you think the current is turned off. If you need to disconnect electrical circuits to determine the source of magnetic fields, you should call a licensed electrician.

There are several techniques that we employ when we *ground* a home. The first thing to understand is that each of us is a unique electrical conduit. We truly are little antennas walking around that filter electrical impulses as energy. A cursory understanding of quantum physics tells us that everything, broken down to its smallest component, is simply energy vibrating at a specific frequency. EMFs disturb our body's own frequencies.

Computers, Electric Blankets, and Waterbeds

EMFs radiate from all sides of the computer and can pose a serious health risk. Thus, you must not only be concerned with sitting in front of the monitor but also if you are sitting near a computer or if a computer is operating in a nearby room, for it is a major generating source of EMFs.

In 1990, the Swedish safety standard specified a maximum of 0.25mG at 50cm from a computer display. Many US-manufactured computers have EMFs of 5-100mG at this same distance. Screens placed over monitors do not block EMFs; even a lead screen will not block ELF and VLF (very low frequency) magnetic fields.

I know that it is almost impossible to live without a computer; I certainly couldn't! Try this: turn it off and unplug it when not in use.

Possibly one of the worst things to own, electric blankets create a magnetic field that penetrates about 6-7 inches into the body. It is not surprising that an epidemiological study has linked electric blankets with miscarriages and childhood leukemia. Just throw it away!

This pioneering work was performed by Dr. Nancy Wertheimer and Ed Leeper who originally discovered that magnetic fields were linked to childhood leukemia. Similar health effects have been noted with users of many electric blankets and waterbed heaters will emit EMFs even when turned off.

Electric Clocks, Fluorescent Lights, and Appliances

Electric clocks sitting on bedside stands across America have a very high magnetic field, as much as 5 to 10mG up to three feet away. It's like sleeping in an EMF equivalent to that of a power line. Think about moving all clocks and other electrical devices (such as telephones and answering devices) at least 6 feet from your bed; or better yet, **not** in the room where you sleep.

Fluorescent lights produce much more EMFs than incandescent bulbs. A typical fluorescent lamp in an office ceiling have readings of 160 to 200mg 1 inch away; that's horrible.

Microwave ovens and radar from military installations and airports emit two types of radiation: microwave and ELF. All microwave ovens leak and exceed safety limits. In addition, recent Russian studies have shown that normal microwave cooking converts food protein molecules into carcinogenic substances.

Electric razors and hair dryers emit EMFs as high as 200 to 400mG for the sort time they are in use. There are just not enough studies that prove whether short-term, high EMF exposure is more or less damaging than chronic exposure to a 2-3mG field. Some EMF consultants recommend that hair dryers not be used on children as the high fields are held close to their rapidly developing brain and nervous system can be a problem.

Telephones and Cell Phones

Telephones, especially cordless telephones, can emit surprisingly strong EMFs from the handset. This is a problem because of course we hold the telephone so close to our head. Place a Gauss meter right against the earpiece and the mouthpiece before buying a phone, or better yet, do **not** use cordless phones in your home. Cell phones have gotten a ton of press regarding EMFs. Surprise, surprise, every study that has shown no ill-effects from cell phones was paid for by the cell phone industry. Always read into the possible biases of scientific studies.

What to *Do*

Dr. Sinatra wrote a book with Clinton Ober and Martin Zucker titled *Earthing*. It goes into details on the need for all of us to remain "grounded" with the earth. I know to most reading this book, these concepts sound more like something out of the hippy generation, but it makes scientific sense. Grounding or Earthing as spoken of in the book I referred to is natural and simple and affects every aspect of your physiology. When you ground yourself, you physically add electrons to your body and thereby increase pH to the tissue; an important concept for those with cancer.

James Oschman, Ph.D., an internationally renowned expert on energy medicine and author of *Energy Medicine; The Scientific Basis*, describes the phenomenon of personal grounding/earthing: "Recently I attended a meeting on the East coast. One of my colleagues came in from the West coast. She had a bad case of jet lag. I told her to take her shoes and socks off and step outside on the grass for 15 minutes. When she came back in, she was completely transformed. Her jet lag was gone. That is how fast Earthing works. Anyone can try this. If you don't feel well, for whatever reason, just make barefoot contact with the Earth for a few minutes and see what happens. Of course, if you have a medical problem, you should see a doctor. There is nothing that comes close to earthing for quick relief. You can literally feel pain draining from your body the instant you touch the Earth."

The human body is mostly water and minerals and is therefore a good conductor of electricity (electrons.) The free electrons on the surface of the earth are easily transferred to the human body as long as there is direct contact. Remember, you are simply an antenna. Unfortunately, synthetically soled shoes made of rubber and plastic act as insulators so that even when we are outside and walking on the ground; we are insulated from the earth's electric field. When we are in homes and office buildings, we are also unable to receive the earth's balancing energies.

Is this "new age?" No, it is simply physics. The Earth's electric field is mainly a continuous direct current (DC) producing field that is a giant transmitter of electrons. By comparison, home wiring systems in the US use 60-cycle per second alternating current (AC) and other forms of man-made environmental electromagnetic fields (EMFs.) Some people are just more sensitive to EMFs than others. Someone may develop cancer due in part to EMF exposure and another family member with equal exposure appears unaffected. Again, this is just one more causative factor!

So, what can you do? There are some simple steps that everyone can take (not just people with cancer) to ground their home and themselves. First, start with looking at your footwear. Standard plastic/rubber or composite soles on your shoes do not conduct the earth's electric energy and can contribute to a host of illnesses. You need leather or hide soles, which used to be the primary footwear materials in the past. Leather itself isn't conductive, but the foot perspires, and the moisture permits conduction of the energy from the earth through the leather and up into the body. In addition, moisture from walking on damp ground or sidewalks could permeate up into the leather-soled shoe. Thickness of the sole can also be a factor, and specifically that very thick leather soles may not allow the moisture through. Moccasins are the best type of natural conductive footwear. Leather isn't quite as good as bare feet on the ground but certainly much, much better than standard soles that are insulating.

There are companies that sell grounding kits and Earthing products around the world. Remember, there is a difference between personally grounding yourself to the earth (Earthing) and grounding your home or office in a protective measure against stray EMFs. In our practice, we sometimes send a team out to the home of cancer patients to make sure their house is as free from EMFs as possible. We also test for hidden mold, fungi, etc. There are lots of things that can make you and keep you sick!

Grounding your home includes physically checking grounding rods that were supposed to be installed to see if they are working properly, installing new rods and connections if this is not done, utilizing special volcanic materials called dragonite (it's a ground basalt) to block stray EMFs as well as other techniques to "clean" the home, and using products from Satic company that are specially designed and tested to reduce "dirty electricity." There are personal products that can also help, like grounding mats that you can stand on, mattress pads, seat cushions, attachments to computers and other things. But start simply by unplugging appliances that are not in use, stop using some of the things I wrote about above, and get the electrical things out of your bedroom.

Grounding material, home, and cell phone protection products may be purchased from our office store: shop.ConnersClinic.com/EMF

What We Use

Hedron 5G Cell Phone Protectors

shop.ConnersClinic.com/hedron-phone

Radiation Free Headphones

shop.ConnersClinic.com/earbuds

shop.ConnersClinic.com/over-ear

Hedron Body Shield

shop.ConnersClinic.com/hedron-body

Satic Home Plug-in

shop.ConnersClinic.com/satic-plug

Satic Whole-Home Protection

shop.ConnersClinic.com/satic-home

Grounding Sheet

shop.ConnersClinic.com/grounding-sheet

I highly recommend the book *Earthing* to all my readers to help them understand the concept. It is easy to explain to my Minnesota patients who love to hunt. I often hear men say something like, "I just love to go sit in the woods next to a tree. I don't even care if I see a deer; I just love being out in the woods." They are grounding themselves, whether they know it or not. They are receiving an abundance of electrons from the earth and alkalizing their bodies and decreasing inflammation. They are healing.

This is exactly what the Rife light is doing for my patients with cancer. The photons dispersed from the Tesla tube act as electron donors and ground the patient by adding electrons and alkalizing and healing the patient. The more specific we can be to the frequency of the tissue treated, the more electrons the body receives.

So, it is with grounding and earthing. The more stray EMFs we can erase from the environment and the more electrons we can receive from the earth, the healthier you will become.

Biotoxins

Biotoxins, in general, are living organisms that disrupt cellular function. Many biotoxins are also neurotoxins in that they adversely affect neurologic function.

Biotoxins can be:

- Bacteria
- Fungi
- Mold
- Virus
- Parasite
- Endotoxins

Fungi

You often hear about fungus being a cause of cancer, and that may be true. The most important mycotoxins are aflatoxins, ochratoxin A, fumonisins, trichothecenes and zearalenone. Aflatoxins are potent carcinogens and, in association with hepatitis B virus, are responsible for many thousands of human deaths per annum, mostly in non-industrialized tropical countries. Ochratoxin A is a probable carcinogen and may cause urinary tract cancer and kidney damage in people from northern and eastern Europe. Fumonisins appear to be the cause of esophageal cancer in southern Africa, parts of China and elsewhere. Trichothecenes are highly immunosuppressive and zearalenone causes estrogenic effects in animals and man. Currently available records and statistics do not reflect the major role played by mycotoxins in mortality attributable to food-borne micro-organisms.

Other fungi, like the one that causes Valley Fever in Southwestern US states, Coccidioidomycosis, reveals an initial infection that is almost invariably in the lungs. Other generalized toxic manifestations associated with this and other fungal infections, such as fever, arthralgia, skin rash, etc., and certain complications such as pulmonary cavitation, hemorrhage, Broncho-pleural fistula, and hydropneumothorax are all possible. If you have such symptoms and seek treatment, it doesn't equate to irradiation of the fungus in the body.

Some fungi, like *C. neoformans* grow as a yeast (unicellular) and replicates by budding. When grown as yeast, *C. neoformans* has a prominent capsule composed mostly of lipopolysaccharides (LPS), similar to other gram-negative bacteria. When effectively killed, LPS is released into the bloodstream and becomes a toxin in itself (an endotoxin.)

How fungi cause cancer is believed to be tied to their ability to infiltrate the cell and disrupt apoptotic CASPASE systems.

Using Medicinal Mushrooms to kill fungi may be the best treatment. Following the philosophy of Hormesis, it makes sense that something from the same genus would be an effective cure. We always recommend being tested!

Helicobacter Pylori

Helicobacter pylori, or *H. pylori*, is a spiral-shaped, gram-negative bacterium that is oral-borne, meaning it enters the body through the mouth. In many people, it can reside in the mucus layer that coats the inside of the human stomach, which would then produce an ulcer. In most, it leaves the stomach causing ***cancer*** and/or ***heart disease***.

To survive in the harsh, acidic environment of the stomach, *H. pylori* secretes an enzyme called urease, which converts the chemical urea to ammonia. The production of ammonia around *H. pylori* neutralizes the acidity of the stomach, making it more hospitable for the bacterium. If a person has adequate HCl production in the stomach, the chance of *H. pylori* being able to take hold and proliferate is slim. Decreased HCl and digestive enzyme production, commonly caused by eating a typical American diet, sets an individual up for a local and/or systemic infection. In addition, the helical shape of *H. pylori* allows it to burrow into the mucus layer, which is less acidic than the inside space, or lumen, of the stomach. *H. pylori* can also attach to the cells that line the inner surface of the stomach.

Although immune cells that normally recognize and attack invading bacteria accumulate near sites of *H. pylori* infection, they are unable to reach the stomach lining. In addition, *H. pylori* has developed ways of interfering with local immune responses, making them ineffective in eliminating this bacterium.

H. pylori have an increased risk of gastric adenocarcinoma. According to the WHO, it is the number one cause of stomach cancer worldwide. The risk increase appears to be restricted to non-cardia gastric cancer. For example, a 2001 combined analysis of 12 case–control studies of *H. pylori* and gastric cancer estimated that the risk of non-cardia gastric cancer was nearly six times higher for *H. pylori*-infected people than for uninfected people.

Additional evidence for an association between *H. pylori* infection and the risk of non-cardiac gastric cancer comes from prospective cohort studies such as the Alpha-Tocopherol, Beta-Carotene (ATBC) Cancer Prevention Study in Finland. Comparing subjects who developed non-cardiac gastric cancer with cancer-free control subjects, the researchers found that *H. pylori*-infected individuals had a nearly eightfold increased risk for non-cardiac gastric cancer.

We have found that *H. pylori*-infected people have a much higher risk for *many* types of cancer!

Histamine

Researchers in Finland, Sweden, and Switzerland have shown how the most aggressive form of brain cancer, glioblastoma, can be stopped in its tracks by an antihistamine drug that triggers a form of cell death caused by leaky lysosomes. Though this was a mouse study, as most initial studies are, it is very promising. Headed by Pirjo Laakkonen, PhD, at the University of Helsinki, the studies demonstrated an association between the fatty acid binding protein mammary-derived growth inhibitor (MDGI) and poorer prognosis in patients.

MDGI shuttles fatty acids into cells where they, among other things, become integral components of lysosomal membranes. Lysosomes are little organelles inside our cells that contain numerous digestive enzymes that remove waste and recycle worn-out cellular parts to help keep a cell alive. Healthy lysosomal membranes enclose these enzymes and release them inside the cell only when necessary. If we could destabilize these membranes, we could spill the content of the lysosomes (the digestive enzymes) into the cell and essentially stimulate apoptosis (cell death.)

The study focused on Glioblastoma, one of the most aggressive brain cancers we face. The team's studies found that blocking the MDGI gene (thereby not allowing fatty acids into the cell as readily) in glioblastoma cell lines disrupted fatty acid transport into cells and their incorporation into lysosomal membranes, which compromised lysosomal membrane composition and integrity, resulting in lysosomal membrane permeabilization (LMP.) LMP is an intracellular cell death pathway triggered when the lysosome contents leak into the cell. The team's subsequent studies in cell lines and in live mice found that treatment with the antihistamine Clemastine (Dayhist, Dayhist Allergy, and Allergy Relief), an older type of antihistamine that can cross the blood-brain barrier, effectively mirrored the effects of MDGI, triggering LMP and causing glioblastoma cell death, without harming healthy cells.

In non-brain tumors where crossing the blood-brain barrier is not an issue, theory may admit that any antihistamine, drug or natural histamine blockers, may illicit the same response in many tumors. Should all cancer patients go on antihistamine medications or histamine blocking nutrients? That remains to be answered with more studies, but this looks very promising!

Through further experiments the investigators showed that MDGI was essential to glioma cell survival. Glioma cells engineered to overexpress MDGI also grew more aggressively and invasively than non-engineered tumor cells following implantation into experimental mice. Conversely, silencing the MDGI gene dramatically reduced the viability of patient-derived glioma cells and blocked cell proliferation. Human glioblastoma cells lacking MDGI were also unable to form tumors when transplanted into mice. "These results demonstrate a dose-dependent effect of MDGI silencing on glioblastoma cell growth and viability."

Read more at ConnersClinic.com/histamine-and-cancer

Histamine's Double-Edged Sword

Our body has two distinct methods of clearing things that could bring it harm: our immune system kills living toxins (bacteria, virus, parasites…) and our detoxification pathways clear non-living toxins (chemicals, heavy metals, drugs…) We have one other system that sits somewhere in the middle between the immune and the detoxification systems that helps with both: the mast cells.

Mast cells make a chemical called histamine, which has numerous, distinct, beneficial roles. As part of the immune response, histamine doesn't kill bad guys itself. It draws fluid to tissues by rendering capillaries more permeable, making it easier for immune killer cells to "ride the waves" to a nasty bacteria to destroy. Histamine's immune and detoxification connection runs deep as its functions vary depending on tissue site and specific receptors on the outside of cells to which it binds.

In the brain, histamine can keep us awake, is involved in our reflex reaction to pain, temperature changes, vibration, and hormone balance. It affects our appetite, helps control gastric secretions helping balance blood pH, and serves as a gatekeeper for neurotransmitters that balance mood, concentration, and focus.[98] [99] [100] [101] This makes sense if you think about it. If exposed to an infection, a chemical irritant, something that stimulates pain, or a dangerous vibration felt in the legs or feet, you would need to wake the brain to increase circulation, and flee such harm, buffer the blood to maintain life, and alert us to possible threat.

Histamine so serves the *flight or fight* mechanism to ensure life. It's role in the periphery demonstrates this as well. If histamine attaches to one receptor (there exists 4 main histamine receptors, H1, H2, H3, and H4, with different functions) it is vasoconstrictive enabling quick movement of blood to extremities to fuel muscles for a quick *getaway*. Attaching to a different receptor, histamine dilates small vessels and constricts the bronchial tubes as an immediate protective *freeze* mode. It enhances a hypersensitivity to harmful stimuli creating its most known response: the histamine rash and itch. This would serve to keep us safe from poisonous fauna and teach us that those berries are possibly not edible.

However, histamine, when created in excess over a period of time, will create an environment of chronic inflammation, disturbing cell-to-cell communication and thereby changing its function. Cell function is dependent on their interaction with the environment. If we think of individual cells as people, an organ could be equivalent to a crowded stadium gathered

---

[98] Panula P, Chazot PL, Cowart M, et al. (2015). "International Union of Basic and Clinical Pharmacology. XCVIII. Histamine Receptors". Rev. 67 (3): 601–55

[99] Wouters MM, Vicario M, Santos J (2015). "The role of mast cells in functional GI disorders". Gut. 65: 155–168. doi:10.1136/gutjnl-2015-309151. PMID 26194403

[100] Blandina, Patrizio; Munari, Leonardo; Provensi, Gustavo; Passani, Maria B. (2012). "Histamine neurons in the tuberomamillary nucleus: a whole center or distinct subpopulations?". Frontiers in Systems Neuroscience

[101] Maguire JJ, Davenport AP (29 November 2016). "H2 receptor". IUPHAR/BPS Guide to PHARMACOLOGY. International Union of Basic and Clinical Pharmacology. Retrieved 20 March 2017

to observe a football game. Communication to your friend seated next to you may be relatively easy during slow play and more challenging when the home team is guarding the one-yard line. The roar lifts, chants of "de-fence" try to drown out the opposing quarterback's play call, and you can barely hear yourself think as you stand, scream, cheer, and cover your ears. A touchdown is scored, and silence calms the saddened crowd. All sit. Equilibrium ensues.

If we could liken this scenario to cells in the milieu of the body with thousands upon thousands of conversations taking place, sodas being ordered from barkers selling cold beer and peanuts, opposing fans arguing, people shuffling between rows and hundreds of other activities, we would need to envision a million stadiums with hundreds of millions of observers to understand the complexity of the human body. Think of how difficult it is to communicate when the opposing team has the ball at the one-yard line, and this is similar to a cell receiving correct information in a chaos of chronic inflammation.

When histamine levels increase both within and between the cells, causing fluid to accumulate, our body responds with an intricate system to remove the water and regain equilibrium. It signals a special gene called the HNMT gene to make an enzyme that quickly drops histamine levels and fluids decrease accordingly. The crowd sits during a lull in the game. So it is, when we are exposed to allergens, histamine is released, bringing a washing of fluid, the HNMT gene makes its histamine-degrading enzyme, and tissues are cleansed, the cells are bathed, and balance is achieved. This cycle of the histamine cleanse helps us get rid of things that we eat and breathe that are not beneficial.

Histamine's relationship with the stress response brings a bit of clarity on how the system can go wrong. In its protective role in the "flight, fight, or freeze" response, histamine is released with an uptick of the sympathetic nervous system (SNS.) The SNS controls adrenal output and cortisol release.

When we perceive danger, SNS stimulation protection raises blood pressure, shunts blood to extremities, and dilates pupils, enabling us to best survive the assault. All functions considered non-essential to survival are suppressed. Our brain conserves energy. You don't need to reproduce when you're being chased by a tiger; shut that down. A tiger is going to eat me, who cares if I die from mercury poisoning in ten years, shut down detoxification! I'm soon to be food to a predator, stop all wasted energy on digestion, immune function, and fighting chronic disease.

By now you're probably understanding how the modern, chronic predators of running a business, raising a family, stressful, abusive relationships, paying the bills and filling out tax forms can influence cell communication and our ability to fight disease. You could argue that modern society has created its own tigers and even rewards the increased productivity gained by the chase. The downfalls of such a system are evidenced in the rise of chronic disease including cancer.

Higher histamine levels, together with its stimulation of the H4 cell receptors, have been reported in many different tumors including melanoma, colon, pancreatic, and breast cancer. Moreover, histamine content increased unequivocally in other human cancer types such as ovarian, cervical, and endometrial carcinoma in comparison with their adjoining normal tissues, suggesting the participation of histamine in carcinogenesis.

Histamine's story worsened when recent studies noted that most malignant cell lines express their own histamine-synthesizing enzyme, L-histidine decarboxylase (HDC) and contain high concentrations of endogenous histamine that can be released to the spaces between the cells.[102]

Why would a cancer cell want to create commotion and disturb communication between itself and the body? You

---

[102] Bartholeyns and Fozard, 1985; Garcia-Caballero et al., 1994; Engel et al., 1996; Rivera et al., 2000; Falus et al., 2001; Pós et al., 2004

might theorize that histamine may regulate diverse biological responses related to tumor growth. Growing cancers require angiogenesis, cell invasion, migration, differentiation, stunted apoptosis, and modulation of the immune response, indicating that histamine may be a crucial mediator in cancer development and progression. Many cancers have even revealed a much higher concentration of histamine receptors on their cell membranes, further suggesting that histamine stimulates proliferation.

This reveals, once again, that no bodily function should be labeled as *good* vs *bad*. An imbalance, usually due to some environmental force acting on the body, creates undesirable circumstances. If the imbalance tips histamine levels towards cancer proliferation, how can we target histamine in cancer therapy? You would immediately think that pharmacological antihistamines might be in order, however antihistamine medications only target H1 and H2 histamine receptors. So, while they may reduce a stuffy nose, they do nothing to help a cancer patient. Novel approaches need to be investigated to help target H4 receptors, alter and their ligands.

Here are a few ideas we are beginning to implement at Conners Clinic:

- The use of DAO enzyme both orally and as a rectal suppository. DAO is the specific enzyme made by the HNMT gene in the tissues as well as the ABP gene in the gut cavity. The problem with oral dosing has been its failure to be absorbed and enact any benefit to the tissues. Genetic aberrations (SNPs) or defects (mutations) may result in a lesser ability to produce such enzyme, a decreased capacity to clear histamine, and a tendency towards histamine-related disorders including (possibly) cancer.

- The DAO enzyme requires flavin adenine dinucleotide (FAD) as its cofactor and FAD requires the B Vitamin riboflavin (B2) for its synthesis. So, adding a whole-food source of B2 may also be in order.

- A novel use of Rife frequencies in an attempt to regain the normal synchronicity of over-productive mast and basophil cells.

- Use of relatively higher dose, unique enzymes (beta glucanase, chitinase, xylanase, alpha galactosidase, phytase, astrazyme, serratiopeptidase, peptidases, and proteases) orally to aide in the reduction of histamine stimulating antigens in the digestive tract, break biofilms (histamine-responsible) surrounding the cancer, and help bond to receptor sites on the cancer.

- Coupling nutritional therapies with Sauna Therapy which has shown to decrease mast cell activation[103]

- Stimulation of parasympathetic receptors to reduce sympathetic dominance and lower histamine release.

- Employing the Fasting Mimicking Diet (FMD) as well as Time Restricted Eating (TRE.)

- Cognitive, mindful meditation and prayer.

- A deeper look at genetic pathways gives us other clues to assist DAO production. The HNMT and ADH genes require supplemental zinc, Vitamin C, magnesium, and thiamine.

- Quercetin, a natural compound found in apples, onions, and capers is a wonderful natural histamine

---

[103] Beneficial effect of sauna therapy on severe antihistamine-resistant chronic urticarial, Eli Magen MD, Leumit Health Services, and Allergy and Clinical Immunology Unit, Barzilai Medical Center, Ashkelon, affiliated with Faculty of Health Sciences, Ben-Gurion University of Negev, Beer Sheva, Israel

reducer. Unfortunately, it is poorly absorbed (about 1%) so use as a suppository may prove more beneficial.

- Holy Basil, Milk Thistle, and EGCg (from green tea extract), Aloe, Bromelain, Stinging Nettle, Pine Bark Extract, Marshmallow Root, Bitter Orange, and Licorice can be helpful as may Ellagic acid found in raspberries, strawberries, walnuts, mango kernel, and pomegranate.

Understanding Detoxification

We Are All Exposed!

Even if we only eat organic and have never used chemicals on our plants or lawn, pesticides and herbicides are ubiquitous. You can run, but you cannot hide! Eat healthy and never use this crap on your lawn, but understand that you still have intracellular toxins!

Detoxification is the key. Let's be clear though, you are always detoxifying, or you'd be dead already. We need to both increase the rate of detoxification as well as assist the specialized pathways at clearing these poisons.

As stated, it is mainly the liver that we need to support. Our liver plays an important role in protecting us from potentially toxic chemical insults through its capacity to convert them into more water-soluble metabolites, which can be efficiently eliminated from the body via the urine, or through the bile into the colon, eventually making it into the toilet.

This protective ability of the liver stems from the expression of a wide variety of enzymes and their ability to create detailed processes known as Phase 1 detoxification (oxidation, reduction and hydrolysis), Phase 2 (conjugation), Phase 2.5 (a termed coined by Dr. Kelly Halderman of Conners Clinic that involves it's binding to bile acids), and Phase 3 (a function of the gut to keep toxins bound so they don't simply reabsorb.)

When you desire to support detoxification (regardless of the chemical in question), you need to begin by supporting Phase 3 and then moving backwards through the process. We don't want to support pulling junk out of the cells to have it simply circulate in the blood stream and be deposited elsewhere nor do we want to support Phase 1 liver detoxification to have a blockage just cause a greater toxicity in the liver. We need to unclog the pipe at the bottom first.

Detoxification Simplified: Phases 6 through 0

When we discuss the Phases of Detoxification, we are usually talking about the three phases of liver detoxification. However, if the ultimate purpose is to remove toxins from the body, we need to expand upon these steps. I like to talk about seven phases of detoxification (Phases 0-6) and tell patients they had better begin with phase 6 and work backwards. Let me explain:

Phase 6: Proper Elimination

Daily bowel movements and healthy urinary habits are the final step in removing toxins from the body. It is one of our cardinal rules that health depends on eliminating wastes and we want everyone to be having a regular bowel movement on a daily basis. It is even better to be having several daily bowel movements. If this isn't happening for you, see the steps below. These are in order of what to try first, second, and so on. It is fine to do more than one of these at the same time. For each approach listed below, try for a day or two. If you have little or no success, add another approach:

Fiber: taking SunFiber or SunSpectrum (the products we usually recommend because they contain the best non-

156

digestible fiber) can be a big help. Also, eating whole fruits and vegetables is so important. Find those products here:

SunFiber

shop.ConnersClinic.com/sunfiber

SunSpectrum

shop.ConnersClinic.com/sunspectrum

Magnesium and Vitamin C: take 500-700mg Magnesium Citrate or Magnesium Malate with 1000-1500mg Vitamin C one to two times per day will loosen the stools. Most people are already deficient in magnesium anyways so taking magnesium can benefit nearly every metabolic pathway. If you take excess magnesium (as in this approach), you tend to dump it in the bowel, drawing water with it, thereby loosening the stool. Make sure you are drinking plenty of water to make this happen.

Magna Clear

shop.ConnersClinic.com/magna-clear

Prune Juice

drinking some good old-fashioned prune juice everyday can often do the trick

Senna Tea: Senna is an herb. Celestial Seasons makes a Smooth Move tea that works well. The longer you steep it, the stronger it is, so be aware of this. Drinking one glass or more before bed usually helps by morning. There are many products on the market with Senna as well. The negative and positive about Senna is in its mechanism of action. It stimulates peristaltic contractions of the intestinal smooth muscles. This is great to create a bowel movement but can be fairly uncomfortable as it gives you a strong cramping. Try it once or twice, everyone is a bit different on how they react.

Dr. Schultz Formula One: this is an herbal formula that works very well to produce a healthy bowel movement. Start with one or two before bed and play with the dosage so you don't get diarrhea.

Coffee Enemas: even if you are already doing these, increasing the number per day can really help. Coffee enemas help cleanse the liver and stimulate the vagal nerve and colon function. You can also do an enema with probiotics, warm water, Epsom salts, and olive oil.

Find more info on coffee enemas here:

ConnersClinic.com/coffee-enemas-1

ConnersClinic.com/coffee-enemas-2

Colonics: visiting a clinic that specializes in colonic therapy can be beneficial to help clean out the gut. However, beware of doing more than just a few sessions regardless of what they are trying to sell you as you can flush your good flora with high colonics as well. Stick to 3-4 sessions to start.

Healthy kidney function is the second part of phase 6. You need to be drinking enough water to be flushing out the kidneys and bladder. If you are not eliminating urine completely (as in prostate, kidney, bladder or urethral cancer), a catheter may be necessary. Kidney function testing can reveal a need for increased water intake as well. Products like our Kidney Korrect have herbs that help.

Sweating, e.g. detoxifying through one's skin, is a helpful way to take pressure off the liver and kidneys. This is one reason that saunas are so beneficial. Doing a sauna several times per week aides in detoxification and can even raise the core body temperature to help kill cancers that are close to the skin surface. Doing foot bath detoxification and things like skin brushing can also help the process.

Phase 5: Add a Gut "Binder"

Binders, in nutritional-speak, are nutraceuticals that have a tendency to bind to toxins to aide in their removal. They are chelators that don't absorb, staying in the gut to grab onto toxins and escort them into the toilet.

One major problem in clearing toxins is the fact that they tend to reabsorb in the gut and recirculate again. One reason this happens is an excessive intestinal transit time (food takes too long to get through the gut.) Going back to phase 6 helps with this. Another reason is an imbalance in hormones. Estrogens, especially *bad estrogens* (quinone estrogens, 4-hydroxy catechol estrogens) are easily reabsorbed in the large intestine, which is never a good thing. Using DIM can help prevent this as well as one or more of the binders listed below.

Some of our favorite binder products include:

Zeolite Complex Binder

shop.ConnersClinic.com/zeolite

Detox Accelerator

shop.ConnersClinic.com/detox-accelerator

GastroMycin

shop.ConnersClinic.com/gastromycin

Phase 3 Complete

shop.ConnersClinic.com/phase-3

Phase 4: Flushing the Gallbladder

The gallbladder is a pocket where your body stores bile. Bile is made in the liver and serves several purposes. It carries the excreted toxins from the liver to the intestinal tract and it is the main way we breakdown fat in the intestine. The reason we have a gallbladder to hold the bile is because of bile's second function. Digestion of fats consumed is extremely important, so bile needs to be in the intestinal lumen when fats are present. The gallbladder holds the bile until we eat fat, thereby causing a contraction of the gallbladder, which squirts the majority of stored bile into the first part of the small intestine.

When we have sluggish bile or stones in the gallbladder, this process is not working efficiently. Less bile is present for fat digestion and worse, there exists a backup of toxins exiting the liver. The liver becomes congested and a cascade of problems can ensue including less liver uptake of toxins from the blood that causes toxins to be stored throughout the cells of the body. The liver may increase production of lower density cholesterol to help lubricate the process, which can contribute to other health issues.

Supporting gallbladder function is essential. You can get clues to gallbladder problems by seeing an elevated bilirubin on blood work, but functional issues can be present long before this occurs. We suggest doing a mild gallbladder flush on a regular basis and supporting its function with products like our product named Gallbladder ND.

Phase 3: Support Bile Excretion from the Liver (Flow)

As you can see, we are working our way backwards. Toxins enter the body through absorption through the gut, skin, or lungs, circulate through the bloodstream and hopefully head out of the liver through the bile to the gallbladder to the gut and to the toilet. Our goal is to aide this process.

Bile exits the liver through the right and left hepatic ducts that then form the common bile duct. Bile leaving the gallbladder exits into the common bile duct as well as do enzymes excreted by the pancreas. Cancers of the pancreas and/or bile duct and liver can interfere with this flow as can cause sluggish production of bile by the liver.

One helpful way to support bile flow is to use heat over the liver/gallbladder area. Castor oil packs with heat can be even more helpful.

Phase 2.5: Bile Production

Phase 2.5 is a term coined by Dr. Kelly Halderman to describe the movement of conjugated toxins from phase 2 into the bile, coupled with the movement of bile salts and phosphatidylcholine. This requires adequate production of bile and necessary substrates present for the liver to do so. Oftentimes this process is not functioning properly due to inflammation, endotoxins from pathogenic intestinal flora, and hormone imbalances. Toxins will then be forced to be excreted back into the blood where they may cause further damage and increase stress on the kidneys.

To support the production of bile, an all-important step in clearing the liver, our favorite products include:

Phosphatidylcholine

shop.ConnersClinic.com/phosphatidylcholine

Phase 2.5 Complete

shop.ConnersClinic.com/phase-2-5

Phase 2: Conjugation

Phase 2 enzymes in the liver are regulated by a transcription factor called Nrf2 (nuclear factor erythroid 2 [NF-E2] p45-related factor 2.) Nrf2 is key to regulating the body's detoxification and antioxidant system in other cells as well. When activated, Nrf2 dissociates from the cytosolic protein,

Keap1 (we talk about this when we look at a person's genes), and *turns on* the genes associated with phase 2 detoxification.

Nrf2-modulation by curcumin, sulforaphane, garlic, catechins (EGCg form green tea extract), resveratrol, ginger, coffee, rosemary, blueberry, pomegranate, ellagic acid, and Astaxanthin has proven to be great nutrients to stimulate phase 2 detoxification.

For example, Sulfur transferase is a phase 2 enzyme that adds sulfur groups to compounds in order to make them more water soluble and less reactive. This process is used on a wide variety of toxic molecules including phenols, amines, acetaminophen, and food dyes. Many chemicals that are able to become airborne are sulfated. Patients with autism have been found to have impaired sulfation ability, which will make these individuals more sensitive to toxins.

Paraoxonase 1 (PON1) is an enzyme that is able to perform paraoxonase activity on substrates. This enzyme is able to hydrolyze and detoxify many different types of organophosphate molecules. PON1 is one of the major pathways that protect people from these types of compounds. Mutations to PON1 could lead someone to be more sensitive to pesticides and increase one's risk for cancer. Infants do not have a lot of PON1 activity.

Phase 1: The P450s

There are numerous enzymes and processes in the phase 1 family but the 58 known cytochrome P450 enzymes are most important. While many things happen, we could summarize the process into their ability to take a toxin from the blood and make it able to be processed to get them out of the body.

For example, one P450, Cyp2C9, is involved with the metabolism of a large number of medications including NSAIDs, warfarin, and tamoxifen. Cyp2E1 is involved with the detoxification of many industrial pollutants, as well as carcinogens. Cyp2e1 also metabolizes ethanol to acetaldehyde and acetate. Cyp2e1 is also responsible for bioactivating a number of carcinogens, including cigarette smoke.

Supporting Phase 1 and 2 liver pathways; this is where understanding one's genetic pathway issues come into play. CYP and PON1 defects help guide product use, but, in general, here are some ideas:

PON1 Assist

shop.ConnersClinic.com/pon1

Liver Health

shop.ConnersClinic.com/liver-health

Liver ND

shop.ConnersClinic.com/liver-nd

CleansXym

shop.ConnersClinic.com/cleansxym

HM-ND

shop.ConnersClinic.com/hm-nd

Phase 0: Pulling Garbage Out of the Cells and Intracellular Spaces

Unfortunately, this is where many people want to start when they think they need to detoxify. It's understandable, we want to "get rid of the mercury from our dental fillings" or "detoxify chemicals we were just exposed to" *but starting here can be very dangerous.*

It's true that we are all toxic. Every day the above phases of detoxification are happening to one degree or another, and to the extent they are hindered is the extent we become toxic.

We are what we eat. More accurately, we are what we absorb. Even better stated, *we are what we don't detoxify*! In a magical fairyland, everything you absorb is quickly dumped into the toilet and all is well. In real life, endless events hinder this, and cells gather poisons to store them away. Hopefully, they stay there until we die at age 120, but this isn't always so. If they happen to interrupt normal cell death apoptosis pathways or worse, affect the replication rate of the nucleus, they are causes of cancer.

The way we pull junk out of our cells and tissues is by using a chelator. A chelator is simply a nutrient that tends to grab onto toxins and escorts them back to the blood where they can circulate to the liver and start phase 1. However, I hope you've come to appreciate the need to make sure phases 6, 5, 4, 3, 2.5, 2, and 1 are working well *first* before we start pulling garbage from the cells or we will just re-deposit them elsewhere!

I rank chelators from mild to strong and believe that you should *not* use strong chelators if you have mercury fillings in your teeth (silver fillings) or metal implants.

Mild Chelators (okay for most people)

Chlora-Xyme

shop.ConnersClinic.com/chlora-xym

PectaSol-C

shop.ConnersClinic.com/pectasol-c

Homeopathic Chelators

Moderate Chelators

Metal-X Synergy

shop.ConnersClinic.com/metal-x-synergy

IP-6

shop.ConnersClinic.com/ip6

Strong Chelators (do *not* use if you have silver fillings)

Chela Clear

shop.ConnersClinic.com/chelex

Note: While all 5 steps *can* be done at the same time, it may be best to **start** with phase 6 and work backwards just as I listed them, progressing slowly over multiple weeks. And, as always, it is best to have a qualified practitioner help you along the way.

Great Foods to Help Detoxify

Diet is something a healthy person can change to help keep healthy. Though those with serious issues may require a more concentrated effort to help detoxify, below is a list of foods that can help the process:

Colorful Produce

You've probably noticed that many foods that support good health are also intensely colorful. Their vibrant colors are produced by the rich abundance of phytonutrients and antioxidants they contain. Blueberries, carrots, and beets are good examples. Beets are especially good detoxifiers for the liver, bile duct, and gallbladder and are full of B Vitamins and minerals, including zinc, crucial for the immune system. Beets are also full of fiber, which help cleanse the digestive tract.

Turmeric/Curcumin

Turmeric is a bright-yellow root commonly used as a spice in traditional Indian cooking. As happens so often with ancient medical practices, scientific research has confirmed the benefits of turmeric. This spice (curcumin, its main active ingredient) have been shown to detoxify the body, improve digestion, protect cellular health, increase antioxidant protection, and enhance immunity, among other benefits. It is a major anti-inflammatory supplement!

Cultured/Fermented Foods

Cultured and fermented vegetables should also be on your spring menu. The fermentation process increases digestibility and boosts nutrient and probiotic profiles significantly. These foods support immunity and aid detoxification. Sauerkraut and kimchee, for example, are sources of probiotics, enzymes, and nutrients that support digestion, detoxification, and overall health. See our blog post on Water Kefir; one of my favorites!

Mushrooms

Since Medicinal Mushrooms is obviously one of my favorites, I must include it here as well. Many culinary mushrooms are rich in antioxidants and compounds that help detoxify the body, boost immunity, reduce inflammation, and even repair damaged tissue. Shitake, Oyster, and Maitake are excellent examples that can be included in soups, sautés, and other savory dishes.

Lemons

Lemon helps the body remove toxins and is also an excellent tonic for both the liver and gall bladder. Here's what we've recommended: a daily dose of an olive oil or coconut oil and lemon mixture during detoxification. Cut an organic lemon into small pieces and blend it with 1¼ cups spring water and a tablespoon of olive oil or coconut oil. Partially strain the mixture, leaving some pulp. (The pectin from the lemon peel helps the digestive tract.) Drink before bed. In addition to supporting detoxification, many of my patients report that this drink helps improve their sleep.

Cruciferous Vegetables

Broccoli, and particularly broccoli sprouts, as well as other cruciferous vegetables such as cabbage, kale, and others, are rich in sulfur compounds like sulforaphane, and other critical phytonutrients such as indole-3-carbinol. (Broccoli sprouts in particular have about 20 times more sulforaphane than regular broccoli.) These important nutrients help remove toxins, protect cellular health, and boost long-term wellness among other benefits. You can add these to a blended juice mix as well.

Cilantro

This common herb helps pull mercury and other toxic metals from organs and tissues, allowing these toxins to attach to binding agents like Modified Citrus Pectin, for safe elimination through the urinary and GI tract. Cilantro also offers support for immunity and other areas of health.

Artichokes

Artichokes support the liver by increasing bile production to help your body metabolize and remove toxins and wastes efficiently.

CHAPTER 3

The Lymph System, Rife, & Autoimmune

"I cannot and will not recant anything, for to go against conscience is neither right nor safe. Here I stand; I can do no other, so help me God. Amen."

— Martin Luther

The Lymph System

The movement of fluid through the lymphatic system is essential in detoxifying the body, supporting the immune system, and maintaining homeostasis (normal healthy function.) The fluid carried by the lymphatic system largely consists of wastes disposed of by the cells. Think of the lymph as the body's garbage collection system. Normally the lymph is pumped through the vessels by the contraction of muscles squeezing the fluid through the vessels that contain check-valves that only allow the waste to flow in one direction. Our body's electromagnetic field and even breathing also aid the motion of waste. A clogged or sluggish lymphatic system prevents the body from circulating vital fluids and eliminating toxic waste and dulls the immune system's response. This makes us vulnerable to swelling, infection, pain, and a whole host of diseases.

In order to be healthy, it is essential to keep the energy and fluids moving so that the body's own natural intelligence may operate in its full healing capacity. In addition, each cell must be enlivened with its own unique frequency and ideal energy-state and be fully connected to the electrical impulses that flow through and are kept balanced by lymph. Lymph is much more than waste; it is the intracellular matrix of enzymes, nutrients, sugars, cytokines, and hundreds of necessary chemicals that make up a healthy slurry that bathes the cells. It's like a healthy river, needing a constant flow of fresh nourishment or it becomes a stagnant pond.

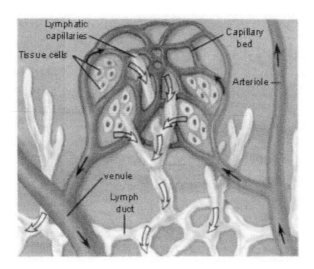

Stimulating the lymphatic system by the use of electrical fields is a well-established and recognized therapy in Canada, Mexico, Europe, and Asia as an effective aid in detoxifying the body while opening and cleansing the lymphatic and circulatory systems.

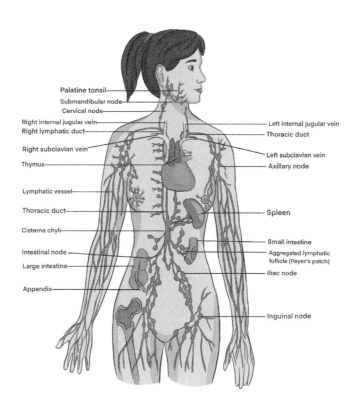

Lymphatic capillaries converge to form lymph vessels that ultimately return lymph fluid back to the circulatory system via the subclavian vein. The presence of one-way valves in the lymph vessels ensures unidirectional flow of lymph fluid toward the subclavian vein.

If excess fluid cannot be returned to the blood stream then interstitial fluid builds up, leading to swelling of the tissues with fluid, which is called edema, and is essentially a sick, stagnant pond.

Lymph nodes are the filters along the lymphatic system. Their job is to filter out and trap bacteria, viruses, cancer cells, and other unwanted substances, and to make sure they are safely eliminated from the body. You can probably start to understand how important it is to keep the lymph system healthy.

Royal Raymond Rife

What if you had spent more than two decades of your life in painfully laborious research, and in doing so you discovered an incredibly simple, electronic approach to helping literally every disease on the planet? That would be great; you'd be a hero, a rich hero! Your discovery would help end the pain and suffering of countless millions and change life on Earth forever. Certainly, you would think, the medical world would rush to embrace you with every imaginable accolade and financial reward imaginable. You would think so, wouldn't you?

Unfortunately, arguably the greatest medical genius in all recorded history suffered a fate literally the opposite of the foregoing logical scenario. In fact, the history of medicine is replete with stories of geniuses betrayed by backward thought and jealously, but most pathetically, by greed and money.

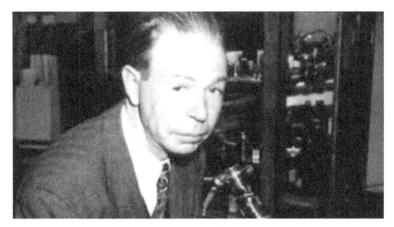

In the nineteenth century, Semmelweiss struggled mightily to convince surgeons that it was a good idea to sterilize their instruments and use sterile surgical procedures. Pasteur was ridiculed for years for his theory that germs could cause disease. Scores of other medical visionaries went through horrible ridicule and even lost their ability to practice simply for challenging the medical status quo of that day. These include such legends as Roentgen and his X-rays, Morton for promoting the "absurd" idea of anesthesia, Harvey for his theory of the circulation of blood, and many others in recent decades (W.F. Koch, Revici, Burzynski, Naessens, Priore, Livingston-Wheeler, and Hoxsey.)

Orthodox big-money medicine resents and seeks to neutralize and/or destroy those who challenge its beliefs. Often, the visionary who challenges it pays a heavy price for his "heresy."

So, you have just discovered a new therapy, which can eradicate any microbial disease but, so far, you and your amazing cure aren't very popular. What do you do next? Well, certainly the research foundations and teaching institutions would welcome news of your astounding discovery. Won't they be thrilled to learn you have a possible cure for the very same diseases they are receiving hundreds of millions of dollars per year to investigate? Maybe not, if it means the end of the "gravy train." These people have mortgages to pay and families to support. A friend of mine, a cancer researcher at a major university once told me that when he questioned his authority about their purpose he was told, "We're not here to find a cure for cancer, we're here to get our next grant."

Regardless of what you may believe, all that the "Walk-for-a-Cure" and cancer fundraising does is feed countless organizations with voracious appetites and no desire to solve the problem that feeds them. Let's get real for a moment: if you owned a drug company and your researchers came to you with a discovery that a new rainforest herb cured lung cancer, an Indian spice that cured brain cancer, a common herb mixture that cures most cancers, and an electrical frequency device that cures all cancers, you'd have a choice: 1) declare it to the world and bankrupt the corporation, putting thousands of individuals with families out of work, turning the entire pharmaceutical industry into an unnecessary entity, or 2) tell them to figure out a way they can synthesize a byproduct that can be patented and thereby make the company extremely profitable and destroy any evidence that may reveal the simplicity of the cure.

I can understand that we live in a capitalistic culture; I understand that profits must be made, and people need to feed their families. I do **not** understand the evil conspiracies to forcefully shutdown and shut-up anything and anyone revealing the truth. Hollywood couldn't write a better story.

Here follows the story of exactly such a sensational therapy and what happened to the man who discovered it. It was a dark time in medical history, when doctors and clinics would claim all sorts of "cures" and new devices popped up to solve all our ills. Many were nothing more than snake oil salesman, attempting to steal from the hurting population, but many were sincere, sacrificing their lives to find help for their patients. Raymond Rife was the later, and his discovery of the benefits of light frequency, a remarkable electronic therapy, was sabotaged and buried by a ruthless group of men who, under the pretense of "protecting the innocent" would squash anything that they could not financially profit from. Rife's work would re-emerge in the underground medical/alternative health world only since the 1970's when it was re-introduced by some physicists. This is the story of Royal Raymond Rife and his fabulous discoveries and electronic instruments.

If you have never heard of Rife before, prepare to be angered and incredulous at what this great man achieved for all of us, only to have it practically driven from the face of the planet.

174

But, reserve your final judgment and decision until after you have read this.

Of course, some may regard this as just an amusing piece of fiction. However, for those who are willing to do some investigating on their own, there will be mentioned several highly respected doctors and medical authorities who worked with Rife as well as some of the remarkable technical aspects of his creation. In the final analysis, the only real way to determine if such a revolutionary therapy exists is to experience it yourself. The medical literature is full of rigged "double-blind" clinical research tests, the results of which are often determined in advance by the vested corporate interests involved.

Royal Raymond Rife was a brilliant scientist born in 1888 who died in 1971. After studying at Johns Hopkins, Rife developed technology which is still commonly used today in the fields of optics, electronics, radiochemistry, biochemistry, ballistics, and aviation. It is a fair statement that Rife practically developed bioelectric medicine himself. He received 14 major awards and honors and was given an honorary Doctorate by the University of Heidelberg for his work. During the 66 years that Rife spent designing and building medical instruments, he worked for Zeiss Optics, the U.S. Government, and several private benefactors, most notable was millionaire Henry Timkin, of the Timkin roller bearing fame. Timken was inducted into the National Inventors Hall of Fame on September 19, 1998.

Because Rife was self-educated in so many different fields, he intuitively looked for his answers in areas beyond the rigid scientific structure of his day. He had mastered so many different disciplines that he literally had, at his intellectual disposal, the skills and knowledge of an entire team of scientists and technicians from a number of different scientific fields. So, whenever new technology was needed to perform a new task,

Rife simply invented and then built it himself, as was necessary for many scientists of his day.

Rife's inventions include a heterodyning ultraviolet microscope, a micro-dissector, and a micromanipulator. When you thoroughly understand Rife's achievements, you may well decide that he had one of the most gifted, versatile, scientific minds in human history. By 1920, Rife had finished building the world's first virus microscope. By 1933, he had perfected that technology and had constructed the incredibly complex Universal Microscope, which had nearly 6,000 different parts and was capable of magnifying objects 60,000 times their normal size. With this incredible microscope, Rife became the first human being to actually see a live virus, and until quite recently, the Universal Microscope was the only one which was able view live viruses.

Modern electron microscopes instantly kill everything beneath them, viewing only the mummified remains and debris. What the Rife microscope can see is the bustling activity of living viruses as they change form to accommodate changes in environment, replicate rapidly in response to carcinogens, and transform normal cells into tumor cells.

But how was Rife able to accomplish this, in an age when electronics and medicine were still just evolving? Here are a few technical details to placate the skeptics.

Rife painstakingly identified the individual spectroscopic signature of each microbe, using a slit spectroscope attachment. Then, he slowly rotated block quartz prisms to focus light of a single wavelength upon the microorganism he was examining. This wavelength was selected because it resonated with the spectroscopic signature frequency of the microbe based on the now-established fact that every molecule oscillates at its own distinct frequency.

The atoms that come together to form a molecule are held together in that molecular configuration with a covalent energy bond which both emits and absorbs its own specific electromagnetic frequency. No two species of molecule have the same electromagnetic oscillations or energetic signature. Resonance amplifies light in the same way two ocean waves intensify each other when they merge together.

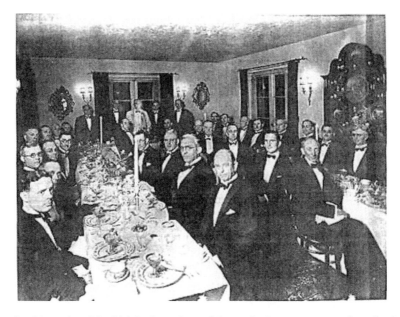

On November 20, 1931, forty-four of the nation's most respected medical authorities honored Royal Rife with a banquet billed as "The End To All Diseases" at the Pasadena estate of Dr. Milbank Johnson.

The result of using a resonant wavelength is that micro-organisms which are invisible in white light suddenly become visible in a brilliant flash of light when they are exposed to the color frequency that resonates with their own distinct spectroscopic signature. Rife was thus able to see these otherwise invisible organisms and watch them actively invading tissue cultures. Rife's discovery enabled him to view

177

organisms that no one else could see with ordinary microscopes.

More than 75% of the organisms Rife could see with his Universal Microscope are only visible with ultra-violet light. But ultraviolet light is outside the range of human vision; it is invisible to us. Rife's brilliance allowed him to overcome this limitation by heterodyning, a technique which became popular in early radio broadcasting. He illuminated the microbe (usually a virus or bacteria) with two different wavelengths of the same ultraviolet light frequency which resonated with the spectral signature of the microbe. These two wavelengths produced interference where they merged. This interference was, in effect, a third, longer wave which fell into the visible portion of the electromagnetic spectrum. This was how Rife made invisible microbes visible without killing them, a feat which today's electron microscopes cannot duplicate.

By this time, Rife was so far ahead of his colleagues of the 1930's that they could not comprehend what he was doing without actually traveling to San Diego to visit Rife's laboratory to look through his Virus Microscope for themselves. And many did exactly that.

One was Virginia Livingston. She eventually moved from New Jersey to Rife's Point Loma (San Diego) neighborhood and became a frequent visitor to his lab. Virginia Livingston is now often given the credit for identifying the organism which can cause human cancer, beginning with research papers she began publishing in 1948.

In reality, Royal Rife had identified a human cancer virus first, in 1920! Rife then made over 20,000 unsuccessful attempts to transform normal cells into tumor cells. He finally succeeded when he irradiated the cancer virus, passed it through a cell-catching, ultra-fine porcelain filter, and injected it into lab animals. Not content to prove this virus would cause one tumor, Rife then created 400 tumors in succession from the same culture. He documented everything with film, photographs, and meticulous records. He named the cancer virus "Cryptocides primordiales."

Virginia Livingston, a physician and cancer researcher, in her papers, renamed it Progenitor Cryptocides. Royal Rife was never given credit nor even mentioned in her papers. In fact, Rife seldom got credit for any of his monumental discoveries. He was a quiet, unassuming scientist, dedicated to expanding his discoveries rather than to ambition, fame, and glory. His distaste for medical politics (which he could afford to ignore thanks to generous trusts set up by private benefactors) left him at a disadvantage later, when powerful forces attacked and finally destroyed him. Coupled with the influence of the pharmaceutical industry in purging his papers from medical journals, it is hardly surprising that few have heard of Rife today.

Note: Though both Rife and Livingston purported that cancer was always caused by an organism, viral or bacterial, I do **not** hold that belief, nor does the American Cancer Society. There are also books written that claim cancer is a fungus. Throughout this book, the reader will see that both my belief as well as the current understanding in medicine is that cancer is a rapid replication of cells **caused** by something disrupting the cell's replication mechanism. While that "something" could be a fungus, bacteria, or virus, there are thousands of other things that can set this in motion. While Rife's belief that cancer was always caused by a specific, identifiable virus may have proved to be incorrect, it no less discounts his contributions to medicine.

Meanwhile, debate raged between those who had seen viruses changing into different forms beneath Rife's microscopes, and those who had not. Those who condemned without investigation, such as the influential Dr. Thomas Rivers, claimed these forms didn't exist. Because his microscope did not reveal them, Rivers argued that there was "no logical basis for belief in this theory." The same argument is used today in evaluating many other "alternative" medical treatments; if there is no precedent, then it must not be valid. Nothing can convince a closed mind. Most had never actually looked though the San Diego microscopes; air travel in the 1930's was uncomfortable, primitive, and rather risky. So, the debate about the life cycle of viruses was resolved in favor of those who never saw it (even modern electron microscopes show frozen images, not the life cycle of viruses in process.)

Nevertheless, many scientists and doctors have since confirmed Rife's discovery of a cancer virus and its pleomorphic nature, using darkfield techniques, the Naessens microscope, and laboratory experiments. Rife also worked with the top scientists and doctors of his day who also confirmed or endorsed various areas of his work. They included E.C. Rosenow, Sr. (longtime Chief of Bacteriology, Mayo Clinic), Arthur Kendall (Director, Northwestern Medical School), Dr. George Dock (internationally-renowned), Alvin Foord (famous pathologist), Rufus Klein-Schmidt (President of USC), R.T. Hamer (Superintendent, Paradise Valley Sanitarium, Dr. Milbank Johnson (Director of the Southern California AMA), Whalen Morrison (Chief Surgeon, Santa Fe Railway), George Fischer (Childrens Hospital, N.Y.), Edward Kopps (Metabolic Clinic, La Jolla), Karl Meyer (Hooper Foundation, S.F.), M. Zite (Chicago University), and many others.

Rife ignored the debate, preferring to concentrate on refining his method of destroying these tiny killer viruses. He used the same principle to kill them, which made them visible: resonance. By increasing the intensity of a frequency which resonated naturally with these microbes, Rife increased their natural oscillations until they distorted and disintegrated from structural stresses. Rife called this frequency "the mortal oscillatory rate," or MOR, and it did no harm whatsoever to the surrounding tissues.

180

This principle can be illustrated by using an intense musical note to shatter a wine glass: the molecules of the glass are already oscillating at some harmonic (multiple) of that musical note; they are in resonance with it, vibrate, and can no longer remain in configuration. Because everything else around it has a different resonant frequency, nothing but the glass's molecular configuration is destroyed. There are literally hundreds of trillions of different resonant frequencies, and every species, tissue, cell, and molecule has its very own.

Understand, when you use a Rife machine, programmed to a frequency of a cancer, you will cause vibration of the cells just like hitting the molecules of a crystal goblet with sound frequencies. The frequencies are not changing the molecular structure nor its properties, however, vibration can have serious healing benefits.

It took Rife many years, working 48 hours at a time, until he discovered the frequencies which specifically helped destroy herpes, polio, spinal meningitis, tetanus, influenza, and an immense number of other dangerous disease organisms. Understand, he was destroying these in test tubes, slides, and petri dishes (in vitro) using light frequencies. Destroying them in someone's body is much more complex, but knowing the correct frequencies is a beginning.

In 1934, the University of Southern California appointed a Special Medical Research Committee to bring terminal cancer patients from Pasadena County Hospital to Rife's San Diego Laboratory and clinic for treatment. The team included doctors and pathologists assigned to examine the patients, if they were still alive, in 90 days. This was obviously a *different age!* I don't believe I'll be seeing the University of Minnesota bringing any patients my way anytime soon. Remember, 1934 was pre-big-money-chemo!

After the 90 days of treatment, the Committee concluded that 86.5% of the patients had been completely cured. The treatment was then adjusted and the remaining 13.5% of the patients also responded within the next four weeks. The total recovery rate using Rife's technology was 100%. Now understand, we do not know how this was determined. No CT scans, PET scans, nor MRIs were available then so we can assume that x-ray was the mode of reassessment. I highly doubt that 100% of the people were cured and I would add that I don't believe that anyone is really every "cured" or "cancer free." While I just might be the biggest advocate of Rife technology currently on the planet, I will be the first to say that it is **not** a magic bullet that cures everyone!

The pre-Big Pharma days were good to Royal Rife. On November 20, 1934, forty-four of the nation's most respected medical authorities honored Royal Rife with a banquet billed as "The End To All Diseases" at the Pasadena estate of Dr. Milbank Johnson. His fame was celebrated, yet short-lived.

By 1939, almost all of these distinguished doctors and scientists were denying that they had ever met Rife. What happened to make so many brilliant men have complete memory lapses? It seems that news of Rife's miracles with terminal patients had reached other ears. Remember our hypothetical question at the beginning of this report: What would happen if you discovered a cure for everything? You are now about to find out that it wouldn't end well.

At first, a token attempt was made to buy-out Rife. Morris Fishbein, who had acquired the entire stock of the American Medical Association by 1934, sent an attorney to Rife with "an offer you can't refuse." Rife refused. We many never know the exact terms of this offer. But we do know the terms of the offer Fishbein made to Harry Hoxsey for control of his herbal cancer remedy. Fishbein's associates would receive all profits for nine years and Hoxsey would receive nothing. Then, if they were satisfied that it worked, Hoxsey would begin to receive 10% of the profits. Hoxsey decided that trusting Fishbein would mean an end to his remedy. When Hoxsey turned Fishbein down, Fishbein used his immensely powerful political connections to have Hoxsey arrested 125 times in a period of 16 months. The charges (based on practicing without a license) were always thrown out of court, but the harassment drove eventually Hoxsey out of the country.

Fishbein must have realized that this strategy would backfire with Rife. First, Rife could not be arrested like Hoxsey for practicing without a license since he had a license. A trial on trumped-up charges would mean that prominent medical authorities working with Rife would introduce testimony supporting Rife, and the defense would undoubtedly take the opportunity to introduce evidence such as the 1934 medical study done with USC. The last thing in the world that the pharmaceutical industry wanted was a public trial about a painless therapy that cured 100% of the terminal cancer patients and cost nothing to use but a little electricity; it might give people the idea that they didn't need drugs! Though the drug industry was still in its infancy in 1934, it was becoming a very naughty teenager by 1939.

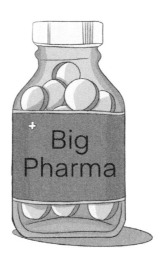

In 1939, a mysterious lawsuit against Beam Ray Corporation, the only company manufacturing Rife's frequency instruments (Rife was not a partner), tied the company up in court and legal expenses in the middle of the Great Depression and ultimately bankrupted the company. Fishbein and the AMA had won; commercial production of Rife's frequency instruments ceased completely.

Often the tactics of our foes involve a character smear; often they use the strong arm of law. The evil can go as deep as their desire to destroy us.

On the other hand, big money was spent ensuring that doctors who had seen Rife's therapy would forget what they saw. Almost no price was too much to suppress it. Remember that, today, treatment of a single cancer patient averages over $300,000. It's *big* business.

Thus, Arthur Kendall, the Director of the Northwestern School of Medicine who worked with Rife on the cancer virus, accepted almost a quarter of a million dollars to suddenly "retire" in Mexico. That was an exorbitant amount of money in the Depression. Dr. George Dock, another prominent figure who collaborated with Rife, was silenced with an enormous grant, along with the highest honors the AMA could bestow. Between the carrots and the sticks, everyone except Dr. Couche and Dr. Milbank Johnson gave up Rife's work and went back to prescribing drugs.

To finish the job, the medical journals, supported almost entirely by drug company revenues and controlled by the AMA, refused to publish any paper by anyone on Rife's therapy. Therefore, an entire generation of medical students graduated into practice without ever once hearing of Rife's breakthroughs in medicine. The magnitude of such an insane crime eclipses every mass murder in history. Cancer picks us off quietly, but by 1960 the casualties from this disease exceeded the carnage of all the wars America ever fought. In

1989, it was estimated that 40% of us will experience cancer at some time in our lives.

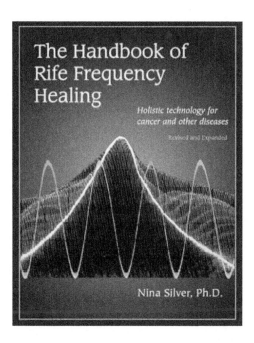

In Rife's lifetime, he had witnessed the progress of civilization from horse-and-buggy travel to jet planes. In that same time, he saw the epidemic of cancer increase from 1 in 24 Americans in 1905 to, partially because his work was squashed, 1 in 3 today.

He also witnessed the phenomenal growth of the American Cancer Society, the Salk Foundation, and many others, collecting hundreds of millions of dollars for diseases that were successfully treated long before in his own San Diego laboratories. In one period, 176,500 cancer drugs were submitted for approval. Any that showed "favorable" results in only one-sixth of 1% of the cases being studied could be licensed. Some of these drugs had a mortality rate of 14-17%.

When death came from the drug, not the cancer, the case was recorded as a "complete" or "partial remission" because the patient didn't actually die from the cancer. It's just absurd!! In reality, it has become a race to see which would kill the patient first: the drug or the disease.

The inevitable conclusion reached by Rife was that his life-long labor and discoveries had not only been ignored but probably would be buried with him. At that point, he ceased to produce much of anything and spent the last third of his life seeking oblivion in alcohol. It dulled the pain and his acute awareness of half a century of wasted effort (ignored) while the unnecessary suffering of millions continued so that a vested few might profit. Profit they did, and profit they do.

I am not so ignorant to think that there are powers that want me destroyed as well. I remain to be a very small fish in a very big pond, and this gives me some protection. However, I know that we are protected by a power greater than ourselves and God alone holds the final say in all of this. In this I find strength.

Fortunately, his death was not the end of his electronic light therapy. A few humanitarian doctors and engineers reconstructed his frequency instruments and kept his genius alive. Rife technology became public knowledge again in 1986 with the publication of The Cancer Cure That Worked, by Barry Lynes, and other material about Royal Rife and his monumental work.

There is wide variation in the cost, design, and quality of the modern portable Rife frequency research instruments available. Costs vary from about $500 to $26,000 with price being no legitimate indicator of the technical competence in the design or performance of the instrument. Some of the most expensive units have serious technical limitations and are essentially a waste of money. At the other extreme, some researchers do get crude results from inexpensive, simple, unmodified frequency generators; but this is just as misguided

186

as spending too much money. Without the proper modifications, the basic frequency generator gives only minimal and inconsistent results. Rife's work was always with **light frequency**. In my opinion, a **real** Rife unit must use a Tesla bulb.

Other theories abound on exactly why and how Rife technology works. Dr. Robert O. Becker, MD, in his book, *The Body Electric*, published by Harper in 1985, gives an exciting report in chapter 15 regarding the fact that photons in light act as an electron "donor" to tissue cells which stimulates mitochondrial function, raises tissue pH, and increases healing. There are dozens of other theories purported by people much smarter than I that explain the success of light therapy.

One day, the name of Royal Raymond Rife may ascend to its rightful place as the giant of modern medical science. Until that time, his fabulous technology remains available only to the people who have the interest to seek it out. While perfectly legal for veterinarians to use to save the lives of animals, Rife's brilliant frequency therapy remains taboo to orthodox mainstream medicine because of the continuing threat it poses to the international pharmaceutical medical monopoly that controls the lives (and deaths) of the vast majority of the people on this planet.

Recent studies on Rife's work have been published in peer-reviewed medical journals. The *Journal of Exp Clinical Cancer Research* 2009 Apr 14; 28: 51, published a paper titled, **Amplitude-modulated electromagnetic fields for the treatment of cancer: discovery of tumor-specific frequencies and assessment of a novel therapeutic approach.** The paper revealed, "CONCLUSION: Cancer-related frequencies appear to be tumor-specific and treatment with tumor-specific frequencies is feasible, well tolerated and may have biological efficacy in patients with advanced cancer."

187

Their results were remarkable: "RESULTS: We examined a total of 163 patients with a diagnosis of cancer and identified a total of 1524 frequencies ranging from 0.1 Hz to 114 kHz. Most frequencies (57-92%) were specific for a single tumor type. Compassionate treatment with tumor-specific frequencies was offered to 28 patients. Three patients experienced grade 1 fatigue during or immediately after treatment. There were no NCI grade 2, 3 or 4 toxicities. Thirteen patients were evaluable for response. One patient with hormone-refractory breast cancer metastatic to the adrenal gland and bones had a complete response lasting 11 months. One patient with hormone-refractory breast cancer metastatic to liver and bones had a partial response lasting 13.5 months. Four patients had stable disease lasting for +34.1 months (thyroid cancer metastatic to lung), 5.1 months (non-small cell lung cancer), 4.1 months (pancreatic cancer metastatic to liver) and 4.0 months (leiomyosarcoma metastatic to liver.)"

Many more articles are coming out on what is now being termed Energy Medicine or Biofield Therapies.[104 105 106 107 108 109 110 111 112]

For more information on Rife and how we use this technology use the search bar at ConnersClinic.com

Cancer is a Th2-Dominant Disorder

Mother Teresa said, "Be faithful in small things because it is in them that your strength lies." It is truly the "small things" that move the masses. When we begin a discussion of our immune system, it is the small things, the chemicals that form the slurries of our defense system that eventually influence much happening in our body.

---

[104] Cancer Journal 2006 Sep-Oct;12(5): 425-31. Complementary medicine in palliative care and cancer symptom management
[105] J Holist Nurs. 2011 Dec;29(4): 270-8. doi: 10.1177/0898010111412186. Epub 2011 Aug 8
[106] Prim Care. 2010 Mar;37(1): 165-79. Biofield therapies: energy medicine and primary care
[107] Ann N Y Acad Sci. 2009 Aug;1172: 297-311. Bioelectromagnetic and subtle energy medicine: the interface between mind and matter
[108] J Altern Complement Med. 2009 Aug;15(8): 819-26. An HMO-based prospective pilot study of energy medicine for chronic headaches: whole-person outcomes point to the need for new instrumentation
[109] Integr Med Insights. 2009; 4:13-20. Epub 2009 Oct 19. Integral healthcare: the benefits and challenges of integrating complementary and alternative medicine with a conventional healthcare practice
[110] Altern Ther Health Med. 2008 Jan-Feb;14(1): 44-54. Six pillars of energy medicine: clinical strengths of a complementary paradigm
[111] Explore (NY). 2006 Nov-Dec; 2(6): 509-14. World hypotheses and the evolution of integrative medicine: combining categorical diagnoses and cause-effect interventions with whole systems research and nonvisualizable (seemingly "impossible") healing
[112] Biomed Sci Instrum. 2006; 42: 428-33. Localized pulsed magnetic fields for tendonitis therapy

If you learn anything from this book may it be to stimulate you to ask one simple question: "why?" Most people, after the devastation of the cancer diagnosis settles in, just accept the fact that they have a grave disease and follow the doctor's orders as to the next step. They may hear a, "We just don't know" or "It's probably genetic" if they are so bold to ask such questions of "why" to their oncologist. Most don't feel qualified to dig for themselves and simply follow in blind faith what is recommended. I beg you to be different!

I come from the philosophy that an effect always has a cause. If something is set in motion, there existed an initial stimulus that propelled it. Cancer, though scary and often deadly, seems to numb most people into a fearful obedience to the culturally accepted treatment plan. After all, it is only human to want someone else to remove the responsibility from us regarding any painful situation. Cancer is serious; cancer isn't to be played with; you need to go to a real doctor.

I am not asking you to trust me or anything in this book; I am asking you to *not* check your brain at the door of the hospital and to demand answers from your doctors or those who will help you through this journey.

The quality of your experience as well as your outcome depends on the quality of the questions you ask. You have the right to receive logical answers; keep asking "why?" Don't stop asking and don't accept any treatment that isn't logically treating the answers to your constant questions of, "Why?"

When we see a person that has a diagnosis of cancer of any name, the goal really is to discover the cause or the reason why the body has allowed or responded in such a way. Is it logical to believe that, though medical intervention *may* be best to slow a fast-growing cancer, finding and correcting the cause would be the best approach to treating any dysfunction?

In this section I will explain the connection between cancer and the immune system as simply as I know how. You'll see that if you don't support and modulate your immune system you will **never** improve your physiology and the cancer will simply progress.

Some very simplified highlight points to know about your immune system:

- Your immune system does one thing and only one thing: it **kills** things

- Your immune system may be separated into two responses: Th1 and Th2 (simplistically, there are more but we'll leave it at that for now)

- Your immune system is supposed to only *turn on* against bio-toxins (living organisms like bacteria, virus, parasites…that is, things that it can kill)

- The Th1 response is the immediate, killer cell response (think of it as the Marine Corps) against the enemy and is the primary killer of antigens and cancer cells. What it *turns on* against is called an antigen in the immune response

- The Th2 response is sent out secondarily and is mainly responsible for making antibodies against the antigen that the Th1 system *turned on* against. The antibodies "tag" that antigen(s) and the Th1 system can then better find it and kill it

- Your immune system assists in the cleaning up of old cells necessary for cancer to **not** develop in the first place. This is primarily a Th1 function

- Both Th1 and Th2 responses are named such because they carry a slurry of different chemicals (chemokines and cytokines) that make up such a response.

An ***autoimmune*** disorder happens when your immune system starts attacking self-tissue. Really, an autoimmune disease develops because your immune system has *turned on* against something it found lodged in self-tissue and now is destroying that self-tissue as well.

Let's expand that a little more so you can fully understand it: If my immune system fires a response against a flu virus I just picked up and it's a particularly virulent virus, a strong Th1 response is released in an attempt to kill the foreign invader and bring me back to health. My "strong Th1 response" is really a collection of different immune (Th1) cells that are looking for a battle; they are seeking an enemy with guns loaded. Let's say they find the flu virus, recognize that it is the enemy they were commissioned to kill, attack it, kill it, and then retreat in victory. The Th1/Th2 system goes back into balance and life is good.

An autoimmune disease begins when, for a multitude of reasons we won't go into here, stray cytokines from a Th1 response didn't recognize the flu virus as the enemy but recognized something that they were never supposed to recognize as an enemy, let's say a heavy metal toxicity in my thyroid. Because I was exposed to a great amount of mercury from amalgams, vaccinations, and just living in a toxic world, mercury had lodged in the fat cells surrounding my thyroid and other tissues. My liver, unable to clear out that which I was exposed to, caused my system to shunt the toxicity to fat storage cells for safe keeping. Never was my immune system supposed to *turn on* against such chemical toxicity!

Is my immune system ever going to be able to kill mercury? Of course not; mercury is an element on the periodic table, not a living organism. If my immune system inadvertently *turns on* against something that cannot or will not die, there will be a lot of collateral damage and I might even begin to start making antibodies against the tissues surrounding the attack. This is an autoimmune disease; it isn't really a disease at all, it is an immune attack on self-tissue because my immune system is firing against something it never should have fired against! Remember, when the immune system *turns on* against something, it does so until it achieves victory; until it kills it.

Summary: An autoimmune disease is when your immune system has created antibodies against your own cells.

What does all of this have to do with cancer? Everything! Remember, your Th1 response not only kills foreign enemies but also helps mop up cells that are supposed to die when they've served out their usefulness. Cancer may be defined as cells **not** dying but instead reproducing a useless cell again and again. If a person has a Th2 dominant autoimmune disorder, their Th1 system will be suppressed. If your Th1 system is suppressed, normal cell death will be hindered.

There are things that suppress the Th1 (killer side) of your immune system other than an autoimmune disease. Stress, for example, is possibly the most common culprit of Th1 immune suppression.

When we look at a person that is not well, one of the first questions needs to be, "what's the mechanism?" With cancer it's no different. Why did you get cancer? What suppressed the immune systems fail-safe clean-up? Could it be that you've had a Th2 dominant autoimmune disorder for years and never even knew it? Could it simply be a stressful event that pushed you into a Th2 dominance long enough for the cancer to get a foothold? We don't **need** to know the full answer to this question, but we **do** need to address the Th2 dominance.

Neither the standard medical nor an alternative healthcare has adequately dealt with autoimmune conditions. Medically, the patient is given steroids, anti-inflammatories that may relieve the symptoms but do nothing to remove the cause; alternative doctors support the organ with glandulars or other supplements. Let's face it, if neither traditional medical nor the alternative models had any great percentage of success treating autoimmune disease, you wouldn't be reading this book because you probably wouldn't have cancer.

Let's reason together: Is it *reasonable* to think that if the part of my immune system responsible for aiding in normal cell death is suppressed, cell replication may proceed? Is it *reasonable* to think that maybe I should be checked for Th2 dominance? Is it *reasonable* that failure to discover the cause of immune dysregulation would lead to further destruction? I think it is *reasonable* that someone "out there" must be able to find out what was causing the dysregulation; and I think that it is *reasonable* that if whatever caused such dysregulation could be evaded, then it is *reasonable* that the damage suffered would at least slow down.

It is important to understand that an autoimmune disease is a *state* that the immune system is in. It is **not** a disease of an organ; and even though it is given a multitude of names depending on the tissue currently affected, it is a **state** of the immune system attacking the tissue it was meant to protect.

Hence, both the traditional medical and the alternative models of care are doomed to failure. The most important battle to fight is to calm down the immune response and stop the destruction, or in the case of cancer, decrease the Th2 response that is causing the Th1 suppression!

The *new model* we are proposing is simply to be more specific. If an autoimmune disease is a hyper-Th2 attack (Th2 dominant) against an antigen, doesn't it make sense to do everything possible to find out what the antigen is, attempt to remove it, and calm down the Th2 dominance? I'm no rocket scientist, but this makes sense to me. It's logical and possible to find the specific biochemical pattern perpetrating the response so we can determine how we treat them.

If you can understand this chapter and the role of the immune system, you can understand how antigens (non-living toxins or nasty, hard to kill virus, mold, candida…) *can* be at the heart of cancer.

A **major** part of my practice is **identifying** and **eliminating** antigens (toxins and biotoxins: virus, bacteria, mold, Lyme, parasites and fungus)! In doing so, the body can return to homeostasis (balance) and miraculously heal itself!

The remainder of the book discusses the need and method of improving your immune system to bring 'your system into balance and help restore health. We'll look at diets that feed and starve cancer and nutraceuticals that strengthen the body and directly kill cancer.

As much as I try to bring clarification to an often-tangled web, I realize support is needed by most. Know that our clinic will be open to care for those who need us.

CHAPTER 4

Diet, Nutrition,
& Blocking the Fuel Source

"Rarely do we find men who willingly engage in hard, solid thinking. There is an almost universal quest for easy answers and half-baked solutions. Nothing pains some people more than having to think."

— Martin Luther King, Jr.

Blocking Cancer's Fuel Source

Reprogramming Cancer's Energy Source

We eat to live. Cancer cells eat to live also. Macronutrients we consume provide many of the compounds required for metabolism, the sum of all the biochemical reactions in the body. You could say that diet and exercise are the primary influencers of cellular metabolism, and reprogramming energy use (particularly in cancer cells) could be an effective way to curb growth.[113]

Some tumor cells seem to thrive on glucose through a pathway called glycolysis. This was first observed by Otto Warburg in the 1920's when he proved that some cancers tend to convert glucose, through glycolysis, to lactic acid and this has been termed, the Warburg effect. He noticed that, in an anaerobic (without oxygen) environment, cancer cells shift the normal endpoint of glycolysis away the Krebs Cycle (formation of Acetyl-CoA) to a less efficient energy source (Lactic Acid.)

This may sound like complicated biochemistry, but it's simple 7th grade biology. Simply put, some cancers gobble up sugar, preferring it as its fuel source. There are several reasons that a growing cancer may prefer lactic acid, ranging from a localized relative hypoxia, genetic alterations that tend to push the production of Lactic Acid, and defects in tumor suppressor and/or tumor oncogenes.

Warburg's original hypothesis suggested that there was a dysfunction in the mitochondria (the organelles inside the cell where all this takes place) of cancer cells; some theories still exist that blame the mitochondria, but more recent research has shown that most cancer cells don't have defective organelles, rather it is the complexity of the metabolic process that can break down for a variety of reasons, including those discussed above.

This video begins to help unravel this complex issue ConnersClinic.com/what-feeds-cancer

Why is it that some people can do so many wrong things, like eat a poor diet, smoke, drink excessive alcohol, take numerous drugs, etc. and still live long, relatively healthy lives, while

---

[113] Cancer is a preventable disease that requires major lifestyle changes. Anand P, Kunnumakkara AB, Sundaram C, Harikumar KB, et al. Pharm Res 2008, 25:2097-2116

others receive a grim diagnosis early in life? I can't tell you the number of patients I see that ask a similar question, "Why do I have cancer? I've eaten organic and lived a clean life for decades."

In the past we've blamed genes, as if we all possess a hidden, inherited code that determines our fate. This has long been debunked, yet unfortunately, while diet and lifestyle play an important role in maintaining health and preventing cancer, life is more complex. To answer my patient's question, I usually point to the plethora of factors involved in disease that go beyond diet: environmental toxins that no one can avoid, exogenous estrogens and hormone disruptors, heavy metals, sub-clinical bacteria and other biotoxins, and yes, genetic alterations in tumor suppressor and oncogenes. Many of these things are beyond our control.

Here is a video that helps breakdown the tumor suppressor gene factor: ConnersClinic.com/understanding-oncogenes

There are many links between nutrient availability and cancer formation and progression that have been peer-review studied. One is the link between Vitamin D and cancer. A precursor to the biologically active Vitamin D can be obtained in the diet or produced in the skin from 7-dehydrocholesterol (note: a healthy cholesterol level must be maintained to produce this product) upon exposure to sunlight. This precursor is first metabolized in the liver to form 25-hydroxyvitamin D (biologically inert) and then in the kidney to form the active form of Vitamin D (1,25-dihydroxyvitamin D.)

When we have adequate store of 7-dehydrocholesterol in the skin, UV rays from the sun accounts for 90-95% of an individual's requirements of Vitamin D. 7-dehydrocholesterol is synthesized from cholesterol which is another reason to rethink what our normal blood cholesterol levels should be and whether artificially reducing such with statin medications is a good idea. While we're at it, we may need to rethink the excessive use of sun-blocking chemicals. You can agree with the health issues associated with the toxic sources in the chemicals contained in them, but here we may argue against the decrease in Vitamin D production. While excessive burning from the sun is cancer causing, sun phobia may be equally damaging.

Numerous studies have revealed that there is an increased risk of several cancers (especially prostate, colon, and breast) in people living at higher latitudes and it has been proposed that Vitamin D deficiency is at least a partial contributor. One study compared the growth of cancer cells in Vitamin D deficient versus Vitamin D sufficient mice. (Tangpricha et al, 2005) Tumors grew 80 % larger on average in the Vitamin D deficient mice.

Current data reveals that Vitamin D is a chemopreventative agent that inhibits cancer growth and induces differentiation and apoptosis through several molecular processes. It can act as a negative ligand (blocking) tumor growth (through the EGFR, epidermal growth factor receptor pathway); it can also directly activate specific tumor suppressor genes such as the BRCA1 and p21 pathways, thereby stimulating cancer cell death.

Vitamin D may be the simplest addition to anyone's cancer protocol.

See more on Vitamin D at ConnersClinic.com/cancer-vitamin-d

There are several types of cancer that can be more directly linked to exogenous hormone exposure. These hormone-related cancers include breast, endometrial, ovarian, prostate, testes, and thyroid.

Breast cancer is the most common type of cancer in women, and estrogens (estradiol and estrone) can play a pivotal role in the initiation and progression.

This video helps explain the correlation: ConnerClinic.com/cancer-hormones

A team from Rice University's Center for Theoretical Biological Physics (CTBP) and the Baylor College of Medicine claims to have created a basic framework of how cancer cells (whether in tumors or as single cells) adapt when their attempts to metastasize are blocked by drugs or the body's immune system. Understanding the cells' strategies could someday help scientists design therapies that keep them in check. This confirms what we've been saying for years: cancer can change its metabolic pathway (the way it feeds) to stay alive, and the more aggressive a cancer is may well be defined (in part) as the speed at which it can change its source of fuel.

Their model shows a direct connection between gene regulation and metabolic pathways and how cancer cells take advantage of it to adapt to hostile environments; a process known as metabolic plasticity.

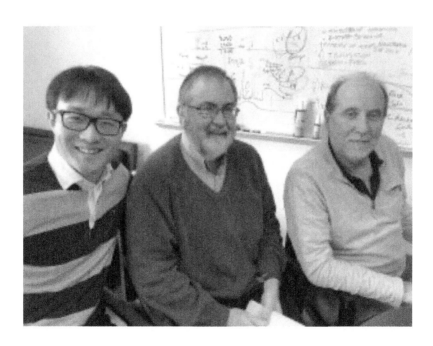

Rice University researchers—from left, Dongya Jia, PhD, Herbert Levine, PhD, and José Onuchic, PhD—detail a direct connection between gene expression and metabolism and how cancer cells take advantage of it to adapt to hostile environments.

Led by physicists Herbert Levine, PhD, and José Onuchic, PhD, and postdoctoral fellow Dongya Jia, PhD, the researchers looked at oxidative phosphorylation (OXPHOS) and glycolysis, metabolic processes that provide cells with the energy and chemical building blocks they need to proliferate. From their model, they detailed for the first time a direct association between the activities of two protein players, AMP-activated protein kinase (AMPK) and hypoxia-inducible factor-1 (HIF-1), the master regulators of OXPHOS and glycolysis, respectively, with the activities of three major metabolic pathways: glucose oxidation, glycolysis, and fatty acid oxidation. These are two genes that we check in all of our patients!

Their theoretical model was experimentally supported by Baylor cancer mitochondrial metabolism researchers led by Benny Abraham Kaipparettu, PhD. The group's study ("Elucidating cancer metabolic plasticity by coupling gene regulation with metabolic pathways") appears in the *Proceedings of the National Academy of Sciences*.

Combination therapy

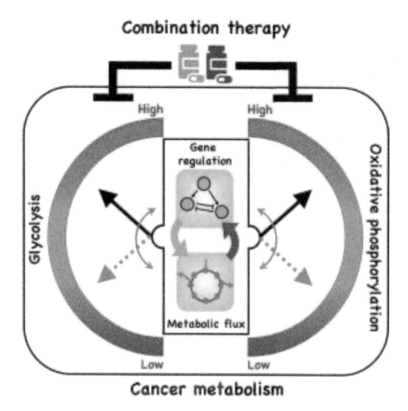

Cancer metabolism

"Metabolic plasticity enables cancer cells to switch their metabolism phenotypes between glycolysis and OXPHOS during tumorigenesis and metastasis. However, it is still largely unknown how cancer cells orchestrate gene regulation to balance their glycolysis and OXPHOS activities. Previously, by modeling the gene regulation of cancer metabolism we have reported that cancer cells can acquire a stable hybrid metabolic state in which both glycolysis and OXPHOS can be used. Here, to comprehensively characterize cancer metabolic activity, we establish a theoretical framework by coupling gene regulation with metabolic pathways," wrote the investigators.

This is precisely why we've begun to experiment with changing a patient's diet, rotationally, with aggressive cancers. You also need to check and change both drug and nutraceutical approaches regularly as well. Fasting and Fasting Mimicking Diets may also be appropriate.

Cancer's Fuel Source and Your Genes

Cancer is a complex disease involving numerous changes in cell physiology, including the metabolic process on how it may be fed. It is defined as cells that are undergoing rapid replication thereby needing a constant source of both energy and byproducts for cell creation.

Looking for genetic variants (or defects) on genes that are responsible for tumor suppression as well as genes that may give a cancer cell more direct access to fuel sources may be important steps to help understand the disease and limit growth. The decreased expression of tumor suppressor genes, our genomic "watchman" involved in sensing and stopping aberrant cell replication, is a part of the problem that may allow cancer to manifest. A better understanding of these genes and learning ways to manipulate their expression is key.

Cancer needs a fuel source, or a supply line. All cells make energy through glucose metabolism, but cancer seems to require greater amounts. A process known as aerobic glycolysis or the Warburg effect[114] is a robust metabolic hallmark of most tumors. Normal cells make energy through a process taking glucose (sugar) through a metabolic chain called glycolysis that makes a chemical called pyruvate. Pyruvate then converts to another chemical in the mitochondria (powerhouse) of the cell to enter a process that produces a lot of energy, the goal of glucose metabolism. Cancer cells are different. They can force pyruvate down a

---

[114] The Warburg Effect: How Does it Benefit Cancer Cells? Maria V. Liberti, et al

different pathway making high quantities of lactic acid in the cytoplasm (the belly) of the cell. There, lactate ferments forming an acid environment and more fuel for cell replication; but it isn't a very efficient system. So, why do cancer cells do this?

The belief has been that cancer cells may have damaged mitochondria that don't allow pyruvate to enter to make energy the way normal cells do. However, recent studies have shown that, though cancer cells need energy for replication, they also need other components.[115] Much like a factory creating shoes might need energy to run the machines; it also needs leather, rubber, and laces. Since cancer cells gobble up glucose through various pathways,[116] their need for it goes beyond simple energy production.

Glucose can enter other metabolic pathways to make other components (leather, rubber, and laces.) Ultimately, the Warburg Effect supports a metabolic environment that allows for rapid biosynthesis of both energy and materials to support growth and proliferation of new cells in cancer.

Although there is no specific gene mutation common to all cancers, nearly all cancers express aerobic glycolysis (the Warburg Effect) as discussed above, regardless of their tissue or cellular origin. Genes for glycolysis are over-expressed and genes that make enzymes to convert pyruvate to Acetyl-CoA in the mitochondria as well as those that help get pyruvate into the mitochondria may be under-expressed. Therefore, it might behoove us to look at such genes in cancer patients.[117]

---

[115] Cancer Undefeated. Bailar JC, Gornik HL; N Engl J Med 1997, 336:1569-1574

[116] Buzzai, M., Bauer, D.E., Jones, R.G., Deberardinis, R.J., Hatzivassiliou, G., Elstrom, R.L., and Thompson, C.B. Oncogene. 2005; 24: 4165–4173

[117] New guardians of the genome. Roth DB, Gellert M; Nature 2000, 404:823-825

Every metabolic process is under the control of genetic factors making enzymes to initiate action. Since cancer may be fueled through excess lactic acid formed when pyruvate fails to take its normal path, would those individuals with variants on the genes responsible to move pyruvate normally into healthy energy production be more susceptible to cancer? Would a patient with cancer be more apt to express defects on genes that might lead to accelerate production of a fuel source preferred by cancer cells? Could we, by assessing such variants in a patient's genes help formulate a plan to help "cut-off" necessary supply lines? These are the questions only time and trials may answer, but ones that I feel are worthy to explore.

Some of the genes in question are the HIF1A, PDH, LDH, KRAS, and PTEN genes. All have been proven to play a part in excess lactic acid production.[118] For instance, the PDH gene, most directly responsible for converting pyruvate to Acetyl-CoA, may be down regulated with genetic variants expressed. Its function is directly hindered by excess HIF-1A expression as well as exogenous sources of toxins suggesting other environmental influences can also be involved. Those with PDH and HIF defects may be more apt to create excess lactic acid, a fuel source for cancer. Dietary considerations in such individuals might be to restrict upstream nutrients that feed that pathway; namely glucose.

In summary, healthy cells take glucose through a process called glycolysis to make pyruvate. This makes some energy necessary for cell function. Pyruvate, through enzymes produced by specific genes (HIF & PDH), then converts to Acetyl-CoA to make much more energy for normal cell health. If you have variants on the genes responsible for such conversions, have variants on genes responsible to aide lactic acid's ability to enter the mitochondria inside the cell, or lack supportive substrates necessary to convert pyruvate to Acetyl-

---

[118] Metabolic Reprogramming: A Cancer Hallmark Even Warburg Did Not Anticipate Patrick S. Ward, Craig B. Thompson. Cancer Cell, Volume 21, Issue 3, p297–308, 20 March 2012

CoA regardless of gene expression, the cell makes excess lactic acid, a known fuel for cancer. Increase fuel equals increased growth.

Our hope is that by better understanding specific metabolic pathways, the genes that drive them, as well as cofactors influencing flow, we can better formulate both a nutritional and dietary plan to help cancer patients. For more information on specific genetic testing, you may contact Conners Clinic at ConnersClinic.com.

See more in our Cancer Diet section on our website and download a free video copy of my book *Cancer Genes* on our site as well at ConnersClinic.com/books

Cancer Diets

The problem with following a diet is knowing if it is right for *you*. There are hundreds of different opinions about diet and cancer and, quite honestly, it is very confusing. For that reason, I personally don't like standard protocols. In our office each patient is tested for individual foods, and the diet recommendations are specific and often less rigid. When we speak to all people, we are forced into a more general approach to diet which, by nature, pigeon-holes people into a protocol that may not be right for them. Unfortunately, there is little we can do to solve this dilemma short of seeing every person in our office, which defeats the purpose of writing a book with a purpose to reach those we can never see.

We hear a lot about the ketogenic diet in recent days. There are even books written that say that *all* cancer patients should be on a ketogenic diet. This is not true! Ketogenic diets are typically high in dairy, an absolute no-no for cancer patients. Dairy makes babies grow (and grow quickly,) doubling their weight in a matter of months because it contains many healthy growth factors. While this is great for babies, it is *not* good for cancer! Ketogenic diets, while eliminating carbohydrates, tend to be higher in protein. Many cancers are fed by protein!

While ketogenic diets may be good for cancers that are completely glycolytically driven, they are horrible for those cancers that are driven by amino acids. While everyone should eliminate simple carbohydrates, not all cancer patients should even consider a ketogenic approach; it can even fuel some cancers!

Others have touted a raw-food, vegan diet for **all** cancer patients. This too could prove disastrous for many patients. A raw-food, high vegetable juice diet tends to be much higher in carbohydrates, feeding a glycolytically driven cancer. Ugh! How do we know which is right for who? In our office we test. For those who could never come to our office, you may either use a trial and error approach (e.g. try a ketogenic-like diet and see if the cancer slows or continues) and make appropriate changes, or do a metabolic diet quiz (do an internet search for this.) The metabolic diet quiz is an older way to get an idea of what diet may be best for you.

We suggest you start with a balanced approach: eating far fewer animal proteins and far, far fewer simple carbohydrates. All diets should **begin** with a thorough understanding of an identical **base step**: understanding whole foods.

The Basic Principles of eating Whole Foods

Making the switch to a whole foods diet is not an overly expensive or difficult change. It will help you to avoid chemicals, hormones, and pesticides that are in our food supply. Whole foods come from natural sources. If you hunted and gathered your foods or owned a homestead hundred years ago or so, you would have the following items, all organic, in your diet: fruits, vegetables, nuts, seeds, honey, water, grass-fed and free-range meats and unprocessed fish, unprocessed unrefined grains (or sprouted grains), and naturally occurring, unpasteurized dairy products.

Think of it: 100 years ago, *everything* was organic!

On this whole food diet, you will be eating primarily whole foods; so that means it is time to clean out your pantry, refrigerator, and freezer from any processed foods. Now, you do not need to eliminate all processed foods, like natural cheeses or whole grain pasta, but if you can't pronounce an ingredient on the label, avoid purchasing the item.

Part of the challenge is to re-think how you eat and make healthier choices. Some easy changes could be:

- **Breakfast**: Less boxed cereal, instant oatmeal, or commercially prepared muffins; rather start with an omelet made with free-range eggs, spinach, cherry tomatoes, and sautéed onions and peppers

- **Lunch or Dinner**: A chicken breast cooked with natural ingredients served with steamed vegetables or a fresh salad instead of chicken nuggets processed with added fats, preservatives, and flavorings

- **Snacks**: A baked sweet potato with fresh chopped onions instead of a bag of potato chips. Or, a freshly made smoothie made from strawberries and blueberries instead of a blue-colored frozen ice drink

We have created a list of acceptable foods and foods to avoid which are good to have handy while grocery shopping:

Acceptable Foods

- Whole foods are those that are as close to their natural form and have not been processed

- Lots of fresh fruits and vegetables

- Whole grains that are **non-GMO** and organic (see information about grains below)

- Seafood (wild caught, *not* farm raised)

- Only locally raised, grass-fed meats such as beef, and chicken; start eating half of the amount you are used to

- Beverages limited to pure water, and naturally sweetened coffee & tea, or freshly made vegetable juices

- Snacks like seeds, nuts, non-GMO popcorn, and organic bars

- All-natural sweeteners including honey, 100% maple syrup, and stevia

- There are now so many great options as compared to a few years ago when the first edition of this book was published. If you can just think about eating things as God created them, it will help you understand a whole food diet

Foods to Avoid

- No refined grains such as white flour or white rice; labels must state whole grain

- You are better off staying away from gluten as it is so highly inflammatory

- Stay away from dairy products of all kinds as they stimulate growth pathways. I realize that typical whole-food diets allow raw dairy and tout its health benefits, but with cancer, things are different. Dairy makes babies grow; it also can make cancer grow!

210

- Avoid pork of all types. Avoid all farmed fish; make sure your fish is wild caught and your meat is grass-fed

- Avoid refined sweeteners such as sugar, any form of corn syrup, cane juice, or any artificial sweeteners such as Splenda

- Avoid foods that come out of a box, can, bag, bottle or package that has more than 5 ingredients listed on the label (this is an easy rule to follow)

- Avoid all deep-fried foods unless you are doing the frying in a healthy oil

- Avoid all fast foods

More Hints to Help Avoid Processed Foods and Refined Sugars

- Read the ingredients label before buying anything. The best indicator of how highly processed a food is found in the list of ingredients. If what you are buying contains more than 5 ingredients and includes a lot of unfamiliar, unpronounceable items you want to reconsider buying that item. Of course, modern labeling laws often require manufacturers to list added nutrients and vitamins in the ingredient list. Become familiar with what these are and occlude these from your "5"

- Shop around the edges of the grocery store where the fresh, whole foods are located. Avoid the center isles where most of the boxed, bagged and canned foods are located. Granted, not all canned (jarred) foods are highly processed and many, many more organic sources are easily found since recent demand has skyrocketed. Just start reading labels!

- Increase your consumption of whole foods, especially vegetables and fruits, since this will help to displace the processed foods in your diet, and will actually make your food selections, in general, very simple. Your only concern is selecting whole foods that are a product of nature instead of a product of industry

- When selecting foods like pastas, cereals, rice, and crackers always choose the whole-grain option. Since gluten-free is often best, there are limited sources of organic, gluten-free options, so you will be limiting this category altogether

- Avoid store-bought products containing high-fructose corn syrup or any other forms of sugar that are listed in the top three ingredients. This is a good indication that the product has been highly processed

- When eating out as a family, do not order off the kids' menu for your children. Most of the selections on a kids' menu are pre-made items that have been highly processed. An easy option is to assemble your own meal from the side options or try sharing a meal

- Visit your local farmers' market where you will find a selection of pesticide-free produce and better-quality, grass-fed meat

- Lower the number of sweet treats and fried foods that you eat. Taking the time to peel, chop, and deep fry potatoes every time you wanted French fries would impact the amount of times you would eat them. Eating junk food such as cakes, sweets, and fried foods as often as you are willing to make them yourself will automatically ensure the frequency is appropriate

Understanding Sugars

Sugar from the sugar cane is highly processed as is high fructose corn syrup. Locally grown honey and 100% maple syrup are more acceptable choices because they are made in nature and less often found in highly processed foods. Sweeteners such as Splenda, Equal, agave syrup, corn syrup, and Sweet-n-Low should never be used. No matter what kind of sugar you decide to use follow these guidelines:

- Consume any and all types of sugar in moderation and try to reserve them for special occasions

- When purchasing store-bought foods, avoid those that have any form of sugar or sweetener listed among the top three ingredients

- Always choose the natural sweetener over the artificial items like aspartame

Spicing Up Your Meals When Eating Clean

Healthy food has an undeserved reputation for being boring or bland. Whole, fresh foods are actually delicious on their own, with no added seasoning. Unfortunately, many of us have been jaded by too much sodium, sugar, and additives in our food. But there are healthy ways to add flavor to clean foods. Here are some herbs and spices you can use in your daily cooking:

Basil

This bright green delicate leaf contains flavonoids that act as powerful antioxidants. It's also high in Vitamins A and K as well as potassium and manganese. Basil grows very well indoors on a sunny windowsill. Basil can be preserved by freezing or drying it. Use basil in tomato sauces, salad dressings, pesto, sandwich spreads, soups, and chicken, beef, and fish dishes.

Marjoram

This herb contains many phytochemicals (including terpenes, which are anti-inflammatory,) lutein, and beta carotene. Plus, it has lots of Vitamin C and Vitamin D. Marjoram is delicious in any dish made using beef and is perfect with vegetables like tomatoes, peas, carrots, and spinach. Together with bay leaf, parsley, thyme, and tarragon, it makes a mix to use in stews and soups.

Mint

Mint can be used to help upset stomachs because it soothes an irritated GI tract. It is also used to ward off cancer cells due to a phytochemical called perillyl alcohol, which can stop the formation of some cancer cells. Mint is a good source of beta carotene, folate, and riboflavin. Use it in teas, in desserts, as part of a fruit salad or lettuce salad, or as a garnish for puddings.

Oregano

Used in Italian dishes, this strong herb is a potent antioxidant with the phytochemicals lutein and beta carotene. It's a good source of iron, fiber, calcium, Vitamin C, Vitamin A, and omega-3 fatty acids. Add oregano to salad dressings, soups, sauces, gravies, meat dishes, and pork recipes.

Parsley

This mild herb is an excellent source of Vitamin C, iron, calcium, and potassium. It's also packed with flavonoids, which are strong antioxidants, and folate, which can help reduce the risk of heart disease. It can be used in salads as a leafy green to rice pilafs, grilled fish, and sauces and gravies.

Rosemary

Rosemary contains terpenes, which slow down free radical development and stop inflammation. Use this strong and piney herb in soups, stews, meat, and chicken dishes. Chop some fresh rosemary to roast a chicken, cook with lamb or beef, or mix with olive oil for a dip for baked sweet potato slices. Rosemary also contains ursolic acid which is a great anti-viral, anti-cancer nutrient.

Sage

Sage contains the flavonoid phytochemicals apigenin and luteolin and some phenolic acids that act as anti-inflammatory agents and antioxidants. Its earthy aroma and flavor are delicious in classic turkey stuffing (as well as the turkey itself), spaghetti sauces, soups and stews, and frittatas and omelets.

Tarragon

Tarragon is a great source of phytosterols and can reduce the stickiness of platelets in your blood. Tarragon is rich in beta carotene and potassium, too. This herb tastes like licorice. Use it as a salad green or as part of a salad dressing or mix it with Greek yogurt to use as an appetizer dip. It is also wonderful with chicken or fish.

Thyme

This herb is a good source of Vitamin K, manganese, and the monoterpene thymol, which has antibacterial properties. It's fresh, slightly minty, and lemony tasting. It is a good addition in everything from egg dishes to pear desserts to recipes featuring chicken and fish.

Cinnamon

Cinnamon can help reduce blood sugar levels, LDL cholesterol, triglycerides, and overall cholesterol levels. Cinnamaldehyde, an organic compound in cinnamon, prevents clumping of blood platelets, and other compounds in this spice are also anti-inflammatory. Cinnamon can be added to coffee and tea, used it in desserts and curries, and sprinkled on oatmeal for a great breakfast.

Cloves

Cloves are flower buds that are a good source of manganese and omega-3 fatty acids. They contain eugenol, which helps reduce toxicity from pollutants and prevent joint inflammation, and the flavonoids kaempferol and rhamnetin, which act as antioxidants. Cloves are a great addition to hot tea and coffee as well as many dessert recipes, including fruit compote and apple desserts.

Cumin

This spice is rich in antioxidants, which may help reduce the risk of cancer. It also has iron and manganese, which help keep your immune system strong and healthy. Cumin can be added to Middle Eastern recipes, rice pilafs, stir-fried vegetables, and Tex-Mex dishes.

Nutmeg

Nutmeg is rich in calcium, potassium, magnesium, phosphorus, and Vitamins A and C. It can help reduce blood pressure, acts as an antioxidant, and has antifungal properties. Sprinkle it into dishes with spinach, add it to hot tea, use it in curry powder, and add it to rice pudding and other desserts.

Turmeric

This spice is one of the healthiest foods on the planet. Curcumin, a phytochemical in turmeric, can stop cancer cells from reproducing and spreading, slow Alzheimer's disease progression, and help control weight. In fact, researchers are currently studying Curcumin as a cancer fighter, painkiller, and antiseptic. Use it in Indian foods, egg salads, sauces, tea, and fish and chicken recipes.

ANTI-INFLAMMATORY FOODS

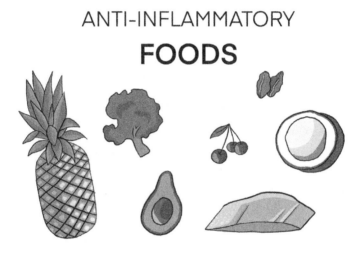

Anti-Inflammatory Foods

Processed sugars and other high-glycemic starches increase inflammation, just as they raise blood sugar and feed cancer cells, according to an article in the *American Journal of Clinical Nutrition*.

Everything that we eat is either pro-inflammatory or anti-inflammatory inside your body. Here are 11 of the best anti-inflammatory foods (because I think that the best way to get your nutrition is through your food):

Cold-Water Fish: including salmon, contain anti-inflammatory fats. Wild salmon have more of these super-healthy fats than do farmed salmon, so never buy farm raised fish of any kind (they are fed processed fish-food.)

Grass-Fed Beef: and other animal foods that are organically raised. As opposed to traditional, grain-fed livestock, meat that comes from animals fed grass contains anti-inflammatory omegas, but in lower concentrations than cold-pressed seed oils. Free-range livestock that graze in pastures build up higher levels of omega-3s. Meat from grain-fed animals has virtually no omega-3s and plenty of poor-quality saturated fat.

Cooking tip: Unless it's ground, grass-fed beef may be tougher, so you're better of slow cooking it.

Olive Oil and Coconut Oil: Olive oil is a great source of oleic acid (omega 9), another anti-inflammatory oil. Researchers wrote in the October 2007 *Journal of the American College of Nutrition* that those who consume more oleic acid have better insulin function and lower blood sugar. Coconut oil is a great oil for everyday use as well!

Shopping tip: Opt for extra-virgin olive oil, which is the least processed, and use it instead of other cooking oils. Other "cold-pressed" or "expeller-pressed" oils can be good sources, too. Use Coconut oil whenever cooking at higher temperatures as it is more stable than olive oil.

Salads: Dark-green lettuce, spinach, tomatoes, and other salad veggies are rich in Vitamin C and other antioxidants, nutrients that dampen inflammation.

Suggestion: Opt for olive oil-and-vinegar salad dressing (vinegar helps moderate blood sugar) and skip the croutons as grains are **very** pro-inflammatory.

Cruciferous Vegetables: These veggies, which include broccoli, cauliflower, Brussels sprouts, and kale, are also loaded with antioxidants. But they also provide another ingredient (sulfur) that the body needs to make its own high-powered antioxidants like glutathione.

Cherries: A study in the April 2006 *Journal of Nutrition* showed that eating cherries daily can significantly reduce inflammation. Cherries are also packed with antioxidants and relatively low on the glycemic index. They are of the *stone fruits* variety (fruits with pits) that are great for diabetic and cancer patients.

Tip: Frozen cherries are available all year long and make a tasty treat when blended in a smoothie.

Blueberries: These delectable fruits are chock-full of natural compounds that reduce inflammation. Blueberries may also protect the brain from many of the effects of aging. Frozen blueberries are usually less expensive than fresh and are just as good for you.

Turmeric or Curcumin: This spice contains a powerful, natural anti-inflammatory compound, according to a report in the August 2007 *Biochemical Pharmacology*. There are perhaps a thousand more studies out on the benefits of Turmeric in cancer and inflammatory disorders. Curcumin has long been part of curry spice blends, used in southern Asian cuisines and is best assimilated in the body when blended with a good fat. Therefore, cooking with this spice greatly increases its absorption. When I recommend it for a supplement (almost every patient with cancer must be on this) I use a brand that is pre-emulsified in a fat (coconut oil) so it is more readily used by the body.

To use in food: I recommend using powdered curry spice (which contains high amounts of turmeric and other spices) as a seasoning whenever you pan fry chicken breasts (of course always use coconut oil when frying.)

Ginger: This relative of turmeric is also known for its anti-inflammatory benefits, and some research suggests that it might also help control blood sugar, heal the stomach and digestive tract, and help breakdown walls of inflammation that surround cancer.

Suggestion: Brew your own ginger tea to sip between juices (juicing vegetables is a must for cancer.) Use a peeler to remove the skin off a piece of ginger, then add several thin slices to a cup, add hot water, and let it steep for a few minutes (vary steep time to taste.)

Garlic: The research isn't consistent, but garlic may have some anti-inflammatory benefits, and it certainly helps increase Th1 responses that are necessary to kill cancer cells. At the very least it won't hurt and makes for a tasty addition to food; you can never use too much!)

Green Tea: Like fruits and vegetables, green tea contains natural anti-inflammatory compounds. It may even reduce the risk of heart disease and cancer. The EGCg compounds found in Green Tea extracts are absolutely essential for every cancer patient. Green Tea is a Th2 stimulant except that it also is of the only compound that reduces the only pro-inflammatory cytokine in the Th2 reaction, interleukin 6 (IL-6.)

Suggestion: Drinking Green Tea is **not** going to give you enough EGCg to greatly reduce IL-6 levels but it certainly helps. I suggest you take Green Tea Extract as a supplement.

Recipes

Honey-Amino Broiled Salmon

This sweet, tangy, and salty mixture does double-duty as marinade and sauce. Toasted sesame seeds provide a nutty and attractive accent. Make it a Meal: Serve with gently steamed broccoli and sautéed red peppers and zucchini slices.

Ingredients

- 1 scallion or green onion, minced
- 2 tablespoons Bragg's brand Aminos
- 1 tablespoon rice vinegar
- 1 tablespoon honey
- 1 teaspoon minced fresh ginger
- 1 pound center-cut salmon fillet cut into 4 portions
- 1 teaspoon toasted or raw sesame seeds or pumpkin seeds

Instructions

1. Whisk scallion, Bragg's Aminos, vinegar, honey and ginger in a medium bowl until the honey is dissolved. Place salmon in a sealable plastic bag, add 3 tablespoons of the sauce and refrigerate; let marinate for 15 minutes. Reserve the remaining sauce.

2. Preheat broiler. Line a small baking pan with foil and coat with cooking spray. Transfer the salmon to the pan, skinned side down. (Discard the marinade.) Broil the salmon 4 to 6 inches from the heat source until cooked through, 6 to 10 minutes. Drizzle with the reserved sauce and garnish with sesame seeds.

Curried Ginger Soup

Ingredients

- 1 teaspoon coriander seeds
- 1/2 teaspoon yellow mustard seeds
- 3 tablespoons coconut oil
- 1/2 teaspoon curry powder
- 1 tablespoon minced peeled fresh ginger
- 2 cups finely chopped red onions
- 1 1/2 pounds organic carrots, peeled, thinly sliced into rounds (about 4 cups)
- 1 1/2 teaspoons finely grated lime peel
- 5 cups organic chicken broth
- 2 cups coconut milk
- 2 teaspoons fresh lime juice
- Plain yogurt (for garnish)

Instructions

Grind coriander and mustard seeds in spice mill to fine powder. Heat the coconut oil in heavy large pot over medium-high heat. Add ground seeds and curry powder; stir 1 minute. Add ginger; stir 1 minute. Add next 3 ingredients. Sprinkle with salt and pepper; sauté until onions begin to soften, about 3 minutes. Add all the chicken broth and coconut milk; bring to boil. Reduce heat to medium-low; simmer uncovered until carrots are tender, about 30 minutes. Cool slightly.

Now you have a choice:

1. Eat and enjoy as is by adding the lime juice and a bit of salt and pepper or…

2. Working in batches, puree in blender until smooth. Return soup to pot. Add more broth by 1/4 cups if too thick. Stir in lime juice; season with salt and pepper. Ladle soup into bowls. Garnish with yogurt and serve.

Chick Pea, Cumin, and Coriander Salad

You can also make this the day before serving to allow all of the aromatic flavors to marinate and blend together (makes 8 servings so you can have it for lunch the next day.)

Ingredients

Dressing:

- 3 tablespoons fresh squeezed lemon juice
- 2 tablespoons white-wine vinegar
- 2 garlic cloves, minced and mashed with 1/4 teaspoon sea salt
- 1 1/2 teaspoons peeled and grated fresh ginger root
- 1 teaspoon ground cumin
- 1/4 teaspoon dried hot red pepper flakes
- 1/2 cup extra virgin olive oil
- Freshly ground black pepper

Salad:

- Four 19-ounce cans chick-peas, rinsed and drained well
- Finely chopped green, red or yellow bell peppers
- Thinly sliced green scallions
- Finely chopped red onion
- 1/2 cup finely chopped fresh coriander
- Lemon wedges
- Mixed organic green leafy lettuce (mixed spinach and spring greens)

Instructions

In a bowl, whisk together the lemon juice, the vinegar, garlic, ginger root, cumin, cayenne, sea salt and freshly ground pepper to taste. Add the oil in a stream, whisking, and whisk the dressing until it is emulsified.

In a large bowl stir together the chick-peas, the bell peppers, scallions, coriander, and the dressing and chill the salad, covered, overnight.

Serve on lettuce leaf and garnish with lemon wedges.

Quinoa-Avocado Salad

Ingredients

- 1 cup quinoa
- 2 cup water or organic chicken broth
- 1 cucumber, chopped up
- 2 avocados, pitted, skinned and chopped
- 1/4 cup dried cranberries
- 1/2 cup slivered almonds
- 1 green onion, finely chopped
- Fresh coriander or parsley, finely chopped

Dressing:

- The juice of one lemon
- 1/4 cup extra virgin Olive oil
- 1 tablespoon apple cider vinegar
- Sea salt
- Dash of Cayenne pepper to taste

Instructions

- Rinse quinoa and cook in broth in a rice cooker or saucepan and wait until it fluffs up, about 15-20 minutes (stirring occasionally)

- Whisk together lemon juice, olive oil, apple cider vinegar, salt and cayenne pepper

- When quinoa is finished cooking, allow to cool slightly

- Add chopped cucumber, avocado, cranberries, green onion, herbs, and lemon juice, stirring to combine well

- Add more salt and pepper to taste, and chill before serving

Roasted Root Vegetables

Ingredients

- 1-2 3 pound butternut squash, peeled, seeded, cut into small pieces
- Several large sweet potatoes, peeled, cut into small pieces
- 1 bunch beets, trimmed but not peeled, scrubbed, cut into small pieces
- 1 large red onion, cut into small pieces (about 2 cups)
- 1 large turnip, peeled, cut into small pieces (about 1 cup)
- Several large carrots, cut into small pieces
- 1 head of garlic, cloves separated, peeled
- 2 tablespoons olive oil

Instructions

Preheat oven to 425°F. Oil 2 large rimmed baking sheets. Combine all ingredients in very large bowl; toss to coat with oil. Divide vegetables between prepared baking sheets; spread evenly. Sprinkle generously with sea salt and pepper. Roast vegetables until tender and golden brown, stirring occasionally, about 1 hour 15 minutes. (Can be prepared 2 hours ahead; let stand at room temperature. Rewarm in 350°F oven 15 minutes.)

Inflammatory Foods to Avoid

The following is a list of inflammatory foods that everyone could consider either avoiding completely or limiting to achieve maximum health. Though I list these as "no-no's" in the cancer diet section, it may be wise to comment on them here.

Dairy (all pasteurized dairy products): *Avoid*

Dairy has other ill-effects for those with cancer as well. It contains factors that stimulate growth pathways and, in general, should be avoided by everyone with cancer. Note, it makes no difference what type of dairy; goat's milk is just as bad as cow's milk and, it makes no difference if the dairy is raw. Dairy has the distinct purpose to make babies grow!

Refined Sugars: *Avoid*

These include white sugar, brown sugar, confectioners' sugar, corn syrup, processed corn fructose, turbinado sugar, etc.

Chemical Sugar Sweeteners & Artificial Sugar Substitutes: *Avoid*

No one, whether they have cancer or not, should ***ever*** use artificial sugar substitutes; ***never ever***!

MSG (Monosodium Glutamate or Hydrolyzed Vegetable Protein): *Avoid*

MSGs can be hidden in foods under labels like "natural and artificial flavorings" so watch out! MSG is a glutamate that both stimulates neurological pathways in ways that are ***very*** detrimental ***and*** has the ability to stimulate cancer growth as a direct fuel! Everyone, everywhere, should avoid MSG.

Alcohol: *Avoid*

Caffeine: *Avoid*

Excess quantities (except in your coffee enema!)

Red Meat: *Reduce or Avoid*

Only eat grass-fed meats

Processed Foods: *Reduce or Avoid*

Grains: *Avoid*

Especially gluten-containing grains (wheat, rye, barley, malt and spelt)

There are times when grains may be recommended. If a person is in a cachexic state with rapid, uncontrolled weight loss, grains such as oatmeal and rice may be an appropriate solution to help keep some weight. There are other times that we allow the use of coffee and alcohol in moderate doses. The above list is to remind us on the foods that typically cause inflammation and should be avoided.

Other Foods to be Cautious Of

Often in regard to Rheumatoid Arthritis and some other autoimmune disorders (including cancers) I advise some patients to avoid the Night Shade Vegetables. This group of foods can be easily tested by avoiding the entire group for a week to a month while monitoring progress. After a period of avoidance, slowly allowing these foods back into the diet, monitoring the effect, will tell you if these are foods that your body can or cannot tolerate. The only problem with testing this food group is, for some reason you may not react immediately, the reaction could be 2-5 days later.

Keep in mind when avoiding this group of foods that if you are eating processed foods, you are not likely to be completely eliminating the night shade vegetables as they are found in most processed foods and sauces.

Nightshade vegetables include eggplant, all white potatoes, all tomatoes, bell peppers (not black pepper) and tobacco.

Other cancer patients can react to other foods as well. Asparagus, for example, can often be reactive to those with Lymphoma. While I stated that gluten is inflammatory, it rarely is a fuel source of cancer. Gluten can cause other issues though. For instance, gluten is a molecular mimic that tends to cause Hashimotos thyroid issues and should be completely avoided for those with thyroid problems. There are just too many variables with food sensitivities that you should get tested if this is expected.

What *Do* Cancer Cells Feed On?

The Basics

Anaerobic (without oxygen) metabolism primarily consumes glucose as a fuel source. More specifically, it consumes the endpoint of glucose (glycolytic) metabolism: lactic acid. Cancer cells respire anaerobically, consuming 7-8 times more glucose than normal cells. Since it is so inefficient compared to aerobic metabolism, cancers have a voracious appetite for glucose to sustain them. This is why excess consumption of sugars tends to promote cancer growth.

Understand, all cells use glucose for metabolic processes. Glucose follows a pathway called glycolysis where it creates a small amount of energy (ATP) and finally exits as two pyruvate molecules. In healthy cells, pyruvate breaks down to Acetyl-CoA and enters the mitochondria into the Krebs cycle where it efficiently produces most of our energy needs.

Cancer cells tend to shunt much of the pyruvate down a different, less efficient path converting it to lactic acid. This is the anaerobic pathway. The HIF-1a gene is also partially responsible for this lactate shunt (see my book *Cancer Genes* on our website as a free download.)

So, generally, all cancer patients should limit carbohydrates. Patients whose cancers are primarily fed through the above glycolytic fuel should consider an even more restrictive, ketogenic-like diet.

This is also why cancer patients may want to limit their type of exercise to more gentle, non-aerobic exercise. Aerobic exercises tend to deplete oxygen (cancers love depleted oxygenation) and produce more lactic acid in the tissue (a major fuel source for many cancers.)

However, as stated, a ketogenic-like diet is **not** best for everyone. Some cancers feed mainly on amino acids.

It is less well known that some cancers have an equally voracious appetite for methionine and glutamine, which are amino acids from proteins. Briefly, glutamine is the most important "nitrogen shuttle" in the blood. It brings the organic nitrogen to the cancer cells so they can use it to make the essential amino acids and thus proteins required to make more cancer cells. As the glutamine supply goes to zero, tumor growth can slow as well.

Patients whose cancers are more amino acid driven do best on vegetarian-type diets. We have found that it is the animal meats (pork, beef, venison, poultry, lamb, etc.) that are primarily responsible for feeding amino acid driven cancers. Often eggs and fish are fine, within reason. We strongly limit simple carbohydrates with these patients as well.

In order for cancer cells to survive, they basically require three conditions:

- Availability of glucose
- Anaerobic surroundings (less oxygen)
- Availability of glutamine, methionine and other amino acids

One avenue to reduce the growth of cancer cells is simply to starve their food sources such as described above, and then increase the amount of oxygen in the blood, which cancers hate.

More on Sugar and Glutamine

I've stated above that the Cancer Diet should decrease sugar and glutamine consumption in general, even in a balanced approach. Again, if you aren't sure if your cancer is fueling one way or another, reduce both. The research that follows here gives us more substantiation.

Researchers at Huntsman Cancer Institute (HCI) at the University of Utah have uncovered new information on the notion that sugar feeds tumors. The findings may also have implications for other diseases such as diabetes and Metabolic Syndrome. The research is published in the journal *Proceedings of the National Academy of Sciences (PNAS.)*

"It's been known since 1923 that tumor cells use a lot more glucose than normal cells. Our research helps show how this process takes place, and how it might be stopped to control tumor growth," says Don Ayer, Ph.D., a Huntsman Cancer Institute investigator and professor in the Department of Oncological Sciences at the University of Utah.

Glucose and glutamine are both essential for cell growth, and it was long assumed they operated independently, but Ayer's research shows they are inter-dependent. During both normal and cancerous cell growth, a cellular process takes place that involves both glucose (sugar) and glutamine (an amino acid.)

Ayer discovered that by restricting glutamine availability, glucose cannot be well utilized by cancer cells. "Essentially, if you don't have glutamine, the cell is short circuited due to a lack of glucose, which halts the growth of the tumor cell," Ayer says.

The research, spearheaded by Mohan Kaadige, Ph.D., a post-doctoral fellow in Ayer's lab, focused on MondoA, a protein that is responsible for turning genes on and off. In the presence of glutamine, MondoA blocks the expression of a gene called TXNIP. TXNIP is thought to be a tumor suppressor, but when it's blocked by MondoA, it allows cancer cells to take up and utilize glucose as its primary energy source, which in turn drives tumor growth.

Ayer says the next step in his research is to develop animal models to test his ideas about how MondoA and TXNIP control cell growth. "If we can understand that, we can break the cycle of glucose utilization which could be beneficial in the treatment of cancer," Ayer says.

So, make sure you are not taking any glutamine in your supplements. Since this is an amino acid, you would most likely find it in a protein powder. Another common source of glutamine would be in products to heal the gut. Glutamine is a primary player in intestinal healing and though healing intestinal permeability issues (leaky gut syndrome) is important for cancer patients, do **not** use a product with glutamine!

Dairy and rbGH

An epidemic rise in one under-publicized category of cancers should sound an alarm for all Americans. There is a powerful link to the dramatic surge in lymphatic cancer: the 1994 approval of the genetically engineered bovine growth hormone (rbGH.) Before 1995, lymphatic cancers were comparatively rare. Today, if you add up the total number of cancer deaths from breast, prostate, lung, pancreatic, and genital cancers, they do not cumulatively equal the number of deaths from lymphatic cancers.

Americans annually consume nearly 180 billion pounds of dairy products that will average out to over 650 pounds per American. Cheese, ice cream, yogurt, and milk will be ingested from hormonally treated cows (cows treated with rbGH.) Most people are unaware that laboratory animals treated with rbGH experienced enormous changes in their lymphatic systems.

The controversial genetically modified cow hormone was approved for human consumption in February of 1994. Cancer statistics have recently been published by the U.S. Census Bureau comparing death rates from cancer by sex and age groups in 1980, 1990, and 1995. These data support evidence of a runaway plague. All of America became a laboratory study for rbGH, which is now in America's ice cream, cheese, and pizza.

There are small increases and decreases in lymphatic cancer rates from 1980 to 1990 depending upon sex and age group. What happened in 1995 represents **the most dramatic short-term increase of any single cancer** in the history of epidemiological discovery and analyses.

DEATH RATES FROM LYMPHATIC CANCER

By Age and Sex (1980-1995)
Deaths per 100,000 population in specified age group

AGE GROUPS	MALE				FEMALE			
	1980	1990	1995	Increase	1980	1990	1995	Increase
35-44	4.3	4.5	36.5	+811%	2.4	2.1	44.0	+2095%
45-54	10.2	10.9	143.7	+1318%	6.6	6.0	140.7	+2345%
55-64	24.4	27.2	480.5	+1767%	16.8	16.7	357.5	+2141%
65-74	48.1	56.8	1089.9	+1919%	34.4	39.5	690.7	+1749%
75-84	80.0	104.5	1842.3	+1763%	57.6	71.2	1061.5	+1495%
85+	93.2	140.5	2837.3	+2019%	63.0	90.0	1249.1	+1588%

The approval process for rbGH was the most controversial drug application in the history of the Food & Drug Administration (FDA.) In order to address that controversy, the FDA published an article in the journal *SCIENCE* (August 24, 1990.)

Data in that paper reveal that the average male rat receiving rbGH developed a spleen 39.6% larger than the spleen of the control animals after just 90 days of treatment. The spleens from rbGH-treated females increased in size by a factor of 46 percent. These are not normal reactions and portray animals in distress. These animals were under attack by the genetically engineered hormone. The spleen is the first line of defense in a mammal's lymphatic system.

Lab animals treated with rbGH developed lymphatic abnormalities. This same hormone causing changes in lab animals was introduced into America's food supply in 1994. As Americans continue to ingest genetically engineered milk and dairy products, lymphatic cancer rates soar. Americans have become laboratory subjects in genetic engineering's experiment, and the resulting data indicates extreme cause for concern.

Lesson: If you stay on the Cancer Diet, you won't have to worry about genetic modification of dairy because you won't be eating dairy. Any dairy consumed, like yogurt, must be rbGH-free!

I could spend the entire book talking about dangerous toxins that have influenced cancer growth, but I want to mention just one more: genetically modifies food (GMO.)

Again, I am **not** a conspiracy theorist, but to think there are **not** financial ties by major industries that financially benefit from GMO and rbGH is absurd! Here is a list for you:

NAME	POSITION AT MONSANTO	POSITION IN US GOVERNMENT	POLITICAL ADMINISTRATION
Toby Moffett	Monsanto Consultant	US Congressman	D-CT
Dennis DeConcini	Monsanto Legal Counsel	US Senator	D-AZ
Margaret Miller	Chemical Lab Supervisor	Dep. Dir. FDA, HFS	Bush Sr, Clinton
Marcia Hale	Director, Int'l Govt. Affairs	White House Senior Staff	Clinton
Mickey Kantor	Board Member	Sec. of Commerce	Clinton
Virginia Weldon	VP, Public Policy	WH-Appt to CSA, Gore's SDR	Clinton
Josh King	Director, Int'l Govt. Affairs	White House Communications	Clinton
David Beler	VP, Gov't & Public Affairs	Gore's Chief Dom. Polcy Advisor	Clinton
Carol Tucker-Foreman	Monsanto Lobbyist	WH-Appointed Consumer Adv	Clinton
Linda Fisher	VP, Gov't & Public Affairs	Deputy Admin EPA	Clinton, Bush
Lidia Watrud	Manager, New Technologies	USDA, EPA	Clinton, Bush, Obama
Michael Taylor	VP, Public Policy	Dep. Commiss. FDA	Obama
Hillary Clinton	Rose Law Firm, Monsanto Counsel	US Senator, Secretary of State	D-NY Obama
Roger Beachy	Director, Monsanto Danforth Center	Director USDA NIFA	Obama
Islam Siddiqui	Monsanto Lobbyist	Ag Negotiator Trade Rep	Obama

Source: OrganicConsumers.org

Dairy and Other Stimulators of mTOR

The mammalian target of rapamycin (mTOR) is a metabolic growth pathway. It has become a much-studied cell-signaling pathway by pharmaceutical researchers attempting to find safe drugs that inhibit it in human cancers. The way mTOR stimulates cancer growth gets more complicated, but you don't need to do know anything other than what stimulates mTOR to help limit its function.

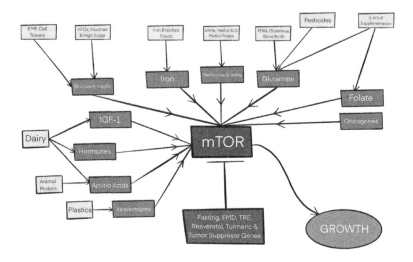

As you study the above chart, you'll see that there are many things (both good and bad) that stimulate mTOR and thereby stimulate growth. Dairy, proteins, iron-enriched foods, bone broth, and methylated nutrients, for instance, are **not** bad things. They are just bad things (contraindicated) for those with cancer!

We **need** mTOR; we need growth. The mTOR pathway is stimulated in healing. It is highly active in children and the cause of growth spurts. It is necessary for life. We only want to suppress it when we have active cancer.

Look at the chart again and see that there are several *bad* things that stimulate mTOR. Harmful EMFs, xenoestrogens from plastics, sugar and high-fructose corn syrup, pesticides, and tumor oncogenes are all negative things that stimulate excessive cell growth and replication.

We might do well to memorize this chart and follow it as best we can to help guide our cancer diet! I refer to it again in my *Cancer Genes* book as there are genes along each pathway that influence just how negatively affected you are by each *stimulator* of mTOR.

Fasting and Fasting Mimicking Diets

Fasting can be one of the best ways to slow mTOR and slow cancer growth. Remember, mTOR is a growth-stimulating pathway spurred on by consumption of dairy, exogenous hormones, excess methyl-groups, iron, sugar, high-fructose corn syrup, proteins, MSG and glutamine, and exposure to plastics and pesticides. These all stimulate the mTOR growth pathway. While this is bad enough, stimulation of mTOR in a rapidly replicating cancer can also stimulate another process called Autophagy.

Autophagy is a cellular clean-up process that removes waste from cells. It is generally thought to be a wonderful, built in, maid service to healthy cells to keep everything tidy.

However, tumor areas can experience episodes of limited nutrient supply due to poor perfusion to the degree that nutrient availability is insufficient for maintaining tumor growth or even survival. This means that growing tumors have a difficulty getting enough parts to make cells.

Also, some tumors tend to be poorly perfused due to low vascularization and high interstitial pressure; a good example of this is pancreatic ductal adenocarcinoma (PDAC).[119]

Unfortunately, this is where the dark side of autophagy plays against us. A well-described alternative mode of nutrient acquisition during these periods of starvation is autophagy or "self-cannibalism."[120] It is a catabolic pathway used by cells to recycle cell content and organelles and reuse their components. The process utilizes autophagosomes (enzymes that gobble-up waste) that eventually fuse with lysosomes (one of the organelles in the cell) for content degradation (sorting and recycling) and the subsequent release of the breakdown products (re-using.)

When a growing cancer, with its ferocious appetite, experiences nutrient starvation (the need for more parts), the breakdown products generated by autophagy (amino acids, fatty acids, sugars, and nucleosides) help sustain energy production and synthesis of essential cellular building blocks. In tumor cells, autophagy has been found to be particularly important for maintaining survival during nutrient stress.[121] *Ugh*!

Although it can support cell survival during episodes of starvation, autophagy is inherently incapable of facilitating tumor growth, as it only recycles or consumes the intracellular biomass. To support proliferation, exogenous (from outside the cell) substrates are also required. Recently, it was found that cancer cells, particularly those with a Ras mutation, can internalize proteins found in the spaces between the cells through a process called micropinocytosis.[122]

This is a process by which extracellular fluid and its components (the matrix between the cells) are engulfed by the plasma cell membrane and, in a sense, gobbled-up by the

---

[119] Koong et al., 2000; Neesse et al., 2011
[120] Rabinowitz and White, 2010
[121] Guo et al., 2011; Yang et al., 2011
[122] Commisso et al., 2013

growing cells.

In a study by Commisso et al., cell consumption of albumin, a blood protein that can be found in extracellular fluid, can be gobbled-up by cancer cells and can reduce the dependence on free glutamine. A later study also confirmed that macropinocytosis occurs commonly in human tumors.[123] Additionally, this process enables pancreatic cancer cells to proliferate in medium lacking essential free amino acids.

From a treatment perspective, we want to do all we can to slow mTOR. To date, nothing pharmaceutical has yet been developed to conquer such a process. Nutritionally, fasting for periods throughout the day (time-restricted eating or TRE), or doing what is called a fasting mimicking diet (FMD) has been an approach that seems to be the most helpful to reduce self-cannibalization to feed a growing cancer. The TRE and/or FMD diet reduces mTOR and can limit autophagy.

In summary, some cancer cells survive and even grow during primary nutrient starvation by maintaining metabolic activity through catabolizing both intracellular and extracellular macromolecules. This metabolic *scavenging* appears important for the growth of a subset of tumors, such as PDAC. Conceivably, it can also form a general mechanism of resistance to antiangiogenic therapies or other nutrient deprivation-based strategies. The use of TRE and/or FMD diets may prove our greatest defense against this process.

Genetically Modified Foods

We discussed GMOs in Chapter 2, but since it is now a nearly unavoidable component of our food supply, we need to address it here as well. Most corn, wheat, beet sugar, soy, and many other vegetables purchased in the United States is GMO food. Proponents argue that there are no ill effects on humans

---

[123] Kamphorst et al., 2015

239

with GMO food, but I and most anyone who has even mildly researched the subject completely disagree. Even if we buy organic, we are still exposed to GMOs as well as pesticides and herbicides through cross-contamination.

Today's GMOs are based on adding new genes to crops like corn, soy, and cotton in order to alter the way the plants function, make them more tolerant to disease and bugs, and able companies to patent the seed and create an endless need for farmers to repurchase, year after year. Gone are the days of saving seeds; it's against the law; Monsanto owns the patent. To say that our food supplies, laced with toxins, filled with additives, colorings and chemicals, and now genetically altered, don't negatively affect our bodies is ludicrous. This book does not contain enough space to discuss these things in detail and I have recommended various books for your personal research, but suffice it to say, removing these poisons from your diet is of the utmost importance.

Bottom line: *Eat only organically grown foods when available*. We need to, at the very least, follow the "Clean 15/Dirty Dozen" lists that are published each year to let us know the most highly contaminated food products (Google this.) Do your own research into the foods you put into your mouth and make sure they are not genetically modified. If we all create a greater demand for good food, the supply will follow; and we see that happening today.

Hormones and BPA (bisphenol A)

"More than 130 studies have linked BPA (bisphenol A) to breast cancer, obesity, and other disorders," concludes a report from President Obama's 2010 Cancer Panel.

BPA is a chemical compound that is practically inescapable in modern American life. It is used in virtually every plastic container, plastic bottles, and coffee cup lids, where it is known to break down and contaminate the liquid contents. It is sprayed inside of the vast majority of our country's canned goods and has routinely been detected in staggering levels in the food it is supposed to be protecting. Cash register and credit card receipts are covered in BPA which give them the slippery feel. In fact, 92% of the food and drinks in the U.S. that come in plastic or metal packaging contain BPA. If you eat *any* prepared foods, even rice and beans that come in plastic bags, you are being exposed.

Why are they bad? BPA's mess with your hormones! Even small amounts of BPA can act as *endocrine disruptors*, altering your body chemistry in alarming ways.

"Hundreds of independent peer-reviewed scientific studies have found harm from low doses of BPA," Laura Vandenberg, a BPA researcher at Tufts University said in a recent statement.

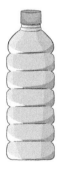 **ALL PLASTICS CONTAIN BISPHENOLS**

The problem is that they are everywhere; you can run but you can't hide from BPA's. But it can be removed from our society. Japan quietly stopped using BPA in the 90's. Canada has banned it from infant toys and bottles, as have a handful of U.S. states. Senator Diane Feinstein has now proposed a much heftier ban of BPA that extends to all food and drink containers used in America, but don't expect the chemical companies (who profit extensively from its use) to quietly surrender.

"I think the outlook is that it's going to be a struggle," Feinstein said of the prospects for passage of the ban. "There's no question about it. There are powerful interests that don't want us to pass this bill."

What to do until a ban will someday be enacted? Here are a few suggestions adapted from Lisa Farino, a writer for MSN Health & Fitness:

Limit Canned Foods & Beverages

The epoxy liners of metal food and beverage cans most likely contain BPA. Vom Saal especially recommends avoiding canned foods that are acidic (tomatoes, tomato-based soups, citrus products, and acidic beverages like soda) and canned alcoholic beverages, since acids and alcohols can exacerbate the leaching of BPA.

The good news: Many foods and beverages can be purchased in glass containers (olive oil, and tomato paste) or frozen (like vegetables.)

Don't Store Foods in Plastic

Glass food storage containers are inert and there are plenty of wonderful Pyrex containers on the market. Just be sure to wash the lids, which are made of plastic, by hand.

Filter Your Drinking and Cooking Water

Since detectable levels of BPA have been found in the water, vom Saal recommends removing it using a reverse osmosis and carbon filter, which generally can be found for less than $200. "In the long run, it's cheaper than buying bottled water, which isn't tested for BPA," he says. If you buy bottled water, you are defeating the purpose if you store it in a plastic container. We have BPA-free plastic water bottles at our office. I believe I ordered them off of Amazon.com

Filter Your Shower and Tub Water

According to vom Saal, the relatively small BPA molecules can easily be absorbed through the skin. BPA can be removed from the water by adding ceramic filters to showerheads and tubs. Just be sure to change them regularly or they just dump contaminates.

Don't Transport Beverages in Plastic Mugs

Instead, opt for an unlined stainless-steel travel mug or glass mug/container. This is especially important when transporting hot beverages, like coffee or tea.

Limit Use of Hard Plastic Water Bottles

Those colorful light-weight plastic bottles may be great for hiking, but unfortunately, they are made of polycarbonate plastic. For everyday use when a little extra weight isn't an issue, choose a stainless-steel water bottle, and make sure it's unlined; some metal water bottles contain a plastic liner that may contain BPA. Again, use stainless steel or glass.

Minimize Hard Plastics in the Kitchen

Hard plastic stirring spoons, pancake flippers, blenders, measuring cups, and colanders regularly come into contact with both food and heat. Fortunately, all of these can easily be replaced with wooden, metal, or glass alternatives.

Skip the Water Cooler

Those hard plastic five-gallon jugs that many companies use to provide their employees and customers with "pure" water are usually made of BPA-containing polycarbonate. Ask if you can order water with non-BPA plastic for a better choice.

If You Must Use Plastic

- Avoid using plastic storage containers for anything that contains acid ingredients, like tomatoes or citrus products

- Avoid putting any warm beverages or citrus products in plastic mugs or travel bottles

- Wait for foods to cool to room temperature before placing in plastic storage containers

- Transfer foods to ceramic or glass before placing in the microwave. Microwaving will break down the plastic, causing it to release BPA into the food

- Wash all plastic containers by hand. The harsher detergents and hotter temperature in the dishwasher will cause the plastic to break down more quickly

- Throw away any plastic food storage containers that are showing signs of age. If the plastic looks hazy or warped, feels sticky, or has any visible lines or cracks, it is beginning to break down and could be releasing even more BPA

- Choose plastics that have the recycling number 2 and 5. These are made out of far less reactive polypropylene and polyethylene

Especially for Kids

Choose BPA-Free Baby Bottles. There are several alternatives to polycarbonate baby bottles. First, there's the old-fashioned, inert glass baby bottle. If you prefer a plastic alternative, check out Born-Free's new line of BPA-free plastic baby bottles.

As with any plastics, you should still avoid harsh detergents, dishwashers, and microwaves.

Choose BPA-Free Sippy Cups. Stainless steel sippy cups, like those by Klean Kanteen, are a great alternative to polycarbonate plastic sippy cups. Klean Kanteen also offers a BPA-free sippy-cup top adapter.

If you prefer a smaller, lighter-weight, totally plastic sippy cup, check out Born Free's line of colorful, BPA-free sippy cups.

Again, it's still wise to avoid exposing plastics to microwaves, harsh detergents, and dishwashers.

Limit Plastic Toys. Unfortunately, polycarbonate plastics are used to make toys, which young kids are so known for chewing on. Since chewing can break down the plastic and release BPA into a toddler's mouth, minimizing plastic toys during the chewing stage is a good idea.

Especially for Pregnant Women

Here's one more reason to keep taking that folic acid. Not only does it help prevent birth defects, it may also help protect a developing fetus from the effects of the BPA you'll inevitably consume even if you take steps to reduce exposure. In pregnant mice, nutritional supplementation with folic acid has shown to protect fetuses against maternal BPA exposure.

Our Integrative Approach

Why I Do What I Do

Always ask the reason why. For anyone who has ever been in my office, that's the big three-letter word with the big question mark behind it that I teach ad nausea. If there is only one thing to learn from me, it would be to ask, "*Why* do I have this problem?" I want you to become a Sherlock Holmes of your own healthcare, desiring to look deeper and say "why?" Never, ever, **ever** be satisfied with a diagnosis.

I am eighth of nine children; born the fifth of five boys with four sisters. From an early age as a grade-schooler, even though I always hated school (there were always too many things to do at home or outside) I always had a great love and curiosity for science.

In about 6th or 7th grade I started getting horrible headaches and body aches. My mom brought me to our family doctor at that time (a medical doctor) and he took x-rays of my head and neck. His conclusion was that I was suffering from "growing pains." I remember walking out of the clinic after the appointment and hearing my mom say, "He's crazy; it doesn't hurt to grow!" We climbed into the car and that was the last time I would go to a medical doctor for almost 25 years.

My symptoms were happening at the same time that my mother was delving into natural health care, having sought help for some issues of her own. A few years earlier she had suffered from Bell's Palsy (a paralysis of cranial nerve 7, your facial nerve, causing one side of your face to droop.) We lived in a town with a population of about 10,000, with only one chiropractor in practice. My mother sought his help and he completely cured her Bell's Palsy.

In effect, my mother asked the right questions, received the right answers and was able to solve her problem. Since then, both of my parents had become believers in natural health care and went to the chiropractor for various issues.

So, abandoning the medical doctor's "growing pains" diagnosis, Mom brought me to her chiropractor and my headaches and body aches were quickly resolved. As my siblings and I grew and became involved in school athletics, we continued to pursue chiropractic care and were always well cared for.

The largest turning-point in my life, career-wise, was when I was in 10th grade. I noticed I excelled in my science classes, but I despised English class; especially when it came to reading. I would receive A's in the rest of my classes but in reading I would be lucky to get a C. I was unable to keep pace with my fellow students and ended up being placed in a remedial English class; extremely embarrassing being down-graded. But I just could not keep up; I couldn't even read through a single page of a book without forgetting everything I had just read.

I finally went to a special kind of chiropractor, one who did some kinesiology work. After some neurological testing he diagnosed me as having mild dyslexia and spent time teaching me some specific brain-based therapies he knew at the time. With the chiropractor's help my dyslexia was miraculously corrected within about 3-5 months, so much so that I was accepted in an Honors History class that required more reading than I ever attempted: James Michener's 900+ page Centennial! I did great and my life slowly changed.

With the healing I experienced through this chiropractor, the direction of my life also changed. I was absolutely intrigued. I thought, "I want to do this, what he is doing", and from that point on I was committed to helping people through this different type of healthcare. By the time I was a junior in High School I had my post-graduate schooling laid out; exactly what courses I needed to take to become a doctor like him. I wanted to figure people out; I wanted to help people who did not have an answer, or worse, didn't even realize they had a problem. I thought that there must be others out there like me, others who didn't know that what they were struggling with was even a problem. I'm sure there are others who think that, like me, "this is just the way that I am, I'm just a horrible reader, I'm just stupid, I'm just fat, I've just been dealt with _____." We can easily think that we are just stuck with a fate in life without any possibility of change. That's what I once thought; but I was wrong.

I went into my whole field, my endeavor/everything that I do, partly based on the experiences I had back then. I have a desire to help people, to dig and figure out the *cause*, even after people and patients and other medical professionals have given up and just settled on a label. Those experiences are what brought me to where I am today, with a relentless drive to find the answers.

There is another thing that drives me: My relationship with Jesus Christ. Years ago, I committed myself to Him, and though I stumble daily and often fail miserably in my walk, He is faithful, always good; and chooses to use me from time to time. I believe that God is sovereign, holy, and sent His Son to become sin and the sacrifice on my behalf. I am forgiven, not because I am good, but because He is good. So, I'll be honest, this is a profession that I chose but how I practice is what He chose for me. It really wasn't my desire to take care of patients diagnosed with cancer; it was God's.

On average, our patients have been to a multitude of doctors (both traditional and alternative) and often can't seem to find satisfactory answers to their problems. We are based in Minnesota, and many of our patients have been to the Mayo Clinic, even *turned away* from Mayo because there's nothing left that can be done to help them. It is then, I believe, that God often sends them to us.

I have to be honest in that sometimes I wish He wouldn't, because it gets to be a little excruciating. Death has not been a stranger in our clinic. Many of our patients are seemingly teeter-tottering on the edge of leaving this world, and it's a dose of reality when some of them do. It is heartbreaking and, in many ways, it makes me furious. But it is also this reality that drives me. It makes me a better person; it makes me a better doctor; and it forces me to do everything I can to figure my patients out.

My belief system is this: If God brings a patient to me, He's going to have to give me the wisdom to figure him/her out, or

He has other plans that are beyond my control. And, it's not like God speaks to me audibly and tells me what's wrong, because He doesn't. He makes me study and He makes me work and He makes me dig. My purpose as a doctor has always been toward constant, never-ending improvement. I believe I can *always* be better than I am right now. I can say it is God's giftedness for me, because I enjoy it and it is my absolute passion, but it is also a serious challenge. Every day I am faced with knowing people are placing their lives, and the lives of their loved ones, in my care. But I do love a good challenge.

It was actually kind of boring for a patient to come to me and say, "I fell down and hurt my knee." It's boring because we already *know* the cause and we can fix it. That's boring. It is much more exciting for a patient to come to me and say, "I have stage 4 cancer, the doctor sent me home to die, I have two weeks left to live, I have never, *ever*, dug in to the possible reasons **why** I have it, I've just followed the medical route to the T, it hasn't worked, and now I'm here." Obviously, it's not "good" considering what the person is dealing with, but it *is* exciting that he/she is in our office and that we have the opportunity to seek God's face and find some answers. Those are the cases that I like: the more difficult, the better.

A few years ago, I held a seminar for doctors called "The Cancer Symposium" which consisted of me lecturing, teaching, and often pleading with doctors to learn how to properly support patients with cancer. I crammed as much of my last 25 years of training into 15 hours of endless speaking as I could. Doctors from around the country (the best of the best) flew to Minnesota right at the time our temperatures dipped to zero degrees. It didn't even faze them!

I love to teach (as I'm sure you could tell by the content on our website as well as this book) but two straight days of talking was exhausting. But it was so necessary! We need more doctors with the knowledge to help people with cancer. A search of the internet reveals pharmaceutical companies advertising their drugs with pretty butterflies and smiling supermodels as if chemotherapy is glamorous. We see non-profit organizations that raise hundreds of millions of dollars for cancer yet do very little to help any individuals but themselves.

We **need** an integrative approach. Sometimes chemo, radiation, or surgery **is** necessary to debulk a rapidly growing tumor, but **none** of them will kill circulating tumor cells (CTCs) or cancer stem cells. Every patient with cancer, even those who have been declared "cancer free" by their oncologists **still** have CTCs and cancer stem cells. This is why it comes back!!

An integrative approach to cancer (one that addresses root causes, requires lifestyle changes, and develops a game-plan that is realistic and self-manageable) is necessary, absolutely necessary, for ultimate patient success. I know we are all going to die, but it just sickens me to see the statistics of what's going on with traditional cancer treatment alone. "We've done all we can," seems to be the mantra of the oncology demi-gods when "all they can" consistently falls short and just ignores alternative therapies that they seem to squash. I am so often reminded of the movie Patch Adams, about a young man of the same name as the title, struggling with his identity, depressed and afraid, checked himself into a hospital, finally realized his purpose in life when he helped a fellow patient; he wanted to be a doctor and help others.

Patch went to the MD that governed the psychiatric institution to demand he be discharged to follow his "calling." The doctor, who ruled with a callous disposition that would rather drug a patient into oblivion then listen to them and feel their pain, was obstinate about letting Patch go, "what is it that you think you want to do with your life," he sneered. "I want to help people; I want to be a doctor," Patch proudly stated. "You can't be a doctor," the MD soured, "I'm a doctor."

"Yeah, but you **suck** at it," Patch pounced back with a simple honest conclusion.

Robin Williams was brilliant in his performance, and if you haven't seen the movie, do so. That line, "Yeah but you **suck** at it" has resounded in my head for years. I do **not** want to be that kind of doctor, but I've personally experienced dozens of them! If you've "done all you can do" then **maybe** there is s**omeone else** who can **do more**!!

Just Another Reason Why I Do This

While I wrote the original edition this book (several years ago), I had a sweet, little angel of a girl (8 years old) with Medulloblastoma. She had surgery to debulk (remove all that the surgeon could) the tumor before her parents brought her to see me. Medulloblastoma is a primary, typically aggressive cancer in the fourth ventricle of the brain, just in front of the cerebellum; a horrible brain cancer that usually attacks young children.

The surgeon believed he "got all the cancer", **but**, the Oncology Department at the University of Minnesota demanded that she still do **full** skull and spine radiation **and full** chemo with 3 chemo drugs (**adult** chemo drugs!!)

The parents were in shock and simply requested some time to think about it. That immediately prompted the Oncologists to call CPS (Child Protective Services) who would forcibly remove the child from the parent's custody should they not proceed with the demands of the demi-gods of medicine. Is it **really** in the "child's best interest"?

I find it amazing that CPS puts abused kids back into the home of the abuser because they went through a few weeks of anger management training, and yet they can remove a child from loving parents because the pharmaceutically controlled monopoly demands blood. If a parent dares to ask, "Hold on, we have to think about that...", we instantly become a police-state where big brother knows better than us lower lifeforms who are unable to make a rational decision. I am afraid of what this country has become!

After speaking to a new oncologist who promised to "work with her," and then two weeks of adjunctive care at my office which included use of a Rife machine at home (what we do for all patients that come to us with cancer) the parents agreed to some medical testing to see if there was any progression. An MRI of her brain and microscopic testing of her cerebral-spinal fluid was next. Prior to the test, the new oncologist called me to ask if I'd help encourage the parents to proceed with the radiation and chemotherapy because she was afraid that if the testing came back clean, the parents would be against proceeding. I cannot even come close to entering into those decisions and asked the oncologist if she was trying to entrap me, for I am not an oncologist and do not treat cancer. She understood but felt that I could help influence the parents. I asked some very pointed questions including why she would want to progress with such harsh treatment which, she was honest about, would produce some potentially horrible side-effects. It all came down to protocol.

I'm all for protocols as long as they work. Dr. Oncologist assured me that 63% of Medulloblastoma patients had a 5-year survival rate at their facility and according to her, the patient had a **zero** percent survival should the parents not follow their protocol. Zero percent is pretty bad, so I asked the same question several different times in different ways and received the same answer; in her professional experience, the patient had a zero percent cure rate if their protocol was not followed!

The next logical question was, "How many Medulloblastoma patients have you had that did **not** follow your treatment?" So, I asked it. "Oh, none," was her answer. Excuse me, did you just say *none*? I'm no mathematician but to claim that a

252

parent is abusive for deciding to **not** follow your recommendations that you claim to have a 37% death rate and **not** have any **real** patients that have opted-out as a comparison is utterly ludicrous. How can they say there is a zero percent survival rate if you do not follow recommendations when they've never had anyone not follow those recommendations? Doesn't that make it a 100% survival rate?

These are the **rubber numbers** used to manipulate you into doing something! I am sick over this! I ended my conversation with Dr. Oncologist (and I at least give her credit for being nice and talking to me) after she said something like, "I believe in praying too and I believe in miracles, but miracles are few and far between." I answered, "Maybe you should come to my office because I see them every day."

The tests came back and there were **no** traces of anything on the MRI or the Cerebral Spinal Fluid!! Hurrah!! It was a short-lived celebration; CPS is at the door and demanding cooperation with the powers that be. Hundreds of hours in prayer, dozens of prayer-chains and multiple conversations with attorneys leaves the parents with little choice: either do what the establishment thinks is best or lose control of their child.

Her mom was beside herself! I was in tears writing this and this poor, little sweetheart of a child suffered at the hands of almighty medicine. We did everything we could to protect her little body from the effects of the powerful drugs and I'm happy to say that she survived and thrived and is still thriving today, many years later.

Understand; I am **not** saying that I know the **best** thing to do **nor** am I saying that chemotherapy and radiation weren't the right thing to do in this little girl's case; they could have been the thing that saved her little life. **I am saying** that the oncologists with their rubber numbers **also** do **not** know. Why can't we let everyone (all professionals) give their **best** recommendation based upon experience, research data, and clinical certainty and then *let the parents decide*.

I know there are those who will argue that the parents just are not smart enough to make such a tough decision so the government must do it for them. Hogwash!

I'm reminded of the Apostle Paul when he heard that new believers were required by some to be circumcised in order to follow Christ. He was outraged: "Look out for those dogs [Judaizers, legalists], look out for those mischief-makers, look out for those who mutilate the flesh," – Philippians 3:2

Our purpose as a clinic is to be a blessing to the people who come to us. We believe we have a responsibility to every person we accept as a patient, a responsibility to dig and figure each person out. We may not *solve* the problem (I want to be very clear about that), but for the most-part we can figure out what's going on or find someone who can.

These are the types of stories we hear on a fairly regular basis since we committed to this type of work, and quite frankly, they drive me! We are in a battle; not against cancer, but against an enemy. Cancer is an outcome; cancer is awful and devastating, but it is not our enemy. Our enemy is alive and active and desires to kill, steal and destroy. Our advocate is also alive and well; He is more powerful than anything the enemy can throw against us and will always, ultimately have victory! The battle may be fierce, but the victory is secure.

Cancer is a disease that sick people get; I hope to take sick people and help them get better and sometimes the cancer, or MS, or seizures, or headaches, or Autism, goes away. It's kind of like the farmer who had a horrible problem with rats that were infiltrating his barn from a giant trash heap near the south pasture. He would spend all afternoon sitting on his tractor with his 22-gage rifle waiting for the little buggers to present themselves and he would gun them down. Several weeks and dozens of hours of hunting later, he asked a young man at the feed mill if he wanted to earn some extra money sitting on his tractor shooting rats. The next day the young man paid a visit and accessed the situation. After about 15 minutes he gave the farmer a proposition, "If I can get rid of all the rats, will you pay me $100?" The farmer agreed and the young man took the farmer's tractor, dug a big hole and buried all the garbage, destroying the very environment that fed and nourished the rat population. The rats were gone forever.

So it is with every disease: we can chase the illusion of destruction, or create a healthy environment that promotes self-healing. Cancer is no different. The purpose of care is to detoxify the body, create a healthy environment, and stimulate the body's immune function.

Is cancer *curable*? Only you can answer that. My job is to help access the dysfunctions that promoted/allowed the disease and to assist with the correction of that. I have earned a Fellowship in Integrative Cancer Therapy through The American Academy of Anti-Aging Medicine and South Florida School of Medicine where I am privileged to crunch ideas with the brightest minds in oncology.

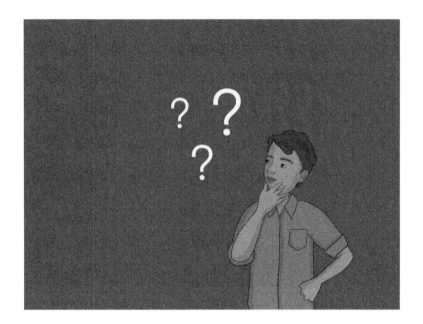

Learning to ask better questions is essential for the successful treatment of any disease. Once a patient receives the dreaded diagnosis, there is a fearful stigma that seems almost stamped on the brain that causes many to follow traditional approaches and surrender all responsibility to a profession that has been less than successful in their treatment. The truth is: according to Oncology, a peer reviewed medical journal, the average cancer patient is worth nearly $300,000 to the hospital and doctors who land the big fish. I hate to paint such a grim picture and must make it perfectly clear that I am *not* against all chemotherapy or radiation, but to ignore and often negate approaches that promote changing the patient's internal environment is malpractice (my opinion, of course.)

My heart cries to hear of young and old dying from cancer that have never even attempted alternative cancer therapy approaches. Surely, we all will die, and some of cancer. God's sovereignty does not preclude the need to seek answers and ask for wisdom.

What We Do

We Build a Protocol Around You

Our first rule of cancer protocols is this: we don't have any! By this we mean that each and every patient is different, which requires us to create a unique protocol specific to **you**.

But remember, we do **not** treat cancer (or any other disease for that matter.) We don't diagnose either. Our mission is to help our Members build their immune system and detoxify in order to help them improve their health.

Our unique Kinesiology and Genetic testing are what set us apart. We believe our success, in part, comes from being as specific as we can be with:

- Determining the **causes**
- Deciding on **best** nutraceuticals
- Defining the optimal **diet**
- Designing the specific care program
- Deciphering your personal genetics
- Specific frequencies for the Rife Therapy

We believe that healing comes from our Heavenly Father and pray that He uses us as His tool. Our purpose is to pray for wisdom (we are promised it should we ask for it with a pure motive), walk in that wisdom, and leave the results to God.

Any care recommended to our Members is Biblically-based, natural, non-invasive, and determined by asking our Heavenly Father for His wisdom.

Our Four Pillars

Pillar 1: Find the Cause

Once your case has been accepted, we begin with a Genetic test to best understand the role of detoxification pathways, tumor suppressor genes, and to give us further hints to both cause and propagation of your particular cancer. We also use Functional Medicine and Kinesiological Testing to help uncover root cause(s) behind *why* you have cancer.

Pillar 2: Address the Cancer

After uncovering what we believe to be the root cause(s), we find the best nutraceuticals for your case, create a personalized diet to aide in cutting off the fuel source of cancer, create your unique in-clinic and take-home therapy plan.

You have a personal care coach every step of the way to help you stay on plan & pray for you along the journey. Examples of different nutraceuticals we may recommend are found in the previous Sections of this book. Remember, less is more!

Pillar 3: Program Your Rife

Through intensive (usually 8+ hours over your initial 2-Day Intensive) scanning, we will determine the exact Rife frequencies that will work best to help your body to begin to fight disease and heal. This is the most important pillar, and what most separates us from any other holistic-minded, alternative cancer clinic. Each patient goes home with what we believe to be the best and most important tool to help you overcome the disease and achieve health.

All our patients use the Rife at night while they sleep. For those that are less able to get up and get out of the house, they use it more. It comes equipped with a foot-bath detox unit to help as well. All programming is complete and tweaked as needed if the cancer progresses. Our promise is to do everything we can to help promote healing.

Pillar 4: Clean the Environment

Your body's **internal environment** has allowed for disease to flourish; whether through your own lifestyle choices or not! Sometimes we can do all the right things (eat organic, minimize sugar and other inflammatory foods, etc.) but still get disease. That's because we live in a toxic world.

We utilize many different types of testing to find out what your body needs (regarding diet, nutritional support, detox, etc.); however, our two primary methods are *Genetic testing* (SNP defects) and *Applied Kinesiology*. Using these we are able to find out specifically what your body needs to help support all your organ systems.

We also address the **external environment** to see what may be negatively influencing your healing process. This includes EMFs, Mold, Toxins, Emotional Barriers, and more.

Ongoing Support

Each care plan includes a lifetime of support. Including:

- Weekly group Zoom calls to answer ongoing questions

- Patients may email questions to be answered on an anonymous video that will be placed on our Blog

- Follow up visits & exams with doctors/practitioners

Interested in our Distance Program?

As an additional add-on, or an alternative option to our in-clinic care plans, you can choose to have one of our Distance Care Coordinators **come to your home** to care for you. We spend two days with you teaching you, your caregivers, and family everything to help you be the most successful in your search for health. In-home visits include some or all of the following services:

- Rife scanning and programming
- Assisting in set up & training of your home therapies
- Personal nutrition coaching, shopping, & meal planning
- Testing your home for dangerous EMFs and other toxins
- Giving you a thorough understanding of everything necessary to achieve your best

Integrative Therapies I May Recommend

First, let me again make one thing perfectly clear: **We do not treat cancer**! In truth, we don't treat anything. Our scope of practice allows me to treat *people*, which makes much more sense. We do not treat diseases, we don't diagnosis, nor do we desire to give any patient a label of *any* disorder. My feeling is this: if more doctors looked at a patient with wonder and curiosity, seeking desperately to figure out *why* they are manifesting such symptoms, worked vigilantly to trace back and correct the mechanisms that brought them to such a state I think we'd get more sick people well. That's our goal!

Below are brief descriptions of some alternative approaches for patients diagnosed with cancer that we use in our office. I do **not** suggest a *shotgun* approach to cancer or any disease! We test patients out with a technique called Applied Kinesiology which, although not perfect, has been a God-send to find the

260

exact nutritional/therapeutic approach that a person's body will best respond to. And of course, we also use specific genetic testing that helps guide care.

I commonly hear patients say that they are *so confused* with the information out there and they don't know who to believe. The truth is that all these approaches **do** work for **some** people. Which approach is going to be best for **you**? That's the question you want to answer; that's the question we try to help you find peace with. I have test kits and supplies for these and many more "cancer cures." Usually a person may test out positive on just one or two; you do not want to guess at the best treatment. There's too much at stake to be playing that game.

Why Everyone Uses Rife Therapy

Rife Therapy, though not proven with peer-reviewed, double-blind studies, is using specific frequencies of light with the goal to help the body heal. The Rife Machine was originally thought to target pathogens or cancer cells by means of matching the correct frequency or range of frequencies to help stimulate an immune attack on those cells. We now believe that Rife Therapy, while **not** a miracle cure or magic wand, can help a person detoxify and heal naturally.

Rife Therapy was the first therapy that we employed when our first patient asked for help in 1999. She had breast cancer in both breasts and was given 3 months to live without chemotherapy. She chose not to do chemo and, with the help of Rife Therapy, lived another 13 years.

While Rife is not a magic wand, God has used it to heal many people. All of our plans include a Rife machine that the patient uses at home, at a minimum every night.

What is it?

Possibly the most impressive method of detoxification ever developed, Rife technology was developed in the 1920s and 1930s by one of the true geniuses of the 20th Century, a microbiologist named Dr. Royal Rife. It involved aiming specific sound frequencies (piggy-backed onto a particular carrier wave for deep penetration) at cancer patients to kill their cancer. The treatment was so easy and non-toxic, it merely involved lying or sitting in front of the light. Documented cancer recoveries that resulted were phenomenal. However, this approach was finally suppressed to the point where it became virtually impossible to find a true Rife Machine that used the exact same technology and specifications of the original creator. Since many machines are being produced today that claim to be authentic, yet are not truly effective, it is important for cancer patients to know about the history and issues revolving around this particular treatment approach (believe me, I've tried many!)

The reason why Rife had his clinics shutdown by the AMA and the FDA was because he was claiming that the light frequency "killed cancer cells." Though this was his belief at the time (and no one could deny his success rate) it is **not** the current understanding of how light frequency works. We believe that since light is a photon, a particle on a waveform, it has different characteristics than other wave forms. Everything, on a quantum physics level, is made up of energy vibrating at a specific frequency. Bombarding cancer or any other particle (toxin, virus, etc.) with its own frequency simply vibrates it, making it recognizable to your own immune system for destruction. Rife technology does not kill cancer, it allows your body to recognize it and do its job in bringing you back to health.

Pulsed Electromagnetic Field Therapy

Having healthy cells is not a passive process. We are, after all, only as healthy as our cells. Imperceptible cell dysfunction that is not corrected early on can lead to disease and, as cell biologist Dr. Bruce Lipton explains, the health of the cell and its membrane is the key to healing.

Cellular *fine-tuning* can be aided using pulsed electromagnetic fields (PEMFs.) In addition, when there is a known imbalance (when symptoms are present) or there is a known disease or condition, PEMF treatments, used either alone or along with other therapies, can often help cells rebalance dysfunction faster.

Pulsed Magnetic fields emit a 3-D dimensional magnetic field into the body, creating an extraordinary effect:

- It delivers harmonic impulses that resonate the entire cell membrane. This ringer effect creates faster results

- It helps to re-energize cells by inducing electrical changes within the cell that helps the body restore the cell to a more normal state

- Cellular Metabolism can be boosted, blood cells can be regenerated, circulation can be improved, and oxygen capacity can be increased

- The immune system can become healthier, the nervous system can relax, bones and joints can become stronger, and the body may begin detoxing

- ***Research has proven faster neurological, physiological, and psychological benefits***

- Even after years of discomfort, positive results can be seen

It can be unbelievable

The cell can change sodium back to potassium (documented in a US Army study) and this reduces pain. Red blood cells separate in minutes, which allows more surface area to transport oxygen. There is a systemic response as though the body's functions have been fine-tuned or turbo charged. Because of this, many problems get better, wounds heal faster. There are currently hundreds of research studies documenting the benefits of PEMF. Though I wouldn't classify PEMF as a "cancer killer," it can help cells heal and function better, help relieve pain, and help with side-effects of chemotherapy such as peripheral neuropathy.

SEQEX Therapy

SEQEX is an innovative electromedical device for magnetotherapy that administers customized, controlled, pulsed, or variable electromagnetic fields at extremely low intensities and frequencies. It is essentially a more controlled, low intensity (low gauss) PEMF.

One benefit of SEQEX is that can be individualized in relation to each patient's wellness goals. Our clinic can also run a scan of a patient, develop a program of frequencies specific to the patient's needs, and treat appropriately.

The importance of the geomagnetic field (GMF) for the optimal health of all living things on our planet is a well-documented fact. It has been established that electromagnetic fields that are similar in intensity and frequency to the GMF can be safely used to promote health and wellbeing.

The SEQEX therapy machine generates electromagnetic fields whose characteristics are compatible to the GMF.

In sickness, your cells' voltage drops. Your electrolytes/ions become unbalanced (calcium, potassium, sodium etc.) The cells communicate through the exchange of ions at an electrical level. If the cell is diseased, this ion exchange drops. Detoxification decreases, as does nutrification. When the cells are not able to work properly, it is because their electrical voltage is decreased. A healthy cell functions at about 75-100mV and a sick cell functions at between 15-25mV.

If the cells were strong enough to perform electrically, they would function optimally and there would be no disease, but because they do not have the energy, they function less than optimally.

Hyperthermia

Directly from the American Cancer Society: "Hyperthermia means a body temperature that is higher than normal. High body temperatures are often caused by illnesses, such as fever or heat stroke. But hyperthermia can also refer to heat treatment: the carefully controlled use of heat for medical purposes. Here, we will focus on how heat is used to treat cancer.

When cells in the body are exposed to higher than normal temperatures, changes take place inside the cells. Warmer temperatures can make the cells more likely to be affected by other treatments such as radiation therapy or chemotherapy. Very high temperatures can kill cancer cells outright, but they also can injure or kill normal cells and tissues. This is why hyperthermia must be carefully controlled and should be done by doctors who are experienced in using it.

The idea of using heat to treat cancer has been around for some time, but early attempts had mixed results. For instance, it was hard to maintain the right temperature in the right area while limiting the effects on other parts of the body. But today, newer tools allow better control and more precise delivery of heat, and hyperthermia is being used (or studied for use) against many types of cancer."[124]

We utilize hyperthermia technology from Japan. As a matter of fact, it is widely used (in nearly 500 hospitals) there for a multitude of diseases.

There are 2 very different ways hyperthermia can be used:

1. Very high temperatures can be used to destroy a small area of cells, such as a tumor. This is often called *local hyperthermia* or *thermal ablation*. This is the safest and is the form that we utilize.

2. The temperature of a part of the body (or even the whole body) can be raised a few degrees higher than normal. It also helps other cancer treatments such as radiation, immunotherapy, or chemotherapy work better. This is called *regional hyperthermia* or *whole-body hyperthermia*.

Local hyperthermia is used to heat a small area like a tumor. A high temperature true-infrared instrument is used to kill the cancer cells by coagulating the proteins in them and destroying nearby blood vessels. In effect, this *cooks* the area that is exposed to the heat. While the damage is done to the cancer, the patient simply feels a warm sensation that is both comfortable and noninvasive.

Recent published study

Hisataka Kobayashi, a chief scientist at the U.S. National Institutes of Health, has developed a new method for treating cancer that uses harmless infrared light, a potentially major breakthrough in the battle against the deadly disease.

---

[124] https://www.cancer.org/treatment/treatments-and-side-effects/treatment-types/hyperthermia.html

In experiments, the treatment cured mice in 80% of cases with no side-effects. The research results were published online in the Nature Medicine magazine in November.

Kobayashi and his team focused on a special chemical that emits heat when exposed to light. They created a drug that combines this chemical with an antibody that connects to proteins (antigens) on cancer cells. The day after the drug is injected, near-infrared light, which easily passes through the body, is shone on the cancer cells to which the drug has adhered, thus creating heat and destroying the cancerous cells.

The harmless infrared light and the ability of the heat-emitting chemical to quickly metabolize in the body make the treatment *very safe*, according to Kobayashi, a graduate of Kyoto University.

In the study, mice with malignant cancer that would normally die within two weeks were injected with the drug. Over the following two days they were exposed to a daily dose of 15 minutes of near-infrared light. Repeating this regimen four times, with treatment performed every other week, completely cured 80% of the mice.

Reportedly, practical application of antibodies has already been employed for treating lung, colon, breast and other forms of cancer. Different drugs for each type of cancer can be made.

"The advantages are that it produces no side-effects and the treatment is repeatable," said Kobayashi. "We want to start clinical trials within the next five years."

Medsonix Sound Therapy

Medsonix acoustic technology is registered with the FDA as a Class 1 Medical Device and has been granted three distinct U.S. patents as a low-frequency acoustic methodology for treating pain. Medsonix Therapy System is a patented pain treatment alternative that is non-invasive, drug free, and therapeutic.

Many people experience an immediate and sustained beneficial effect after just one Medsonix treatment, although the maximum benefit is realized with routine treatment as needed. University pilot studies indicate over 85% of Medsonix therapy recipient's experienced symptomatic improvement and no negative side effects, with only one treatment.

Each session is 30-60 minutes in duration. Patients are placed in a relaxed environment, with headphones providing calming music to you. Healing sound waves are delivered during this time, using the music to filter out the actual pitch of the sound waves, making them barely audible.

Medsonix uses low frequency/high pressure acoustic sound waves to break up infectious colonies within damaged tissues caused by disease, allowing for increased blood flow to the damaged tissues. Blood circulation previously blocked by these colonies can now flood the damaged tissues and restore normal functionality. The body can then begin to heal itself by clearing out toxins, calming inflammation, and decreasing pain.

Some individuals may feel a slight tingling sensation throughout the body as the sound waves begin stimulating blood circulation. After treatment many individuals feel energized by the increased circulation and dilation of the blood vessels. The detoxification effects of Medsonix treatments are observed with patients reporting an increased frequency to urinate and more frequent bowel movements.

Medsonix treatments decrease inflammation of damaged tissues, relieving symptomatic pain, while also speeding up the healing process of disease.

While we don't believe that sound therapy will heal or even beneficially affect everyone, it is another tool to help those desiring to decrease pain, increase circulation and oxygenation to tissues, and speed healing.

There are plenty of testimonies of those that have experienced benefits from Medsonix, and though some may claim it may be from placebo, we really don't care as long as it works.

The Medsonix projects a 360° omnidirectional beam pattern. When operated, a range of low frequency electrical signals between 400-800 Hz are sent to the transducer and converted into acoustic energy. This produces waves that flow through the liquid medium and are transferred through air into the patient's body.

The waves extend up to 20 feet but are most effective within one to eight feet of the device.

Intravenous Vitamin C

Vitamin C has long been touted as a powerful antioxidant with abundant benefits including immune enhancement, protection from viruses and bacteria, cardiovascular protection, eye diseases, and even skin wrinkles. What many people may not know, however, is that in high-doses, IV Vitamin C may also help kill cancer cells.

Put simply, high-dose Vitamin C (available only through an IV) works with metals in the body to create hydrogen peroxide, an oxidative process. Whereas normal cells have the ability to reduce the effects of hydrogen peroxide, cancer cells do not. The high concentration of the resulting hydrogen peroxide damages the DNA of the cancer cells, cuts off their energy supply, and can help kill them. Vitamin C, even in very high doses, is toxic only to the cancer cells yet does not harm the healthy cells in your body.

Vitamin C IV is a very popular therapy that we offer at our clinic. While we believe that it is best used in combination with a multitude of therapies to boost your immune response and help your body recover from disease, we offer it in its own package to local patients. In the past we've hesitated to offer this therapy since the majority of our patients travel here from out-of-state or out-of-country, and practicality prevailed. However, we are seeing more and more patients that need this beneficial addition, whether it be just a quick immune boost or a prolonged, steady therapy, the addition of IV Vitamin C can be a fantastic addition to an alternative cancer treatment protocol.

In addition to its benefits as a non-toxic chemotherapeutic agent, intravenous Vitamin C also boosts immunity. It can stimulate collagen formation to help the body wall off the tumor. It inhibits hyaluronidase, an enzyme that tumors use to metastasize and invade other organs throughout the body. It induces apoptosis to help program cancer cells into dying early.

Light Beam Generator Therapy

Each human body is unique. Born with a unique combination of cells (and each cell with its own energy), no two human beings are the same. This is our blueprint; our electromagnetic signature.

Our electromagnetic signature is our body's method of control; a control from within that affects the mind, the body, and our well-being. Cells in the body have a natural polarity that when balanced places our blueprint in a restored state of health and optimal well-being. Combining safe and non-invasive, scalar technology with the harmonic sweep of frequencies, the Light Beam Generator (LBG) Lymph

Drainage Equipment assists the body in its natural process of moving stagnant lymph pathways.

Proper lymphatic drainage removes debris and proteins from the body to help create a protective barrier to health-related issues. As a result of re-establishing our electromagnetic signature, our blueprint is brought to life.

The LBG assists in restoring the natural polarity of our electromagnetic signature, which is essential for optimum immune response.

The LBG

- Uses electric signals known to influence the energetic pattern of virus, fungus, and bacteria to inhibit their development in cells that are stagnant

- Helps with the removal from the interstitial space of unnatural additives in our food, including steroids that mimic hormones and attach to proteins

- Aids in proper lymphatic drainage: rapid movement of waste material within the cells can occur, which greatly increases the delivery of waste material to the organs responsible for body waste disposal

- Helps bring stagnant lymph pathways to life, building an immunological barrier to disease

- Uses SpectraSweep technology, complementing the electromagnetic field to bring the body into a tranquil state, which can be felt even during the first use

Hyperbaric Oxygen Therapy (HBOT)

Hyperbaric Oxygen Therapy is a medical treatment that can

be traced back to the 1600's. In 1662, the first renowned chamber was built and operated by a British clergyman named Henshaw. He erected a structure titled, the Domicilium, that was used to treat a variety of conditions. In 1878, Paul Bert, a French physiologist, discovered the link between decompression sickness and nitrogen bubbles. Bert later identified that the pain could be ameliorated with recompression. The concept of treating patients under pressurized conditions was continued by the French surgeon Fontaine, who later built a pressurized mobile operating room in 1879. Fontaine found that inhaled nitrous oxide had a greater potency under pressure, in addition to his patients having improved oxygenation.

In the early 1900's Dr. Orville Cunningham, a professor of anesthesia, observed that people with particular heart diseases improved better when they lived closer to sea level than those living at higher altitudes. He treated a colleague who was suffering from influenza and was near death due to lung restriction. His resounding success led him to develop what was known as the *Steel Ball Hospital* located along the shore of Lake Erie. The six-story structure was erected in 1928 and was 64 feet in diameter. The hospital could reach 3 atmospheres absolute. Unfortunately, due to the depressed financial status of the economy, it was deconstructed in 1942 for scrap.

Subsequently, hyperbaric chambers were later developed by the military in the 1940's to treat deep-sea divers who suffered from decompression sickness. In the 1950's, physicians first employed **HBOT** during heart and lung surgery, which led to its use for carbon monoxide poisoning and other oxygen-depletion scenarios, such as gangrene, in the 1960's. It was thus shown to increase not just blood oxygen levels but also tissue oxygen as well as improve tissue healing. Since then, over 10,000 clinical trials and case studies have been completed for numerous other health-related applications with the vast majority of results reporting resounding success.

There are now many other illnesses and conditions for which the idea of increasing cellular oxygen load is accepted as having significant benefits, for example ulceration (caused by radiotherapy, diabetes, and so on), brain damage after accidents, and plastic surgery. Brain disorders such as Alzheimer's and Parkinson's have been shown to have favorable results with HBOT. Also, Autism and the other disorders on the spectrum have wonderful results larger due to the fact that the brain has a greater call for oxygen than any other tissue.

Using HBOT for cancer is based on the fact that most cancers, at their center, lack oxygen and multiply in a hypoxic environment. Oxygen has shown to aide in the body's ability to kill the cancer.

Otto Warburg

In 1931 Otto Warburg won a Nobel prize for explaining that oxygen was the enemy of the cancer cell. It kills them. Indeed, cancer cells thrive in an environment where oxygen is depleted (Hypoxia.) The abnormal blood supplies created by tumors feature "hypoxic pockets" where there is no oxygen and lower pH (a more acidic environment.) These "hypoxic pockets" seem to protect the cancer cell from the outside world, leaving it alone to burn glucose (glycolysis) and flourish. The pH inside such tumors is highly acidic, around 6.2 pH.

Since Warburg's discovery, many alternative cancer experts have pondered over ways of delivering oxygen to cancerous tissue in the hope of killing the cancer cells and restoring the tissue to a normal state. HBOT can be a wonderful tool to aide in the detoxification, healing, and recovery process.

Why Do We Test Genetic SNPs?

Cancer patients have distinct genes that we want to review.

273

There are cancer suppressor genes that, if defective, we want to support; there are genes that hint at what a person's cancer may be feeding on, thereby helping us more effectively govern their diet.

Each person has a set of genes, about 20,000 in all. The differences between people come from slight variations in these genes. For example, a person with defects (variants) on their genetic detoxification pathways may have a greater difficulty ridding their body of pesticides, giving them an increased risk of health issues.

Your body contains 50 trillion cells, and almost every one of them contains the complete set of instructions for making you. These instructions are encoded in your DNA.

Looking at genetic SNP tests help us shape your specific treatment protocol to best aide your ability to recover from disease. Variants (or defects) affect function, your strength to fight cancer, your ability to detoxify, and your ease of healing.

While we don't *treat the defect*, we **do** support the pathway. Every gene makes an enzyme with a specific duty. When we know the minor flaws that contribute to cancer, we can better adjust therapy to your unique situation. While your genes may "tell your story," **you** get to write the ending. It is what you do with the information that makes the difference.

Note: Dr. Conners' new "living eBook" format of his book *Cancer Genes* will be ever-evolving and constantly growing. For those who know him, they'll testify that he never stops learning; and this eBook simply could not be printed as it will be added to on a very regular basis.

Your genes are **so** important and knowing how they function can be the hidden key to turning the corner and getting well.

Download *Cancer Genes* for free at ConnersClinic.com/books

If You're Thinking of Care with Us

In our clinic, everyone starts with what we call a Case Review. This is usually done over the phone or via a Skype or Zoom call for those outside of the United States. It consists of a 30-minute consultation with me or one of our practitioners to discuss your case and offer some direction. We will not offer direct care suggestions like which supplements to take or directions to go as we need a proper examination for that, and we would have yet to decide on you becoming a patient.

Most people ask if they need to come to Minnesota to receive care. The answer is **no**. At this writing, we are in the middle of a perceived epidemic and most patients are choosing a distance plan. Our Level 2 Distance Plan is less expensive and still includes most everything involved with our in-clinic plan including a programmed Rife machine, genetic testing, nutraceutical plan, dietary program, etc. We address all of our Four Pillars of care no matter which care plan you choose.

Please visit our website ConnersClinic.com to access all necessary information about our care plans as well as links to complete the required online paperwork. You'll find that we believe in full disclosure of all our fees, there is nothing hidden! You will not find a more transparent clinic. Regardless of where you choose to receive care, our desire is that you find peace in your decision.

Always know that we will be praying for you!

CHAPTER 5

Nutraceuticals: "Natural Chemotherapy"

"Rarely do we find men who willingly engage in hard, solid thinking. There is an almost universal quest for easy answers and half-baked solutions. Nothing pains some people more than having to think."

— Martin Luther King, Jr.

This section of the book covers my favorite nutraceuticals. A nutraceutical may be described as a natural pharmaceutical. Vitamins, herbal remedies, minerals, homeopathic remedies, and other natural products would fall into this category. I list them by number and, while the first few might be my most favorite, I firmly believe that testing for which particular product (including a specific brand/manufacturer) is **best** for **you** is of the utmost importance. That stated, I realize that not everyone will be able to do this, and you will need to make the best decision possible. I recommend people pray about their decision with care, and that also includes which nutrients to use. Remember, too much of a good thing is a bad thing. Don't take too many things!

Polysaccharides

It's no doubt that polysaccharides are my favorite cancer killer but, like anything else, they don't work for everyone.

Personally, I take these daily for my cancer. I use the Evolv Immun Acemannan product listed below. In combination with other nutrients, it has served me well.

What are Polysaccharides?

A polysaccharide is a large molecule made of many smaller *monosaccharides*. Monosaccharides are simple sugars, like glucose. Special enzymes bind these small monomers together creating large sugar polymers, or polysaccharides. Depending on their structure, polysaccharides can have a wide variety of functions in nature. Some polysaccharides are used for storing energy, some for sending cellular messages, and others for providing support to cells and tissues. We are more interested in the types of polysaccharides that stimulate immune function. Let's see how that's done.

Their Effects on Immune Function

People hear "saccharide and sugar" and immediately get scared that it may feed their cancer. Think again. Polysaccharides have many different functions, but they do not stimulate cell reproduction. Certain polysaccharides have been called "immunomodulators" because they have been identified to have profound effects in the regulation of immune responses during the progression of infectious diseases and even cancer. They influence innate and cell-mediated immunity through interactions with T cells, monocytes, macrophages, and polymorphonuclear lymphocytes. In short, specific polysaccharides are wonderful at stimulating immune responses.

What are the *Best* Polysaccharides?

Poly = many, as in a chain of saccharide molecules. The number of saccharides in each chain are what defines the molecule and determines how it works in the body. The inner leaf of the Aloe plant has the greatest concentration of beneficial polysaccharides yet discovered. The immune-stimulating, cancer-killing component of Aloe was determined to be an acetylated polymannan called **Acemannan**. Acemannan works by stimulating the body's own immune system to help it heal itself!

Recently published in the American Society of Gene and Cell Therapy, cell therapy is defined as "the administration of living whole cells for the patient for the treatment of a disease." When treating cancer, this has largely meant immunotherapy medication with T cells, both engineered and not. But that is changing. As our understanding of the innate immune system (TH1 response) catches up with our understanding of the adaptive immune system (TH2 response), natural killer (NK) cells are emerging as an alternative to T cells in eliciting an immune response to tumors. This is what natural immune system stimulation has been all about for years!

At the *Innate Killer Summit* held recently in San Diego, scientists in industry and academia described the approaches they are using to improve cell therapies. Some of the scientists are engineering NK cells, as a drug, to use in cancer treatment. Robert Igarashi, PhD, the co-founder and CSO of CytoSen Therapeutics, a pharmaceutical company attempting to patent a drug to stimulate NK cells, says, "Normal adults have one to two million circulating NK cells." The company is attempting to duplicate and stimulate an immune attack on the cancer.[125]

There are numerous ways to stimulate NK Cells naturally. Mushrooms such as shiitake, maitake, Coriolus, and others boost NK cell activity courtesy of beta-glucans, a polysaccharide known for its immune-boosting and cancer-

---

[125] Polysaccharide Immunomodulators as Therapeutic Agents: Structural Aspects and Biologic Function. Arthur O. Tzianabos Clinical Microbiology Reviews Oct 2000, 13 (4) 523-533; DOI: 10.1128/CMR.13.4.523

fighting activities. As noted in a 2007 study in the journal *Medicine*:

"[B]eta-glucans (a polysaccharide)…increase host immune defense by activating complement system, enhancing macrophages and natural killer cell function. The induction of cellular responses by mushroom and other beta-glucans is likely to involve their specific interaction with several cell surface receptors, as complement receptor 3, lactosylceramide, selected scavenger receptors, and dectin-1 (betaGR.) Beta-glucans also show anticarcinogenic activity. They can prevent oncogenesis due to the protective effect against potent genotoxic carcinogens. As [an] immunostimulating agent, which acts through the activation of macrophages and NK cell cytotoxicity, beta-glucan can inhibit tumor growth in promotion stage too."

See more info here: ConnersClinic.com/nk-cells

Acemannan

The Problem, and Solution, with Acemannan

Numerous studies have been published about the benefits of Acemannan and the Aloe plant. As usual, when this happens, sales of Aloe rise to consumers wanting the immune-stimulating benefits. The problem is that the Acemannan (the active, beneficial component) is **not** stable! **Ugh**! Millions of dollars a year are spent on Aloe products that, though other benefits may still avail, the immune-stimulating, cancer-killing properties simply no longer exist (due to Acemannan's instability).

However, thank goodness, a research team discovered not only how to stabilize Acemannan so that it can be capsulized and utilized by the body, but they also discovered the best chain length (50-400) of polysaccharides to give the most immune-stimulating properties. Evolv Immun holds the patent on the only stabilized, correct-chain polysaccharide available for human consumption.

Evolv Immun

shop.ConnersClinic.com/evolve-immun

An Animal Study

Forty-three dogs and cats with spontaneous tumors were treated with the immunostimulating polysaccharide Acemannan by intraperitoneal and intralesional routes of administration. Tumors from 26 of these animals showed histopathological (microscopically looking at the cells) evidence of immunological attack as shown by marked necrosis or lymphocytic infiltration. In lay-man's terms, this means that, as the tumors were viewed under the microscope, the tumor cells were dying. Thirteen showed moderate to marked tumor necrosis (tumor cell death) or liquefaction. Twenty-one demonstrated lymphoid infiltration (the immune system was beginning to attack the tumor), and seven demonstrated encapsulations (the body walled-off the tumor.) Twelve animals showed obvious clinical improvement as assessed by tumor shrinkage, tumor necrosis, or prolonged survival; these included five of seven animals with fibrosarcoma (quite serious, aggressive cancers.) "It is believed," said the scientists that published the study, "that Acemannan exerts its antitumor activity through macrophage activation and the release of tumor necrosis factor, interleukin-1, and interferon." This means that Acemannan helps the body kill the tumor by stimulating the main killing mechanisms of the immune system.[126]

---

[126] Efficacy of acemannan in treatment of canine and feline spontaneous neoplasms. https://www.altmetric.com/details/13929345

A Human Study

Most human cancer studies will only get their funding if the study couples chemotherapy along with the natural substance. But, that's okay, it still gives us wonderful data. A study on the polysaccharides from aloe on 240 patients with cancer revealed, "the analysis of tumor immunobiology suggest the possibility of biologically manipulating the efficacy and toxicity of cancer chemotherapy by endogenous or exogenous immunomodulating substances."

The Polysaccharides in Aloe make it one of the most important plants exhibiting anticancer activity and its antineoplastic property is due to at least three different mechanisms, based on antiproliferative, immunostimulatory and antioxidant effects. The anti-proliferative action is determined by anthracenic and antraquinonic molecules, while the immunostimulating activity is mainly due to acemannan.

Patients and Methods: A study was planned to include 240 patients with metastatic solid tumor who were randomized to receive chemotherapy with or without Aloe. According to tumor histotype and clinical status, lung cancer patients were treated with cisplatin and etoposide or weekly vinorelbine, colorectal cancer patients received oxaliplatin plus 5-fluorouracil (5-FU), gastric cancer patients were treated with weekly 5-FU and pancreatic cancer patients received weekly gemcitabine. Aloe was given orally at 10 ml thrice/daily.

Results: The percentage of both objective **tumor regressions** and **disease control** was significantly higher in patients concomitantly **treated with Aloe** than with chemotherapy alone, as well as the percent of 3-year survival patients.

Conclusion: This study seems to suggest that Aloe may be successfully associated with chemotherapy to increase its efficacy in terms of both tumor regression rate and survival time.[127]

My Experience

I will be writing more on this subject, as this product has been partly responsible for helping me achieve remission in my Stage 4 Cancer.

Father Romano Zago's Aloe "Cure"

Father Romano Zago is a Franciscan Friar, born in Brazil in 1932. He was appointed professor of the seminary of Taquari, but in 1991 he was sent to Israel where discovered the healing power of the aloe used by poor people. The aloe vera, present in abundance in the region, is the raw material on which he focused all his attention in his free time. "I already knew the plant in Brazil," he declared. "My mother gave it to us as a soothing agent when, as children, we used to get hurt while playing or for other physical problems. However, at that time, I had never suspected that such a small and diffused plant could have such great healing powers."

Once back in Brazil in 1995, Father Romano Zago further refined his formula and dedicated himself to experimentation; he apparently helped many people with numerous problems including cancer. Convinced by the numerous extraordinary recoveries, he assembled all his experiences in one book, *O Cancer Tem Cura* (One can recover from cancer, Italian edition, Adle, Padova), in which Father Romano exposes, in the simplest and clearest of manners, the practice of cure from the "disease of the century " through his drink based on aloe.

---

[127] A Randomized Study of Chemotherapy VersusBiochemotherapy with Chemotherapy plus Aloe arborescens in Patients with Metastatic Cancer, PAOLO LISSONI, FRANCO ROVELLI, FERNANDO BRIVIO, et al. In Vivo January-February 2009 vol. 23 no. 1 171-175

"Since some have cured themselves through the use of this simple and economic method, why not offer this same opportunity to more persons? This is my only objective," he explains in his book. He also relates various witness accounts of people who underwent perfect recovery through the use of the above-mentioned mixture. In 1993 Father Romano Zago conceded the authorization to a Brazilian industry to produce his aloe-based mixture under his name. This gave rise to the original drink according to the father's ingredients, which were then commercialized in many countries.

The problem that many have faced in trying to reproduce Father Romano's results speak to the more recent discoveries on the instability of the healing nutrients in aloe. It has been shown that the immune-stimulating properties contained in the aloe plant are the long-chain polysaccharides unique to the plant. Polysaccharides have been long known to benefit immune function. They are also found in various medicinal mushroom varieties used in natural healing. But, like the polysaccharides found in mushrooms, the polysaccharides in aloe are extremely fragile. This instability explains the frequent lack of benefit found by many using over-the-counter preparations.

See more about Father Romano here:

ConnersClinic.com/father-romano

Medicinal Mushrooms

Watch some of my videos on Medicinal Mushrooms:

ConnersClinic.com/cancer-medicinal-mushrooms

ConnersClinic.com/cancer-and-fungi

Since we are talking about mushrooms, I must tell you that I love to use them to stimulate the immune system. Here are some of my favorites:

Agaricus Mushroom: Agaricus mushroom is a Brazilian rainforest herb that is among the premier immune system tonics of all known natural substances. It is the richest source in the world of a type of polysaccharide known as *beta-glucans (see the section on this)*, which has been solidly established to be among nature's most potent immune potentiating substances. Agaricus has *double-direction activity* on the immune system. In other words, it may be used to bolster a deficient immune system, as occurs in cases involving infections, or Agaricus may be used to moderate an excessive system, as occurs in cases of autoimmune disease and allergies. This means it is an immune modulator. In cancer patients, it helps suppress a hyper-active Th2 system and increase a Th1 response! Agaricus may therefore be used by anyone. In Japan, Agaricus is considered a "cure-all" herb.

Cordyceps Mushroom: Cordyceps is one of the major players of the Chinese tonic herbal system and is a *hit* in dealing with cancer. It is an extremely effective and powerful life-enhancing agent, boosting energy and vitality. Because it is rare, potent, and highly treasured, like Deer Antler, good cordyceps can be expensive. It is a mushroom that consumes the body of a particular type of caterpillar in mountainous regions of China, Mongolia, and Tibet. It has enormous renown as a *supertonic* in Chinese herbal circles, and is said to build sexual and physical power, mental energy, the immune system, and is universally believed in the Orient to prolong life.

Cordyceps is used to strengthen and stabilize the body and mind at a fundamental level. It is said to be able to increase the "primary motive force for life activities" which can be lost following a grim diagnosis. Some people walk into my office with a complete loss of hope; cordyceps is one tool that can give people a renewed desire to live. Because it contains both *Yin* and *Yang* (Chinese medicine for a balance in force) it can be used by anyone safely and over a long period of time. It replenishes the deep energy expended as a result of excessive exertion, adapting to extreme stress (the real killer in cancer patients) or from aging.

Medicinal Mushrooms

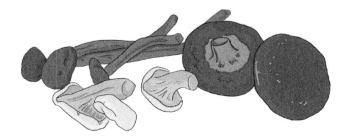

Cordyceps is also used for the purposes of strengthening the Kidney functions and kidney detoxification, which also includes sexual function, brain power (decreasing Th17 activity that causes inflammation in the brain), structural integrity, and healing ability. Consistent use of Cordyceps helps to strengthen the skeletal structure, and specifically benefits the lower back region, the knees, and ankles. It can be great for patients with metastatic disease to the bones.

Cordyceps is also a major Lung tonic. It can be used to strengthen respiratory power in those who require extra energy in order to perform physical work (e.g. labor, sports, or exercise) or it can be used by those who suffer from deficiency of Lung strength due to cancer, asthma, Mesothelioma, etc. It is especially beneficial to those who suffer chronic Lung weakness with coughing, wheezing, or shortness of breath. It is highly regarded in China as a tonic for those who are

286

recovering from an illness or an operation, or after giving birth. In these cases, the Cordyceps helps the patient more quickly recover their physical power, to improve their appetite, and to protect the body from infection.

Maitake Mushroom: Maitake mushroom has gained a place in tonic herbalism due to its broad-spectrum tonic benefits similar to Agaricus and Reishi. Like Agaricus, it is primarily beneficial to the immune system, having double-direction activity on the entire immune system. It is often called the *king of mushrooms* and though only a legend, it has been said that Japanese monkeys who commonly consume large quantities of Maitake have no known cancer and other diseases.

Clinically, Maitake has proven itself to be an effective tool for cancer patients. In lab tests, powdered Maitake increased the activity of three types of Th1 immune cells (macrophages, natural killer (NKC) cells, and T cells) by 140, 186, and 160 percent, respectively. A Chinese clinical study established that Maitake treatment reduces the recurrence of bladder surgery from 65-33%. Researchers have found that Maitake, when combined with the standard chemotherapy drug mitomycin (Mutamycin), inhibits the growth of breast cancer cells, even after metastasis. (Note: most studies on alternate products like this **must** be done "in conjunction with standard pharmaceutical drugs" to get funding!)

Maitake also protects the liver. Chinese doctors conducted a controlled trial with 32 patients who had chronic hepatitis B. The recovery rate was 72% in the Maitake treatment group, compared with 57% in the control group. Hepatitis antigens disappeared in more than 40% of the Maitake patients, indicating the virus had been purged from the liver. Laboratory studies also show that Maitake protects liver tissue from hepatitis caused by environmental toxins such as carbon tetrachloride and paracematol. These compounds go through a two-step process in the liver in which they are first activated into toxic forms and then deactivated into harmless forms. Since Maitake helps the liver handle chemical poisons in both steps, it protects this organ against a broad range of potential toxins. Finally, Maitake provides nutritional support by enhancing the colon's ability to absorb micronutrients, especially in its help to balance copper and zinc.

Reishi Mushroom: Reishi mushroom (*Ganoderma lucidum*) is the most revered herbal substance in Asia, ranking as the elite substance for the attainment of radiant health, longevity, and spiritual attainment. It ranks with Asiawith Ginseng, Deer Antler, Rhodiola, and Cordyceps as a pre-eminent tool in the attainment of radiant health. It has maintained that position for at least 3000 years, and its reputation and value are only increasing. Numerous legends provide a rich and extensive record of Reishi in Asian society.

Reishi has traditionally been used as (and recent studies confirm the benefits) an anti-aging herb and has been used for many diseases and disorders as well. It has long been a favorite tonic by the Chinese Royal family and virtually anyone who could obtain it. Reishi was particularly revered by the followers of the Taoist tradition as the "Elixir of Immortality." Taoists have continuously claimed that Reishi promotes calmness, centeredness, balance, inner awareness, and inner strength. They have used it to improve meditative practices and to protect the body, mind, and spirit so that the adept could attain both a long and healthy life and "spiritual immortality" (enlightenment.) Due to its rarity in the past, the common people could rarely obtain a Reishi mushroom, and it was popularly revered as a greater treasure than any jewel.

Reishi is said to be capable of building body resistance, and to be powerfully detoxifying to the cells and tissues. Reishi is slightly sedative on an immediate basis but builds energy over time; it is universally believed in Asia to prolong life and

288

enhance intelligence and wisdom. Since Reishi has been known to have many functions, it has been the subject of a great deal of research in recent years. It is absolutely safe for everyone and is completely non-toxic.

Use in cancer patients centers around Reishi as a profound immune modulator. It has been found to significantly improve the balance of the immune system whether the immune system is deficient or excessive. Many chemical constituents play a role in Reishi's immune modulating capacity. The polysaccharide components in particular seem to play an important role in attacking cancerous cells, while simultaneously strengthening the body's overall immune functions. The polysaccharides appear to help the body attack microbial invaders such as viruses, bacteria, and yeast.

Another group of chemicals found in Reishi known as the ganoderic acids help fight autoimmune diseases by inhibiting histamine release, improving oxygen utilization, and improving liver functions. Ganoderic acids are also potent antioxidant free-radical scavengers.

Our Medicinal Mushroom blend consists of:

- Elderberry fruit
- Fermented Soy
- Magnolia bark
- Red Clover
- Reishi mushroom
- Mistletoe
- Moringa Oliefera
- Chaga mushroom
- Coriolus mushroom
- Maitake mushroom
- Cordyceps mushroom

Chaga Mushroom: I list Chaga separately because I'm such a big fan. Chaga is another of the few that really helped me personally and I take it separately as a tea. Actually, though I'm told I can't really taste things because of my nasal polyps, I think ground Chaga, mixed with hot water, tastes a lot like coffee. Often, I add a teaspoon to my coffee to give an earthy, woody flavor.

From *The Truth About Cancer*:

"The mysterious Chaga mushroom (*Inonotus obliquus*) is a non-toxic, medicinal mycelium with a propensity for birch bark. If you were to spot it while roaming through a birch forest in the Northern hemisphere, you'd probably assume (based on its rather unappealing appearance), that it was some kind of tree infection. But Chaga is a whole lot more than just an unsightly forest blemish. ***The chaga mushroom is actually a treasure trove of science-backed healing potential that's been a prominent feature in folk medicine for thousands of years***.

Chaga's reputation as a powerful natural remedy for everything from gastrointestinal disease to tuberculosis to cancer spans at least as far back as the 16th century when botanical artisans are said to have figured out that it could be steeped as a tea for a variety of therapeutic purposes.

The historical record suggests that, even prior to this, natural healers in Asia were likely among the first to document Chaga's medicinal potential more than 4,600 years ago. They observed that the strange fungus has a unique ability to extract nutrients from its hosts and concentrate them into itself. Hence the chaga mushroom's incredible density of B Vitamins, antioxidants, trace minerals, enzymes, and more.

Since these ancient times science has taken our understanding of Chaga to a whole new level, and the West is finally catching on to what this amazing mushroom is capable of. ***Just in the*** *last century the Chaga mushroom's antiviral, antimicrobial, anti-inflammatory, cardio-protective, anti-hyperglycemic, and anti-cancer properties have become more widely known.*

Prominent authorities, including the International Society for Mushroom Science (ISMS), have declared it to be a worthwhile dietary supplement that may be useful as a first-line nutraceutical remedy. This means it's a functional food that exhibits significant medicinal and/or tonic qualities from which humans can derive benefit."

How Chaga Supports a Vibrant Immune System

You probably already know that the primary means by which the human body avoids disease is through the immune system; a complex network of organs, cells, and proteins that actively wards off foreign invaders. *Without an immune system, our bodies would quickly succumb to harmful pathogens* like bacteria, viruses, parasites, and malignant fungi, leading to serious illness and eventually death. This is why it's critically important to support the immune system with immuno-modulatory nutrition like the kind found in Chaga.

A natural Biological Response Modifier (BRM), Chaga mushroom is rich in a class of polysaccharides known as Beta-D-Glucans that help to balance the body's immune system response, boosting or slowing it as needed for optimal function. *Chaga also possesses key nutrient compounds that give it the ability to activate an array of immune cells*, including lymphocytes, macrophages, and natural killer cells. These cells allow the body to suppress the formation of chronic health conditions like autoimmune disease, allergies, and cancer.

The immuno-modulatory effects of Chaga appear to extend

even further than this, with investigatory research suggesting benefits in the remediation of both food and asthma allergies, atopic dermatitis, inflammation (including autoimmune inflammatory conditions such as rheumatoid arthritis), atherosclerosis, thrombosis, human immunodeficiency virus (HIV), listeriosis, septic shock, and perhaps most prominently, cancer.

While science has yet to uncover every precise mechanism behind how Chaga performs these functions, it's clear from what's already been uncovered that *Chaga is a powerful potentiating and immune enhancing "superfood" with vast healing potential*.

Inflammation is No Match for Chaga Mushroom

In addition to Beta-D-Glucans, Chaga mushrooms contain a variety of other polysaccharides that have been scientifically shown to help boost energy levels and promote mental clarity, while protecting the various organs of the body against damaging inflammation. Particularly in the area of cardiovascular health, *Chaga exhibits a type of soothing effect that's been shown to help relax blood vessels and improve blood flow*. This in turn delivers more oxygen throughout the body.

Patients suffering from chronic pain, neuropathy, and even diabetes are strong candidates for Chaga's use in this regard, as the mushroom's constituents have further been shown to help modulate platelet aggregation.

Heart disease is another area where Chaga has shown pronounced benefits. It contains high levels of a triterpene substance known as betulinic acid, as well as its precursor betulin, that studies show is a powerful weapon against high cholesterol. Researchers from Jiangnan University in China found that a culture broth containing dry matter of Chaga extract exhibited both anti-hyperglycemic and anti-lipid peroxidative effects, helping to break down damaging LDL (low-density lipoprotein) cholesterol in the bloodstream.

Chaga's diverse antioxidant profile is even more impressive, as it bears the highest ORAC score of any known superfood (ORAC is a measure of antioxidant potency.) According to research compiled by Tufts University, Chaga has 3x the antioxidant power of wolfberries (aka goji berries), which is the next strongest known food. *One could argue that this makes Chaga the world's number one source of inflammation-fighting antioxidants*.

Chaga mushroom contains high amounts of Super Oxide Dismutase (SOD), a powerful class of enzymes that contributes to its robust antioxidant defense against oxidation and free radical damage. *Chaga's natural black pigmentation is indicative of its high content of melanin, a polyphenol-rich "super" antioxidant that protects against DNA damage*. Melanin is the same antioxidant naturally found in human skin that protects against sun damage.

Chaga and Cancer: A Potential Natural Alternative to Drugs and Surgery?

Where Chaga really shines is in the area of cancer. *Dozens of scientific studies (and counting!) suggest that Chaga exhibits strong apoptotic, anti-proliferative, and chemo-protective benefits*. Its full spectrum of phytosterols, including lanosterol, inotodiol, ergosterol, and fecosterol, are among the many Chaga constituents that have been shown both in vivo (inside a living organism) and in vitro (in a laboratory model) to directly inhibit the growth and spread of cancer cells.

In tumor-bearing mice, extracts of Chaga showed significant

tumor-suppressive effects, the supplementation of which resulted in an impressive 60% reduction in tumor size, on average. The same research found that Chaga helped to increase tumor agglomeration as well as inhibit tumor vascularization, further inhibiting the growth and spread of cancer in these mice. Related research demonstrated Chaga's anti-cancer potential as it pertains to the downregulation of certain cell pathways associated with cancer, including in colitis-induced human colorectal cancer.

Our Chaga is grown in Alaska at 60 degrees latitude, harvested off of living birch trees. Though I have patients that often harvest their own Chaga, you need to learn how to identify it.

Researchers from Russia have been actively studying the benefits of Chaga and other similar mushrooms that grow throughout their country and in nearby Siberia, taking a particular interest in how these mushroom constituents affect cancer. Among their discoveries are the therapeutic benefits of Chaga's bioactive triterpene compounds (primarily those containing OH group at C-22 and a side chain unsaturated bond) which these researchers found have the ability to directly inhibit the growth of a number of cancer cell lines, as demonstrated both in vitro and in vivo.

Chaga also possesses hepatoprotective properties that are particularly relevant not only to liver injuries but also to liver cancer. Studies have found that even when taken at relatively low doses, Chaga actively scavenges the free radicals that cause oxidative liver injury, effectively blocking the formation of liver disease and liver cancer.

All of this and more is why *one study dubbed Chaga as a premier "natural anti-cancer ingredient in food,"* suggesting that it may, in fact, be a safe and effective treatment and preventative protocol for cancer. This sentiment is further

294

reflected by David Winston, RH, AHG, Dean of the Center for Herbal Studies in Broadway, New Jersey, and an herbal practitioner with more than 40 years of experience under his belt, who's convinced that Chaga is the most powerfully anti-cancer medicinal mushroom in existence.

It all makes sense when you consider the incredible nutrient profile of Chaga, which is virtually unmatched in the natural world. Even with all that we know it can do, there's still so much more to learn about the wonders of the Chaga mushroom, which is why this powerful superfood will continue to be the focus of scientific research involving functional foods for many years to come.

AHCC: AHCC (Active Hexose Correlated Compound) is a supplement made from medicinal mushrooms that have been fermented in rice bran. It is currently being used in 700 hospitals and clinics in Japan to treat a wide range of health conditions, from minor ailments such as colds and flu, to serious diseases such as cancer, hepatitis, diabetes, and cardiovascular disease.

AHCC works as a Th1 stimulator (increasing the strength of your immune system.) The common underlining factor in *all* cancers is compromised immunity. As a biological response modifier, AHCC turns the dial up on your natural immune response, helping you fight all kinds of threats to your health.

Remember the Key Players of the Th1 Immune Response: Your First Line of Defense

- **Cytokines**: Chemical messengers that help immune cells communicate and coordinate an immune response

- **Natural killer (NK) cells**: Specialized white blood cells (WBCs) that recognize and destroy infected or abnormal cells by injecting granules into them, causing them to explode

- **Macrophages**: WBC that engulf and ingest bacteria, virus, and other cellular debris

- **Dendritic cells**: WBC that present foreign substances to B and T cells, initiating an adaptive response

Proven Benefits of AHCC

In vivo and human clinical trials have shown that AHCC increases the Th1 immune response by:

- Increasing the production of cytokines
- Increasing the activity of NK cells by as much as 300-800%
- Increasing populations of macrophages, in some cases doubling them
- Increasing the number of dendritic cells
- Increasing the number of T cells by as much as 200%

AHCC has been used in Japan with great success in cancer patients. Data from the treatment of over 100,000 individuals with various types of cancer have shown AHCC treatment to be of benefit in 60% of cases. That doesn't mean the cancer disappeared; it means it helped. AHCC has been shown to be particularly effective for liver, lung, stomach, colon, breast, thyroid, ovarian, testicular, tongue, kidney and pancreatic cancers.

One landmark AHCC trial enrolled 269 patients with liver cancer. Following surgery, about half of the patients took AHCC and about half did not. The results were dramatic: At the end of the ten-year study, only 34.5% of the AHCC patients experienced a recurrence in their cancer, compared with 66.1% of the control group that did not take AHCC.

Similarly, while 46.8% of the patients in the control group had died at the end of ten years, less than half that amount (20.4%) of those in the AHCC group had. Another study found that AHCC not only prolonged survival of advanced liver cancer patients, it also improved various parameters of quality of life, including mental stability, general physical health status and the ability to have normal activities.

Beta 1,3D Glucan Mushroom: I list this product separately as well because it is sold separately and so often spoken of in this form. However, beta-glucans are a polysaccharide. The Department of Urology, New York Medical College recently published a study entitled, "*Induction of apoptosis in human prostatic cancer cells with beta-glucan (Maitake mushroom polysaccharide)*" that was pretty exciting. I always get excited over current medical research that proves what herbalists have already known for centuries. It's even comical when they "discovered" something that we've been already using for decades and the Chinese have used for thousands of years before Christ.

The purpose of the study was to "explore more effective treatment for hormone-refractory prostate cancer." They investigated the potential antitumor effect of beta-glucan, a polysaccharide of the Maitake mushroom, on prostatic cancer cells in vitro. Beta-glucans are found in a variety of sources and as I've already stated; they are a pivotal complex found in Medicinal Mushrooms.

The above study treated human prostate cancer PC-3 cells with various concentrations of the highly purified beta-glucan preparation. The "dose-response study" (increased doses increased results) showed that almost complete (>95%) cell death was attained in 24 hours.

Interestingly, they also simultaneously tested various anticancer drugs that "showed little potentiation of their efficacy." Their conclusion revealed, "A bioactive beta-glucan from the Maitake mushroom has a cytotoxic (cancer killing) effect, presumably through oxidative stress, on prostatic cancer cells in vitro, leading to apoptosis (cell death)...therefore, this unique mushroom polysaccharide may have great a potential as an alternative therapeutic modality for prostate cancer."

We use Beta-glucan alone as a supplement as well as in our Medicinal Mushrooms; both are great and really have no side effects.

What We Use

Evolv Immun

shop.ConnersClinic.com/evolv-immun

Dr. Conners Medicinal Mushroom Blend

shop.ConnersClinic.com/mm

Chaga Powdered Mushrooms

shop.ConnersClinic.com/chaga

Coriolus Super Strength

shop.ConnersClinic.com/coriolus

Enzyme Therapy

Dr. William Kelley's Enzyme Therapy

Dr. Kelley made most of his discoveries when he cured himself of metastatic pancreatic cancer after he was given two months to live. He studied Dr. Beard's work (published in the early 1900's) and discovered the benefits of high dose enzyme therapy. The wonderful thing about this type of therapy is that, not only does it **work** but also it has neither side effects nor contraindications. Two physicians in New York (who were some of **my** teachers in my Integrative Cancer Therapy Fellowship program), Dr. Gonzalez and Dr. Isaacs, are working together to treat cancer patients with this approach and are having great results. The treatment centers around taking high doses of special enzymes that could once only be gotten from these physicians; we now have full access to this approach! Though I do **not** advocate all of Dr. Gonzalez's work, the enzyme portion of his therapy derived from Dr. Kelley's work is one that we readily incorporate, involving strict diet based on Sympathetic or Parasympathetic dominance, high-dose enzymes, and regular coffee enemas. While we do not adhere to Dr. González' "mega-vitamin" approach, we do believe enzyme therapy has proven itself clinically.

Understand, if we have the ability to test the patient on the correct supplementation and dosage, we can greatly reduce the number of supplements and thereby the cost of care. It is common to see our patients with previously diagnosed cancer to be on no more than a few supplements!

Dr. Nicholas Gonzalez's Enzyme Therapy

Dr. Gonzalez was one of my instructors in the Fellowship program through the American Academy of Anti-Aging Medicine. He is featured in Suzanne Somers book on cancer and was on the TV program 20/20. This interview is excerpted from the November 1999 *Clinical Pearls News*:

Kirk Hamilton: What is your educational background and current position?

Nicholas J. Gonzalez: I graduated from Brown University, Phi Beta Kappa, Magna Cum Laude with a degree in English literature. I did my premedical work as a postgraduate student at Columbia University, and received my medical degree from Cornell University Medical College in New York. I subsequently completed a year of internship in internal medicine, and a fellowship in immunology.

KH: Where did you come up with the idea at all to use pancreatic enzymes in cancer and what is the theoretic mechanism?

NJG: I didn't come up with the idea to use pancreatic enzymes to treat cancer. The Scottish embryologist, John Beard, who worked at the University of Edinburgh at the turn of the century, first proposed in 1906 that pancreatic proteolytic enzymes, in addition to their well-known digestive function, represent the body's main defense against cancer. He further proposed that pancreatic enzymes would most likely be useful as a cancer treatment. During the first two decades of this century, a number of physicians, both in Europe and in the United States, used injectable pancreatic enzymes to treat advanced human cancer, oftentimes (depending on the quality of the product) with great success. I have collected a number of reports from that time in the major medical journals documenting tumor regression and long-term survival in patients treated with enzyme therapy. In my first article, I mentioned that in 1911, Dr. Beard published a monograph entitled *The Enzyme Therapy of Cancer*, which summarized his therapy and the supporting evidence (available through New Spring Press.)

After Dr. Beard's death in 1923, the enzyme therapy was largely forgotten. Periodically, alternative therapists have rediscovered Dr. Beard's work, and used pancreatic proteolytic enzymes as a treatment for cancer.

I began researching the use of oral pancreatic proteolytic

300

enzyme therapy as a treatment for cancer after completion of my second year at Cornell University Medical College in 1981. My research advisor at the time supported and directed my early work, and later supported me during my formal immunology fellowship. In terms of the theoretical foundation, the exact mechanism of action has never been demonstrated. After Beard's death, the enzyme therapy was largely forgotten and certainly never generated any significant research effort until recently with the funding of my work. There are several studies from the 1960s showing, in an animal model, that orally ingested pancreatic enzymes have an anti-cancer effect, and might work through immune modulation, but these studies were preliminary and were never followed-up. Dr. Beard believed enzymes had to be injected to prevent destruction by hydrochloric acid in the stomach. However, recent evidence demonstrates that orally ingested pancreatic proteolytic enzymes are acid stable, pass intact into the small intestine and are absorbed through the intestinal mucosa into the blood stream as part of an enteropancreatic recycling process.

It is clear from our extensive clinical experience that pancreatic proteolytic enzymes have a profound anti-neoplastic effect, but we do not know how they work. We have not had the resources to support basic science research, but with appropriate funding we do not believe it would difficult to set up animal models to explore the molecular action of the enzymes against cancer cells.

KH: *Why did you choose a vegetable-based diet, low in red meat and poultry, with a little fish and occasional dairy products?*

NJG: We divide patients into different metabolic categories, depending on each patient's particular genetic, biochemical and physiological make-up. In this model, patients with solid epithelial tumors, such as tumors of the lung, pancreas, colon, prostate, uterus, etc. do best on a largely plant-based diet. Such patients have a metabolism that functions most efficiently with a specific combination of nutrients that are found in fruits, vegetables, nuts, whole grains and seeds, and with minimal to no animal protein.

On the other hand, patients with the blood or immune based malignancies such as leukemia, myeloma and lymphoma do best on a high-animal protein, high-fat diet. Such patients do extremely well with a diet based on animal products with minimal to moderate amounts of plant-based foods, the particular design of the diet again depending on the individual patient's metabolic make-up. We find patients with pancreatic cancer always do best with a largely plant-based diet that emphasizes fruits, vegetables and vegetable juice, nuts, seeds and whole grains. Allowed protein includes fish one to two times a week, one to two eggs daily and yogurt daily, but no other animal protein. In our therapy, we use diets specifically because of the effect of food on the autonomic nervous system. This system consists of the sympathetic and parasympathetic branches and ultimately controls all aspects of our physiology, including immune function, cardiovascular activity, endocrine function and the entire action of our digestive system. The sympathetic and parasympathetic systems have opposing actions on the target organs and so can adjust our physiology depending on needs and demands, enabling our bodies to react to any situation, condition or stress. We believe disease, whatever the form, occurs because there is an imbalance in autonomic function. For example, we find solid tumors, such as tumors of the breast, lung, pancreas, colon, uterus, ovaries, liver, etc. occur only in patients who have an overly strong sympathetic nervous system and a correspondingly weak, ineffective parasympathetic nervous system. We believe that blood-based cancers, such as leukemia, lymphoma and multiple myeloma, only occur in patients that have an overly developed parasympathetic nervous system, and a correspondingly weak sympathetic nervous system. Previous research, such as Dr. Francis Pottenger's research during the

1920s and 1930s proposed that much if not all disease has autonomic imbalance as at least one of the major causes.

We have found that specific nutrients and foods have specific, precise and predictable effects on the autonomic nervous system. For example, a vegetarian diet emphasizes fresh fruits and vegetables, particularly leafy greens, and contains large doses of minerals such as magnesium and potassium. It has been shown in many studies that magnesium suppresses sympathetic function, while potassium stimulates parasympathetic activity. Furthermore, a largely vegetarian diet tends to be very alkalinizing, and the neurophysiologic research documents that in an alkalinizing environment, sympathetic activity is reduced, and parasympathetic activity increased. So, whatever other effect a vegetarian diet has, in terms of autonomic nervous system function, such a diet will reduce sympathetic activity and stimulate the parasympathetic system.

A meat diet is loaded with minerals such as phosphorous and zinc, which tend to have the opposite effect. A high-meat diet stimulates the sympathetic system and tones down parasympathetic activity. Furthermore, such a diet is loaded with sulfates and phosphates that in the body are quickly converted into free acid that in turn stimulates the sympathetic nervous system while suppressing parasympathetic activity.

So, by the careful use of diet, we are able to effect major changes in autonomic function and bring about balance in a dysfunctional nervous system. We find, further, as the autonomic system comes into greater harmony and balance, when the autonomic branches are equally strong, all systems (from the immune system to the cardiovascular system) work better regardless of the underlying problem. In essence, we are using diet to bring about greater physiological efficiency. For cancer patients, long experience has taught us that it is not enough to load patients with enzymes; the question of autonomic imbalance must also be addressed. In terms of pancreatic patients specifically, a plant-based diet provides all the nutrients to correct autonomic dysfunction.

KH: Can you describe the vitamin and mineral supplement regimen you used? Was it megadose or a basic nutritional support?

NJG: All of our patients, whether they have cancer or some other problem, consume specific combinations of vitamins, minerals, trace elements, amino and fatty acids, and animal-derived glandular and organ concentrates. We use such supplements very specifically, in very precise doses and combinations as we use diet, to manipulate autonomic function and to bring about balance to an imbalanced system. Certain vitamins, minerals and trace elements, such as many of the B vitamins and, as mentioned above, magnesium and potassium, tone down the sympathetic nervous system and stimulate the parasympathetic nerves. Other nutrients, particularly calcium, phosphorous and zinc, stimulate the sympathetic system but weaken the parasympathetic system. By the use of precise combinations of vitamins, minerals and trace elements, along with diet, we are able to bring about balance to the autonomic system. And, again, when the autonomic branches come into balance, the patients, whatever the underlying disease, do better.

KH: What is the role of coffee enemas in this particular treatment and what is the history of coffee enemas in traditional medicine?

NJG: When I first began my research efforts, I was very surprised to find that the coffee enemas, often portrayed as one of the most bizarre aspects of alternative medicine, came right out of the *Merck Manual*, a revered compendium of orthodox treatments. When I was completing my immunology fellowship, I had an interesting correspondence with the then editor of the *Merck Manual*, who confirmed that the coffee enemas had been advocated in the *Merck Manual* from about

1890 right up until 1977, when they were removed more for space considerations than anything else. Most nursing texts for the better part of the century recommend coffee enemas. Particularly during the 1920s and 1930s coffee enemas were used in the US and abroad to treat a variety of conditions, and I have put together a library of articles from that time discussing the wide-ranging effects on patients. Coffee enemas were frequently recommended because patients, whatever their underlying problem, tended to feel better after a coffee enema. I have followed thousands of patients over the years who have done coffee enemas in some cases for decades: virtually all patients report an increase sense of well-being. I have done them myself daily since first learning about them in 1981.

There is research going back to the earlier part of the century that indicated that coffee enemas stimulate more efficient liver function and gallbladder emptying, and we believe that is the primary therapeutic benefit. Particularly with cancer patients, who often have a very large tumor burden, as the body repairs and rebuilds and as tumors break down, enormous amounts of toxic debris can be produced, much of which must be processed in the liver. The coffee enemas seem to enhance this processing of toxic metabolic waste. Interestingly enough, in *Hospital Practice* (August 15, 1999 page 128), a very orthodox journal of internal medicine, I read a summary of an article showing coffee seems to enhance gallbladder and liver function.

KH: *Is it possible that the positive effects from the coffee enemas are a result of a "caffeine high" versus a metabolic benefit?*

NJG: The issue of caffeine high is often raised. I don't believe this is the case at all. First, patients almost universally report a relaxing effect, not the stimulation you find with coffee taken orally. Many patients, in fact, fall asleep while doing the enemas. I, myself, have never been able to tolerate drinking coffee because coffee, when drunk, causes in me an amphetamine like response. However, I always feel relaxed when I do a coffee enema and often fall asleep. Something completely different is going on with the enemas.

KH: Can you describe your study and the basic results?

NJG: In July 1993, the then Associate Director for the Cancer Therapy Evaluation Program at the National Cancer Institute, Dr. Michael Friedman, invited me to present selected cases from my own practice as part of an NCI effort to evaluate non-traditional cancer therapies. I prepared for presentation 25 cases with poor prognosis or terminal illness who had either enjoyed long-term survival or tumor regression while following my program. After the session, Dr. Friedman suggested we pursue a pilot study of our methods in 10 patients suffering inoperable adenocarcinoma of the pancreas, with survival as the endpoint. Because the standard survival for the disease is so poor, an effect could be seen in a small number of patients in a short period of time.

Nestec (the Nestle Corporation) agreed to fund the trial, which began in January 1994. The study has been completed and was published in z*Nutrition and Cancer,* June 1999;33(2.) Of 11 patients followed in the trial, eight of 11 suffered stage four disease. Nine of 11 (81%) lived one year, five of 11 lived two years (45%), and four of 11 lived three years (36%.) Two are alive and well with no signs of disease, one at 3.5 years and one at 4.5 years. In comparison, in a recent trial of the newly approved drug gemcitabine, of 126 patients with pancreatic cancer not a single patient lived longer than 19 months.

As a result of the pilot study, the National Cancer Institute approved $1.4 million over five years for a large scale, randomized clinical trial comparing my nutritional therapy against gemcitabine in the treatment of inoperable pancreatic cancer. This study has full FDA approval and is being conducted under the Department of Oncology and the Department of Surgical Oncology at Columbia Presbyterian Medical Center in New York. The trial is the outgrowth of a Congressional hearing last summer encouraging intensive government evaluation of promising alternative cancer treatments and is currently up and running.

KH: *Were there any side effects to this high dose (130 and 160 capsules per day) of pancreatic enzymes? It seems like that would cause some significant gastrointestinal irritation.*

NJG: The only side effects I have noticed in 12 years of treating cancer patients with high dose porcine-based pancreatic enzyme therapy are intestinal gas, occasional bloating, and occasional indigestion. Frankly, the side effects tend to be very minimal. The enzymes we use are made especially for my patients in New Zealand. I believe most pancreatic enzymes available either as a prescription or over the counter in health food stores are not effective against cancer. We actually had to develop a manufacturing process to produce what I think are the appropriate enzymes, and they are not available except to my patients. Until we prove the benefit of my work, I don't think it is appropriate to mass market the enzymes. I also don't think it appropriate for cancer patients to try and treat themselves.

KH: *How compliant were your patients to this regimen?*

NJG: Pancreatic cancer patients are notoriously medically unstable, and some patients in the study were so weak they had difficulty complying fully at times, although many of the patients did comply well. Generally, we find that the better the compliance, the better the effect of the treatment. Patients in the trial came from all over the country, and because our approach is still alternative, patients were not allowed to continue the treatment when hospitalized. In the Columbia study, all patients are going to be treated aggressively for underlying medical problems and will be encouraged to continue their therapy at all times.

KH: What would you like to see in the future with regard to evaluating this protocol as far as studies go?

NJG: As above, we are involved in a large scale, NCI-funded, FDA-approved randomized clinical trial at Columbia University.

KH: What feedback have you gotten from the traditional oncology community with regard to your work?

NJG: The attitude is changing; for example, I have sent you a very supportive article about my work that appeared in the magazine *InTouch*, a news style magazine that is sent to more than 90,000 orthodox physicians, including all oncologists in this country. The oncology newspaper *Oncology News International* had a very nice piece about my research efforts, and I have sent you a copy of that story. I have also sent a copy of a press release in support of our work sent out from Congressman Dan Burton, Chairman of the Committee on Government Reform.

What We Use

Digestxym+ Fermented Enzymes

shop.ConnersClinic.com/digestxym

Pancreatin 8x Plus Enzymes

shop.ConnersClinic.com/pancreatin-8x

Bloodroot Products

Bloodroot is an historic "Cancer Killing" herb used throughout the centuries as a tonic by numerous people groups. We strongly caution people about its topical application as it can be very caustic and requires supervision by a trained practitioner. Taken orally, along with **graviola, burdock root, and chaparral**, it can have wonderful healing benefits, especially for cancers in the digestive tract.

Personally, our Black Salve Bloodroot capsules have been a literal lifesaver for me, so I need to place this product in one of my "favorites" categories. We've seen patients with all types of cancers benefit from it.

What We Use

Black Salve Bloodroot Capsules

ConnersClinic.com/black-salve-bloodroot

CBD and THC

General Info

Cannabinoids from hemp and marijuana plants typically fall into two categories: CBD and THC. CBD does not have any psychoactive properties and is therefore legal to use everywhere. As for THC, due to its mind/mood altering effects, it is *not* legal in all states.

There are many other types of cannabinoids, but for our discussion we'll concentrate on these two. Cannabinoids interact with what is known as the endocannabinoid system (ECS) in our body, which consists of the endocannabinoids, their receptors on our cell membranes, as well as specific enzymes that *turn on* and interact with to change function and

309

help us heal.

A "receptor" is typically defined as an intracellular protein molecule that receives and responds to extracellular chemical signals, ultimately producing a cellular cascade of events. Cannabinoid receptors (CBs) are the primary targets of the ECS, bound by lipid signaling molecules called endocannabinoids (eCBs) that are produced on demand in response to elevated intracellular calcium levels in neurons. After eCBs bind a receptor to inhibit the release of neurotransmitters and exert a particular effect on the body, they are degraded via metabolic enzymes in a process called hydrolysis.

While eCBs are endogenous to the human body, there are two other types of cannabinoids that can bind CBs: phytocannabinoids (plant-based chemicals) and synthetic cannabinoids (designed specifically to interact with the ECS.) Two of the most-studied eCBs include N-archidonylethanolamide (anandamide, AEA) and sn-z-archidonoylglycerol (2-AG).

There are two main types of CBs, which vary in their chemical structure and thus perform different functions in terms of diet, lifestyle, and nutrition:

Cannabinoid Receptor 1 (CB1) is associated with psychoactive, neuromodulatory, and analgesic effects due to its activation by a lipid called tetrahydrocannabinol (THC.) CB1 is mostly expressed in the brain, adipocytes (fat cells), hepatocytes (liver cells), and musculoskeletal tissues.

Cannabinoid Receptor 2 (CB2) is associated with anti-inflammatory and immunomodulatory effects but no psychoactive effects. CB2 is expressed in body cells controlling immune function and (potentially) the central nervous system (CNS.) Additionally, research suggests that secondary metabolites from phytonutrients in plant-based foods enhance the activity of CB2 receptors and confer healthy inflammatory responses.

Hemp, also known as the fiber and seeds from the Cannabis sativa L. plant species, contains a negligible amount of THC. Instead, the phytocannabinoids found in hemp largely activate CB2, thus exerting positive, non-psychoactive effects on the human body. However, a balance of targets and specific receptor activators is more beneficial than non-selective activation.

CBD

How to Choose a good CBD Hemp Oil

For the best results, look for:

- Organically grown
- How it is extracted
- What delivery system is utilized
- Ensure there is 0.0% THC
- Enhanced absorption (bioavailability)
- Enhanced Entourage effect
- Symbiotic immune support

What are the Key Extraction Processes?

When extracting Hemp Oil from the Hemp Plant, there are 2 processes that are commonly used:

1. **Solvent**: Most economical but can damage beneficial terpenes and can leave a chemical residue. Used primarily to extract CBD isolates

2. **Supercritical CO2**: A clean extraction process that protects the heat sensitive terpenes and flavonoids

What are the Different Types of Hemp-Derived CBD Oils?

- **CBD Isolates**: 99.9% pure crystallized cannabinoids with no terpenes or flavonoids

- **Full Spectrum Hemp**: Contains over 100 naturally occurring compounds including cannabinoids (THC at 0.3%), terpenes and other nutrients

- **Broad Spectrum Hemp**: Same as full spectrum with 0.0% THC

See more info here:

ConnersClinic.com/ecs

Research studies are showing that incorporating whole plant (full-spectrum) cannabinoids into a natural treatment regimen may improve anti-tumor effects in both hormone-sensitive and triple-negative breast cancers.

Hormone-sensitive breast cancers are classified using two biomarkers: hormonal receptors (estrogen receptor and progesterone receptor) and the HER2 oncogene. In a patient's diagnosis this is denoted as ER+, PR+ and HER2+, with any combination of biomarkers possible.

In triple-negative breast cancer, which is a more aggressive malignancy, neither hormonal receptors nor the HER2 oncogene are expressed. This means that the cancer has no specific ties or drivers, so the patient is not a candidate for hormone or gene-specific treatments.[128]

A study conducted on each of these cancer types found that THC-rich oil (whole plant cannabinoids) had more

---

[128] Andia, Alex. THC Versus Breast Cancer. Project CBD. [Online] March 18, 2019. [Cited: July 30, 2019.] https://www.projectcbd.org/medicine/thc-versus-breast-cancer

pronounced anti-tumor effects than single-molecule THC. The anti-tumor effect or "Entourage Effect"[129] refers to the natural synergy between multiple cannabis compounds which, when combined, have a therapeutic impact much more powerful than the sum of cannabis' individual components.

Specifically, in hormone-sensitive breast cancers, whole plant cannabinoid oils have an average 15-25% greater anti-proliferative effect than single THC extracts.

The research study focused on 1:1 THC:CBD ratios, along with measurable amounts of CBG, THCa, caryophyllene, humulene, nerolidol, linalool and pinene.

Although I prefer patients seek individualized testing to determine which forms, brands, and dosages of cannabis are the best for them, I am comfortable recommending that any breast cancer patient consider incorporating some form of full-spectrum cannabinoid into daily supplement regimens. As always, strive to find organic sources.

Conners Clinic has several full-spectrum CBD products available online:

CBD Gold Premium Hemp Oil (sold in an oral applicator): 120mg/serving

>   shop.ConnersClinic.com/cbd-gold

Premium CBD Oil (liquid bottle): 33mg/serving

>   shop.ConnersClinic.com/premium-cbd-oil

---

[129] Blasco-Benito, S, et al. Appraising the "entourage effect": Antitumor action of a pure cannabinoid versus a botanical drug preparation in preclinical models of breast cancer. NCBI. [Online] June 27, 2018. [Cited: July 30, 2019.]
https://www.ncbi.nlm.nih.gov/pubmed/29940172

Premium CBD Capsules: 25mg/serving

> shop.ConnersClinic.com/premium-cbd-caps

Pure CBD Capsule (zero THC): 25mg/serving

> shop.ConnersClinic.com/pure-cbd-caps

Evolv Entourage2: CBD liquid with acemannon (this is what I take)

> shop.ConnersClinic.com/entourage

Conners Macrophage Activating Factor (contains whole CBD oil)

> shop.ConnersClinic.com/MAF

Note: At this time, recreational cannabis is not legalized in Minnesota, so all THC-dominant cannabinoids must be purchased through a licensed medical professional.

THC

When we talk about using THC with cancer patients, we are usually referring to what is known as Rick Simpson's Oil (RSO.) RSO is a concentrated THC paste that we will discuss in more detail. Other uses of THC would be the use of marijuana as an edible or smoking it to reduce pain, increase appetite, reduce anxiety, increase sleep, and reduce nausea. These are all great reasons to use THC products, understanding that responsible use of this God-given herb is much better than using pharmaceutical drugs to alleviate the same symptoms.

We legally do not and cannot distribute any THC products, but our freedom of speech allows us to discuss it and we'll let you make up your own mind.

Rick Simpson Oil is another treatment altogether. As stated, it is highly concentrated and will make you feel extremely "loopy," so we suggest you start at a **very** low dose. Rick Simpson, a Canadian engineer, whose name gives us "Rick Simpson Oil", was working in the hospital boiler room covering the asbestos on the hospital's pipes with potent aerosol glue. The boiler room was poorly ventilated, and the toxic fumes caused a temporary nervous system shock, causing Simpson to collapse off his ladder and hit his head. He was knocked unconscious and when he awoke, he managed to contact his colleagues to take him to the emergency room.

He continued to suffer from dizzy spells and a ringing in his ears for years after the accident, but his prescribed medication had little effect, even making his symptoms worse. After seeing a documentary highlighting the positive benefits of using cannabis, Simpson inquired about medical marijuana; but his doctor refused to consider it as a course of treatment. He ended up sourcing cannabis of his own accord and saw a significant improvement in his tinnitus and other symptoms.

As his story goes, in 2003, three suspicious bumps appeared on Simpson's arm. The doctor agreed that the bumps appeared to be cancerous and took a sample for a biopsy. Sure enough, the bumps turned out to be basal cell carcinoma, a form of skin cancer.

Simpson had successfully treated his other symptoms with cannabis in the past, and he had heard about a study from the *Journal of the National Cancer Institute* in which THC was found to kill cancer cells in mice. He made the decision to treat his skin cancer topically, applying concentrated cannabis oil to a bandage and leaving the cancerous spots covered for several days.

After four days, he removed the bandages and the cancerous growths had disappeared. Although his physician refused to acknowledge cannabis as a treatment alternative, Simpson was now a true believer in the medicinal powers of cannabis. From then on out, he began cultivating his own cannabis and harvesting the plants to create his own specialized form of cannabis concentrate, now known as Rick Simpson Oil, or RSO.

I won't spend anymore ink on RSO since it must be purchased through a THC-legal state or through channels that are "undisclosed." You only need to search YouTube for detailed directions and instructions on how to make your own, but that chore is not for the faint of heart.

While more and more research is coming out on CBD/THC, most of it gets buried. The drug companies do **not** want it legalized as it would drastically cut into their profits; CBD/THC may be an excellent substitute for anxiety medication, pain medication, seizure meds, ADD/ADHD meds, and the list goes on.

Research on CBD/THC

It doesn't take a scientist to realize that the use of cannabis is on the rise. Nearly 10% of cannabis users in the United States report using it for medicinal purposes.[130] As of August 2019, 33 states and the District of Columbia have initiated policies allowing the use of cannabis or cannabinoids for the management of specific medical conditions. Yet, the federal government still classifies cannabis as illegal, complicating its medical use and research into its effectiveness as a treatment for the various conditions purported to benefit from cannabis pharmacotherapy and hindering public opinion. Because of this conflict and restrictions on cannabis research, evidence of the efficacy of cannabis to manage various diseases is often lacking (though more and more studies are being published).

---

[130] Compton WM, Han B, Hughes A, Jones CM, Blanco C. Use of marijuana for medical purposes among adults in the United States. JAMA. 2017;317(2):209-211. doi:10.1001/jama.2016.18900

The following article appeared in *JAMA* in August, 2019, that strongly influences physicians into believing that, since studies have yet to prove the beneficial role of cannabis in various disorders, one should refrain from recommending it. What should be stated is that the majority of patients using cannabis medicinally have already tried standard pharmaceutical approaches and failed. While some may jump to alternative approaches first, for most it is a *last attempt* for some relief. To conclude that since, "Insufficient evidence (currently) exists for the use of medical cannabis for most conditions," one should avoid it, restricts novel attempts to help the sick. Though I don't think the author is attempting to steer physicians away from its use, it certainly conveys a spirit of contempt against cannabis:

From *JAMA*, 2019:

"This article updates a review published in the June 23, 2015, issue of *JAMA*[131] and describes newer evidence regarding what is known and not known about the efficacy of cannabis and cannabinoids for managing various conditions:

Indications for Therapeutic Use Approved by the US Food and Drug Administration

Cannabis has numerous cannabinoids, the most notable being tetrahydrocannabinol, which accounts for its psychoactive effects. Individual cannabinoids have unique pharmacologic profiles enabling drug development to manage various conditions without having the cognitive effects typically associated with cannabis. Only a few cannabinoids have high-quality evidence to support their use and are approved for medicinal use by the US Food and Drug Administration (FDA.) The cannabinoids dronabinol and nabilone were approved by the FDA for chemotherapy-induced nausea and

---

[131] Hill KP. Medical marijuana for treatment of chronic pain and other medical and psychiatric problems: a clinical review. JAMA. 2015;313(24):2474-2483. doi:10.1001/jama.2015.6199

vomiting in 1985, with dronabinol gaining an additional indication for appetite stimulation in conditions that cause weight loss, such as AIDS, in 1992. Recently, a third cannabinoid, cannabidiol (CBD), was approved by the FDA for the management of 2 forms of pediatric epilepsy, Dravet syndrome and Lennox-Gastaut syndrome, based on the strength of positive randomized clinical trials (RCTs).[132] [133]

Other Medical Indications

Cannabinoids are often cited as being effective for managing chronic pain. The National Academies of Science, Engineering, and Medicine examined this issue and found that there was conclusive or substantial evidence that cannabis or cannabinoids effectively managed chronic pain,[134] based on their expert committee's assessment that the literature on this topic had many supportive findings from good-quality studies with no credible opposing findings. The panel relied on a single meta-analysis of 28 studies, few of which were from the United States, that assessed a variety of diseases and compounds. Although they concluded that cannabinoids effectively managed pain, the CIs associated with these findings were large, suggesting unreliability in the meta-analysis results.

A more recent meta-analysis of 91 publications found cannabinoids to reduce pain 30% more than placebo (odds ratio, 1.46 [95% CI, 1.16-1.84]), but had a number needed to

---

[132] Devinsky O, Cross JH, Laux L, et al; Cannabidiol in Dravet Syndrome Study Group. Trial of cannabidiol for drug-resistant seizures in the Dravet Syndrome. N Engl J Med. 2017;376(21):2011-2020
[133] Thiele EA, Marsh ED, French JA, et al; GWPCARE4 Study Group. Cannabidiol in patients with seizures associated with Lennox-Gastaut syndrome (GWPCARE4): a randomized, double-blind, placebo-controlled phase 3 trial. Lancet. 2018;391(10125):1085-1096
[134] National Academies of Sciences, Engineering, and Medicine. The Health Effects of Cannabis and Cannabinoids: The Current State of Evidence and Recommendations for Research. Washington, DC: National Academies Press; 2017

treat for chronic pain of 24 (95% CI, 15-61) and a number needed to harm of 6 (95% CI, 5-8). While a moderate level of evidence supports these recommendations, most studies of the efficacy of cannabinoids on pain are for neuropathic pain, with relatively few high-quality studies examining other types of pain. Taken together, at best, there is only inconclusive evidence that cannabinoids effectively manage chronic pain, and large numbers of patients must receive treatment with cannabinoids for a few to benefit, while not many need to receive treatment to result in harm.[135]

There is strong evidence to support relief of symptoms of muscle spasticity resulting from multiple sclerosis from cannabinoids as reported by patients, but the association is much weaker when outcomes are measured by physicians. There is insufficient evidence to support or refute claims that cannabinoids provide relief for spinal cord injury–related muscle spasms.[134]

Recent Clinical Trials

Two multicenter, international trials with substantial numbers of patients (n = 120 and n = 171) demonstrated the efficacy of CBD as an add-on drug to manage some seizure disorders. Over 14 weeks, 20mg/kg of CBD significantly reduced the median frequency of convulsive seizures in children and young adults with Dravet syndrome as well as the estimated median difference in monthly drop seizures between CBD and placebo in patients with Lennox-Gastaut syndrome.[132] [133] Although promising, these results were found in relatively uncommon disorders and the studies were limited by the use of subjective end points and incomplete blinding that is typical of

---

[135] Stockings E, Campbell G, Hall WD, et al. Cannabis and cannabinoids for the treatment of people with chronic noncancer pain conditions: a systematic review and meta-analysis of controlled and observational studies. Pain. 2018;159(10):1932-1954

cannabinoid studies because these drugs have readily identifiable side effects.[132] [133]

Numerous other medical conditions, including Parkinson disease, PTSD, and Tourette's syndrome have a hypothetical rationale for the use of cannabis or cannabinoids as pharmacotherapy based on cannabinoid effects on spasticity, anxiety, and density of cannabinoid receptors in areas implicated in development of tics, such as the basal ganglia and cerebellum. The strength of the evidence supporting the use of cannabinoids for these diseases is weak because most studies of patients with these diseases have been small, often uncontrolled, or crossover studies. Few pharmaceutical companies are conducting cannabinoid trials. Thus, it is not likely that additional cannabinoids will be approved by the FDA in the near future. Public interest in cannabis and cannabinoids as pharmacotherapy continues to increase, as does the number of medical conditions for which patients are utilizing cannabis and CBD, despite insufficient evidence to support this trend.

Neurologic Adverse Effects Are Better Defined Than Physical Adverse Effects

Acute cannabis use is associated with impaired learning, memory, attention, and motor coordination, areas that can affect important activities of daily living, such as driving. Acute cannabis use can also affect judgment, potentially resulting in users making risky decisions that they would not otherwise make. While there is consensus that acute cannabis use results in cognitive deficits, residual cognitive effects persisting after acute intoxication are still debated, especially for individuals who used cannabis regularly as adolescents.[136]

---

[136] Scott JC, Slomiak ST, Jones JD, Rosen AFG, Moore TM, Gur RC. Association of cannabis with cognitive functioning in adolescents and young adults: a systematic review and meta-analysis. JAMA Psychiatry. 2018;75(6):585-595

Chronic cannabis use is associated with an increased risk of psychiatric illness and addiction. There is a significant association (possibly a causal relationship) between cannabis use and the development of psychotic disorders, such as schizophrenia, particularly among heavy users.[137] Chronic cannabis use can lead to cannabis use disorder (CUD) and contributes to impairment in work, school, and relationships in up to 31% of adult users.[138] Regular cannabis use at levels associated with CUD (near-daily use of more than one-eighth ounce of cannabis per week) is associated with worsening functional status, including lower income, greater need for socioeconomic assistance, criminal behavior, unemployment, and decreased life satisfaction.[137] Cannabis use is associated with adverse perinatal outcomes as well; a 2019 study showed the crude rate of preterm birth was 12.0% among cannabis users and 6.1% among nonusers (risk difference, 5.88% [95% CI, 5.22%-6.54%]).[139]

Inadequate Evidence Supporting the Use of Cannabinoids for Many Medical Conditions

The quality of the evidence supporting the use of cannabinoids is suboptimal. First, studies assessing pain and spasticity are difficult to conduct, in part because of heterogeneity of the outcome measures used in these studies. Second, most RCTs that have evaluated cannabinoid clinical outcomes were small, with fewer than 100 participants in each, and small trials may overestimate treatment effects. Third, the timeframe for most studies is too short to assess the long-term effects of these medications. Fourth, tolerance, withdrawal, and potential for

---

[137] Volkow ND, Baler RD, Compton WM, Weiss SR. Adverse health effects of marijuana use. N Engl J Med. 2014;370(23):2219-2227

[138] Hasin DS, Saha TD, Kerridge BT, et al. Prevalence of marijuana use disorders in the United States between 2001-2002 and 2012-2013. JAMA Psychiatry. 2015;72(12):1235-1242

[139] Corsi DJ, Walsh L, Weiss D, et al. Association between self-reported prenatal cannabis use and maternal, perinatal, and neonatal outcomes. JAMA. 2019;322(2):145-152

drug-drug interactions may affect the usefulness of cannabis, and these phenomena are not well understood for cannabinoids. The lack of high-quality evidence results in outsized claims of the efficacy of cannabinoids for numerous medical conditions. There is a need for well-designed, large, multisite RCTs of cannabis or cannabinoids to resolve claims of efficacy for conditions for which there are claims of efficacy not supported by high-quality evidence, such as pain and spasticity.

Conclusions

Insufficient evidence exists for the use of medical cannabis for most conditions for which its use is advocated. Despite the lack of evidence, various US state governments have recommended cannabis for the management of more than 50 medical conditions. Physicians may be appropriately reticent to recommend medical cannabis for their patients because of the limited scientific evidence supporting its use or because cannabis remains illegal in federal law. Cannabis is useful for some conditions, but patients who might benefit may not get appropriate treatment because of insufficient awareness regarding the evidence supporting its use or confusion from federal law deeming cannabis illegal."[140]

Corresponding Author: Kevin P. Hill, MD, MHS, Division of Addiction Psychiatry, Beth Israel Deaconess Medical Center, 330 Brookline Ave, Rabb 2, Boston, MA 02215 (khill1@bidmc.harvard.edu)

Berberine

There is an inflammatory enzyme called cyclooxygenase-2 (COX-2) that is abundantly expressed in colon cancer cells. It also plays a key role in colon tumorigenesis (new cancer growth.) Therefore, compounds inhibiting COX-2

---

[140] Published Online: August 9, 2019. doi:10.1001/jama.2019.11868

transcriptional activity (gene RNA replication) potentially have a chemopreventive property. Finding natural compounds to inhibit COX-2 pathways should prove exciting and promising.

In a recent study, an assay method for estimating COX-2 transcriptional activity in human colon cancer cells was established using a β-galactosidase reporter gene system. The study examined effects made of various medicinal herbs and their ingredients for an inhibitory effect on COX-2 transcriptional activity.

They found that berberine, an isoquinoline alkaloid present in plants of the genera *Berberis* and *Coptis* from Oregon grape root and Bayberry, effectively inhibits COX-2 transcriptional activity in colon cancer cells in a dose- and time-dependent manner at concentrations higher than 0.3 μM. These findings may further explain the mechanism of anti-inflammatory and anti-tumor promoting effects of berberine.

Our Berber Clear (I personally take 1-4/day) supplies high potency berberine combined with alpha lipoic acid to help support optimal blood sugar and insulin levels, cardiovascular health, and liver health. Berberine is an alkaloid compound found in the roots, rhizomes, stems and bark of several plants commonly used in botanical and Chinese medicine, such as goldenseal, Oregon grape, barberry, and Berberis aristata.

Lipoic acid is best known for its antioxidant properties and its ability to support healthy insulin secretion and sensitivity. It is also a key cofactor for mitochondrial enzymes involved in cellular metabolism and energy (ATP) production. Made with non-GMO ingredients.

Metastasis and angiogenesis is to be avoided at all cost. There is increasing evidence that two chemicals, urokinase-type plasminogen activator (u-PA) and matrix metalloproteinases (MMPs) play an important role in cancer spread and vascularization. Inhibition of u-PA and MMPs could suppress migration and invasion of cancer cells. Berberine reported to have anti-cancer effects in different human cancer cell lines by inhibiting u-PA and MMPs according to another study.

Autophagy is a relatively new term applied to the biochemistry of the cells. It refers to the body's need and efficiency in cleaning up or taking out the trash. Trash may be described as the debris from dying cells, waste products of cell metabolism, and general extracellular detoxification. It is a necessary function.

Cancer patients may require an even heightened autophagy response: paying overtime for waste management. One of the hindrances that our immune system experiences in attempting to kill a growing cancer, is to plow through the waste that surrounds a tumor. Cancer, by definition, is rapidly replicating cells. This rapid replication produces a greater amount of waste that can form a protective barrier limiting T-cell and macrophage attack.

Enter autophagy.

There are a few things we can do to stimulate autophagy and more that can inhibit things that inhibit it. We'll talk more about this, but several nutrients are stimulators: berberine and lithium to name a few. I have stated in several videos on the subject that inhibiting mTOR, a major growth pathway, is the best way to also stimulate autophagy. This is one reason why Curcumin is so beneficial to cancer patients.

What We Use

BerberClear

shop.ConnersClinic.com/berber-clear

Gerson Therapy

Regardless of the critics' comments, Dr. Max Gerson helped many people with cancer. His main opponents were deep in the American Medical Association at a time when anyone using anything other than pharmaceuticals was shunned. Dr. Gerson helped people by recommending a strict, low-protein (essentially vegetarian) dietary regimen based on great quantities of fresh vegetable juice, supplements, and systemic detoxification. Charlotte Gerson, his daughter, explains in *The Gerson Therapy*:

"Dr. Gerson found that the underlying problems of all cancer patients are toxicity and deficiency. He had to overcome both these difficulties. He found that one of the important features of his therapy had to be the hourly administration of fresh vegetable juices. These supply ample nutrients, as well as fluids to help flush out the kidneys. When the high levels of nutrients re-enter tissues, toxins accumulated over many years are forced into the bloodstream. The liver then filters out the toxins. The liver is easily overburdened by the continuous release of toxins and is unable to release the load."

"Dr. Gerson found that he could provide help to the liver by the caffeine in coffee, absorbed from the colon via the hemorrhoidal vein, which carries the caffeine to the portal system and then to the liver. The caffeine stimulates the liver/bile ducts to open, releasing the poisons into the intestinal tract for excretion."

Why is There an Issue in the Medical Community Regarding Diet?

Ignorance and arrogance make a bad combination, and modern medicine has been guilty of both for decades. Political physicians did not heed the advice of people like Dr. Gerson. In fact, they publicly condemned him. The news media have been their willing accomplices since they receive the majority of their income from pharmaceutical commercials.[141]

Since standard oncology (with their chemotherapy, radiation and surgery) are such unbelievably huge moneymakers, things will not be changing any time soon. A nutritional approach to cancer has shown, for over six decades, to improve both quality of life and length of life in the sickest, the most hopeless, of cancer patients. Many people have experienced dramatic healing naturally and **none** have experienced the side effects that modern approaches produce.

Our Modified Gerson

Our Modified Gerson program is tailored to each patient personally. We've seen what it can do for terminally ill cancer patients who, without hope, began a healthy diet and slowly turned their life around. Since we believe that cancer's fuel source can be different with every individual and that its fuel source can change throughout the course of the disease as it is trying everything to stay alive, we modify our diet approach for each patient.

To be clear: I believe that a Gerson-type diet is great for cancers that are primarily feeding on proteins, glutamates, glutamine, methionine and such. However, I believe it is contraindicated in cancers feeding primarily through glycolysis (through the breakdown of glucose.) Therefore, we test everyone; and then we test them again, throughout the course of care.

To better understand our approach to diet and to get an idea if a Gerson diet is best for you, visit our website where we have over a dozen blog posts and as many web pages describing its benefits as well as warnings.

---

[141] https://www.trueactivist.com/robert-f-kennedy-jr-says-70-of-news-advertising-revenue-comes-from-big-pharma-t1/

Coffee Enemas

We cannot discuss Max Gerson without talking about the wonderful benefits of coffee enemas. Dr. Gerson certainly didn't invent the coffee enema; the benefits of this therapy were spattered through nearly every reputable medical textbook in the early 1900's, however they disappeared (along with most herbal remedies) when the Rothchild family started funding pharmaceutical approaches at most major medical schools.

What Max Gerson did was reintroduce the benefits of coffee enemas for cancer patients. So, why would anyone want to do a coffee enema and what does caffeine do in the human body? Let me begin by saying that I've heard it all. Initial patient reactions to coffee enemas range from shock to disdain. Some comments come quickly while others surface from experience. Learning to jest about a seemingly unpleasant experience can be not only helpful but healing in itself. Some call it their morning coffee time, others their crap-uccino.

Three reasons to consider coffee enemas:

1. Coffee enemas detoxify the liver and bile ducts
2. Coffee enemas help clean out the colon
3. Coffee enemas stimulate the parasympathetic nervous system and stimulate an immune response

Of the above three reasons, I believe the stimulation of the parasympathetic nervous system is the most important. Our autonomic (think automatic) nervous system unconsciously controls all our organ function. It is divided into two opposing factions: Sympathetic and Parasympathetic. The Sympathetic is our fight, flight, or freeze system which controls protective features during stressful and emergency situations. Our Parasympathetic controls liver detoxification, tissue healing, hormone balance, bowel flow, lymph cleanse, and just about everything you could think of needing to help heal from any disease.

When you are dealing with a serious disease such as cancer, it's safe to say that stress is usually elevated (which means the Sympathetic nervous system is elevated.) The opposite side of the autonomic nervous system teeter-totter, the Parasympathetic, is then depressed, slowing detoxification, bowel function, and generally making matters worse. Coffee enemas stimulate the Vagus nerve (Cranial nerve X) in the rectum where it comes in direct contact with intestinal cells. The Vagus nerve is the primary Parasympathetic carrier, and its stimulation helps bring the teeter-totter back into balance.

Details on how to do coffee enemas are available on our website, simply search "coffee enemas." The specific instructions and helpful hints will help make your experience more pleasant.

Personally, I do coffee enemas only when my pain ramps up. Daily enemas could certainly become a priority for me, but I'll be the first to admit that, while I've done enough to find them pretty simple and often very pain-relieving, I just don't take the time to do them regularly.

Typically, we recommend daily enemas, especially when people are feeling poor. As health begins to return, you can certainly back off and use them like I do, as needed. Some of our patients are doing several per day to help reduce pain and help with detoxification.

Michelle, my trusted colleague, is our resident expert on coffee enemas and you will benefit greatly from her detailed videos on our blog: ConnersClinic.com/blog

Turmeric and Curcumin

Turmeric

Even though most research has been focused on the curcurminoid portion of the turmeric herb, we would be amiss to not talk about whole-food turmeric as a separate beneficial approach. Through the years, I've tried to use whole-food nutrition as much as possible. By this I mean to use the whole plant with the understanding that there are ingredients that God placed in the entire herb that synergistically benefit one another even though we may not yet have discovered how.

Research has been hyper-focused on the Curcumin (curcuminoids) portion of turmeric. Recently, new studies are proving what we "whole-food" advocates have long believed: there is benefit in whole-plant turmeric. The *complete turmeric matrix* (CTM) has been found to maintain the intestinal alkaline phosphatase (IAP) at the GUT border and help balance the endotoxin effect. CTM also supports the abundance of beneficial bacteria (our microbiota) and reduce inflammatory chemicals like IL-6, TNF-alpha, and Nf-kB. These studies are exciting for those in the field and very positive for cancer patients.

Our product, Turmero Clear, is a patented, full-spectrum turmeric that contains all the compounds found in the whole-plant including Curcumin, Turmerone, Turmerin, Curcumol, Cyclo-Curcumin, Curdione, ajd Beta-Elemene.

What We Use

TurmeroClear

shop.ConnersClinic.com/turmero-clear

Curcumin

Curcumin is the active form of the herb turmeric. While it has often been touted as a favorite to reduce inflammation and pain, recent studies have been shown it to interfere with multiple cell signaling pathways, including cell cycle (cyclin D1 and cyclin E), apoptosis (activation of caspases and down-regulation of anti-apoptotic gene products), proliferation (HER-2, EGFR, and AP-1), survival (PI3K/AKT pathway), invasion (MMP-9 and adhesion molecules), angiogenesis (VEGF), metastasis (CXCR-4) and inflammation (NF-κB, TNF, IL-6, IL-1, COX-2, and 5-LOX.) In short, it can help kill cancer.

The activity of Curcumin reported against leukemia and lymphoma, gastrointestinal cancers, genitourinary cancers, breast cancer, ovarian cancer, head and neck squamous cell carcinoma, lung cancer, melanoma, neurological cancers, and sarcoma reflects its ability to affect multiple targets. Thus an "old-age" disease such as cancer requires an "age-old" treatment.

Curcumin has long been one of my favorites as it helps with so many issues, not just the cancer itself. There is more research proving the benefits of Curcumin than any other natural cancer-killing supplement. One simply cannot ignore all the great information. I've made multiple videos on Curcumin, see them at ConnersClinic.com/cancer-and-curcumin

A new research report from Uppsala University suggests that down-regulating synthesis of new ribosomes, an organelle inside our cells that create new proteins that serve as building blocks for cell replication, may slow cancer growth. It is known that the metastatic process is helped by the synthesis of new ribosomes, as this increase in number is necessary for continued growth.

The study results open the possibility for new treatment strategies for advanced cancers, according to the scientists whose study (*"Ribosome biogenesis during cell cycle arrest fuels EMT in development and disease"*) appears in *Nature Communications*.

"Ribosome biogenesis is a canonical hallmark of cell growth and proliferation. Here we show that execution of Epithelial-to-Mesenchymal Transition (EMT), a migratory cellular program associated with development and **tumor metastasis, is fueled by upregulation of ribosome biogenesis** during G1/S arrest," the investigators wrote.

As tumors progress towards advanced stages with continual growth, they dedifferentiate (losing their specialized characteristics), become more aggressive, and lose the cellular functions of the origin tissue. They also acquire the migratory capacity that allows the tumor to metastasize to distant sites in the body, eventually causing patient death. "Until recently, ribosomes have been considered to play only passive roles during the production of proteins. Our study shows that ribosomes potentially have complex, active roles and suggests that more attention should be given to understanding how ribosomes contribute to cell physiology in health and disease states," said Theresa Vincent, PhD, group leader at the department of immunology, genetics, and pathology at Uppsala University.

The study demonstrated that by inhibiting the formation of new ribosomes, aggressive and hormone insensitive tumors could be partially reverted to a benign and non-metastatic type. "We used a small molecule called CX-5461 to inhibit ribosome biogenesis in mouse models of human tumors. We found that primary tumors reverted from an invasive type to a non-invasive type as well as potentially regaining sensitivity to hormonal therapy. Importantly, CX-5461 treatment also resulted in a marked reduction in the number of lung metastases. This suggests that treatment with CX-5461 may enhance hormone therapy responsiveness in patients where this kind of treatment doesn't work anymore. We find this to be a remarkable breakthrough and we are currently pursuing a number of additional validation studies," said Vincent.

It is known that some chemotherapy drugs inhibit ribosomal synthesis but don't distinguish cancer cells from healthy cells.

Other studies suggest that Curcumin, the active form of turmeric, also may inhibit ribosomal synthesis. If we can take away the cancer's building blocks, we discourage growth.

See more at ConnersClinic.com/curcumin-cancer-therapy

What Type of Curcumin is Best?

Conners Clinic Originals *Curcu Clear* is a patent pending, highly bioavailable curcuminoid formulation. It contains a unique combination of three bioactive, health-promoting curcuminoids: curcumin, bisdemethoxy curcumin and demethoxy curcumin, along with turmeric oil. The three curcuminoids are the strongest, most protective and best researched constituents of the turmeric root. The proprietary process uses all-natural ingredients, including Vitamin E, medium chain triglycerides (MCT) and lecithin without the use of potentially harmful surfactants.

It is simply the finest available curcumin that is currently on the market!

What We Use

CurcuClear

shop.ConnersClinic.com/curcu-clear

Essiac Tea

A secret herbal tea, Essiac was first obtained from a Native American healer in Canada. Based on age-old traditions, this combination of herbs has proven successful for thousands of people with cancer over many decades. It was eventually rigorously tested and endorsed in the United States by President Kennedy's personal physician, Dr. Charles A. Brusch. As the story goes, many herbal supplements began with trial and error cures:

"In 1922, a kindhearted nurse of Haileybury, Ontario, noticed a female patient with a severely scarred and disfigured breast. Asking the woman about her scars, she was told an amazing story of how years earlier the woman had been diagnosed with breast cancer. Canadian doctors had told the woman she must have her breast removed immediately. However, in desperation, the woman turned to a more natural route that had been told to her by an Ojibwa Indian medicine man.

The Indian medicine man told her of a combination of herbs to brew into a tea and drink daily. He told her this would cure the cancer in her breast and not require it to be removed. She did as the medicine man instructed and as she sat telling her nurse the story years later, she obviously had not had the surgery and yet she had no recurrence of the cancer!

The nurse asked the patient for the formula for the tea and wrote it down but never really pursued making it. A few years later when her aunt was diagnosed with inoperable cancer, Rene began giving the tea to her aunt. After two months of drinking the tea daily, the aunt rallied and lived an additional 21 years with no recurrence of cancer just as the lady with breast cancer had done!

In her desire to help the sick, the nurse began to give the tea to others with wonderful results. People with various kinds of cancer, diabetes and more seemed to improve with the use of this tea. She decided the unique combination of these particular herbs somehow seemed to cause the different organs in the body to "normalize" helping the body's own immune system to fight and correct whatever was wrong.

This amazing formula, made up only four simple herbs, is believed to normalize body systems by cleansing the blood, purging toxic build up, promoting cell repair and aiding in effective assimilation and elimination. While incredibly simple, when combined with each other, these four herbs and their separate individual effects are greatly enhanced.

The nurse decided to call the tea Essiac, her last name spelled backwards. As time went on, Rene Caisse continued to treat those considered terminally ill with very positive results. Health officials vacillated back and forth between a love/hate attitude toward her. While she never openly claimed the tea would cure all cancers it did seem to have a definite effect on many and it undeniably promoted wellness, general good health and strengthened the immune system.

Her desire was to make the tea available to everyone. She operated a Cancer Treatment Clinic in Canada using her tea for many years, but never charging for any services. She used the herbal tea herself every day and finally died in 1978 at the age of 90.

Her desire was never for financial gain but rather that the formula for this old Indian herbal tea could be used to help mankind. Rene did not want to sell her formula to drug companies since she did not want it to get tied up in bureaucratic red tape or shelved and discredited like so many other natural remedies. However, as she grew old, she finally sold the rights to this formula for only $1. She did this hoping the tea could be developed and made easily available to the public. Now many companies are using a combination four herb formula and making it available to everyone."

Essiac is currently mass-produced in a variety of forms and by a variety of companies. Many people have continued to experience success with it for cancer, but as with any mass-produced herbal treatment, finding a good quality product is extremely important. Combining Essiac with some other alternative cancer approaches has also proven helpful for many cancer patients (however, it cannot be combined with Protocel.)

What We Use

Essiac

shop.ConnersClinic.com/essiac

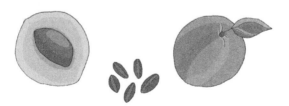

LAETRILE

God's Natural Cancer Killer

Laetrile: B17/B15

This alternative treatment for cancer is possibly the most

misunderstood by the public, as a result of massive misinformation propagated by the cancer industry and press decades ago. However, it is still being successfully used to treat cancer in Mexico as well as in a few places in the U.S. Intravenous treatments along with other nutritional supplementation (and sometimes other adjunctive treatments) is usually combined for best results.

The following was adapted from CancerTutor.com:

How It Works

Laetrile (e.g. amygdalin or Vitamin B17) therapy is one of the better-known alternative cancer treatments. It is very simple to use and is very effective if used in high enough doses and if the product is of high quality and *if it is combined* with an effective cancer diet and key supplements (in other words, you need to do your homework to maximize its benefits).

Laetrile is theorized to work by targeting and killing cancer cells and building the immune system to fend off future outbreaks of cancer. It involves a strict diet (as do all cancer treatments) and several supplements.

How to Obtain Laetrile or Vitamin B17

The FDA has made the purchase of laetrile supplements difficult to obtain, even though it is a perfectly natural and safe supplement. In order for a doctor to use laetrile supplements, they must have a patient sign a statement that the treatment is solely for detoxification and **not** to cure cancer. In other words, all "treatment for cancer," **not** just Laetrile, are effectively illegal unless you are an oncologist.

Fortunately, Laetrile is available over the internet either as apricot kernels, pills, or in some cases in liquid form. I personally believe that the apricot kernels are the best form as they are in more of a "whole food" form.

In the middle of a peach or apricot is a hard shell. If you break open the hard shell with a nutcracker, pliers, or hammer, you will find a small seed/kernel in the middle that looks like an almond. However, it is much softer than an almond and certainly does not taste like an almond (it is bitter and not very tasty.) It is this seed that is rich in natural laetrile.

If you search for "apricot kernels" (use the quotes) on Google, you will be able to find a lot of vendors of apricot kernels. Be advised, however, that apricot kernel sites cannot legally make any medical claims about laetrile being used to treat cancer.

Most experts will recommend a **daily** dose of apricot kernels from between 24 kernels a day up to 40 kernels a day, spread throughout the day. For a person in remission, 16 apricot kernels a day should be used as a minimum.

Other things rich in laetrile are millet grain and buckwheat grain. Breads made with these grains, however, generally do not contain a high percentage of millet or buckwheat or else they would be too hard.

Also, the seeds of berry plants such as red and black raspberries are rich in laetrile. Red raspberries also have a second cancer killer in their seeds: Ellagic Acid, a phenolic. About four dozen foods have Ellagic Acid, but Red Raspberries have the highest concentration. Strawberries also have Ellagic Acid.

This means that when you buy berry jelly or jam, make sure you buy preserves that have the seeds. Basically, the seeds of any fruit, except citrus fruits, have laetrile. I have always eaten apples including the core and seeds; it's the best part!

Of course, apricot kernels are the best source of laetrile. Those who do not yet have cancer might want to plant a few apricot or peach trees in their back yard for a long-term source of lactrile. The kernels can be frozen while still in the shell.

The Theory

When the lactrile compound molecule comes across a cancer cell, it is broken down into 2 molecules of glucose, 1 molecule of hydrogen cyanide and 1 molecule of benzaldehyde. In the early days of lactrile research, it was assumed that the hydrogen cyanide molecule was the major cancer cell killing molecule, but now it is known that it is the benzaldehyde molecule that is by far the major reason the cancer cell is killed.

The reason lactrile therapy takes so long to work, in spite of the marvelous design of the lactrile molecule, is because the lactrile molecule must chemically react with the enzyme of a non-cancerous cell (e.g. rhodanese), before it reacts with the enzyme of a cancerous cell (beta-glucosidase); the rhodanese will break apart the lactrile molecule in such a way that it can no longer kill a cancer cell. Thus, you have to take enough lactrile molecules, over a long enough time, that enough lactrile molecules coincidently (as far as we know) hits all of the cancer cells first.

The Basic Treatment Plan

The specific therapy that I discuss comes from the Binzel book *Alive and Well*. There are other sources of a lactrile diet, but I would compare any other diet with the Binzel diet if you want to use another diet.

As with any cancer treatment, the place to start is with the diet, meaning the foods you can and cannot eat. The Binzel diet is very similar to the Raw Food diet. This is interesting because he was taught by Dr. Krebs himself, thus the lactrile diet probably dates back over 60 years.

338

It is critical **to take the pancreatic or proteolytic enzymes during the laetrile therapy!!**

Note that zinc is also one of the most critical parts of this therapy:

"Zinc is the transportation mechanism for laetrile and nitrilosides in the body. Biochemists and researchers have found that you can give Laetrile to a patient until its coming out of the ears of the patient, but, if that patient did not have sufficient level of Zinc, none of the laetrile would get into the tissues of the body. They also found that nothing heals within the body without sufficient Vitamin C. They also found that magnesium; selenium, Vitamin A, and B, all played an important part in maintaining the body's defense mechanism. This is why it's important to understand that cancer is best treated with a total nutritional program consisting of diet, vitamins, minerals, laetrile and pancreatic enzymes."[142]

Warning #1: Laetrile May Cause Low Blood Pressure

This is an important message I (Cancer Tutor) received by email: "Laetrile ingestion may occasionally cause a temporary low blood pressure reaction due to formation of thiocyanate, a powerful blood pressure lowering agent. In metabolism, nitriloside is hydrolyzed to free hydrogen cyanide, benzaldehyde or acetone and sugar. This occurs largely through the enzyme beta-glucosidase produced by intestinal bacteria as well as by the body. The released HCN (hydrocyanide) is detoxified by the enzyme rhodanese to the relatively non-toxic thiocyanate molecule."

Normally, lowering blood pressure is not an issue, however, for those who are already taking blood pressure medications,

---

[142] http://www.thefountainoflife.ws/cancer/zinc.htm

or have heart issues which would be made worse by a drop in blood pressure, be advised that laetrile can lower blood pressure.

Warning #2: Proteolytic Enzymes May Act as Blood Thinners

Because many people on laetrile also use proteolytic enzymes (e.g. pancreatic enzymes), it is important to know that proteolytic enzymes are blood thinners. Proteolytic enzymes, such as Vitalzym, should **not** be used in conjunction with prescription blood thinners unless the medical doctor understands they are being used.

Also, high doses of proteolytic enzymes should not be taken, just as too high of a dose of any blood thinner should never be taken. **See the bottle for maximum doses**.

Warning #3: Do Not Take Laetrile with Probiotics

From an email: "It was our experience that taking laetrile with high strength probiotics may also increase the amount of free hydrogen cyanide and thus could create adverse side effects."

Space out probiotic use at least 30 minutes from eating any apricot kernels.

Warning #4: Combining Laetrile with Other Alternative Cancer Treatments

Whenever a person combines two or more alternative cancer treatments together, it is critical to do your homework. For example, Vitamin C should be taken with laetrile, however, high-dose Vitamin C should **not** be taken with Protocel, graviola, hydrazine sulfate, etc.

In other words, if you are taking a second or third alternative cancer treatment with laetrile, or if laetrile is being used to supplement another treatment, be careful to watch the warnings on each treatment.

What We Use

Whole Apricot Seed Capsules: contain whole, ground seeds so they are a lower concentration of B 17 but they have B 15 contained.

shop.ConnersClinic.com/apricot-seed-caps

B 17 100mg Capsules: These are a good dose to start.

shop.ConnersClinic.com/b17-100

B 17 500mg Capsules: These are a higher dose per capsule.

shop.ConnersClinic.com/b17-500

B 15 capsules:

shop.ConnersClinic.com/b15

IP-6

IP-6 works by increasing your body's Natural Killer Cell activity. These NK cells have two primary roles: they target cells that have made significant change and become cancerous as well as targeting enemy invaders like virus, bacteria, fungus and molds. The NK cells are a part of the Th1 immune system, which is commonly depressed in cancer patients. Bill Sardi, in his article entitled, *"The Overlooked Cancer Cure from Japan"* writes (adapted):

Nature's most effective iron-chelating molecule is inositol hexaphosphate (IP6), found naturally in seeds and bran. IP6 is a selective agent against cancer cells. Because cancer cells are high in iron content, IP6 directs most of its attention to abnormal cells since IP6 acts as a selective iron chelator. IP6 selectively removes iron from tumors cells (stealing one of its major food sources), which deprives them of their primary growth factor. IP6 does not remove iron from red blood cells which are tightly bound to hemoglobin. Unlike cancer drugs, healthy cells are not affected with IP6, so IP6 has very low toxicity.[143]

There have been numerous lab dish and animal studies that conclusively prove IP6 is an effective and non-toxic anti-cancer molecule. But the National Cancer Institute has never seen fit to conduct a human trial even though IP6 made it on a list of promising anti-cancer agents.[144]

As an alternative to chelating drugs, IP6 has been shown to desirably alter the expression of proteins produced by the p21 and p53 genes (cancer suppressing genes that control cancer growth) but goes unused as a cancer treatment.[145]

IP6 enhances the anti-cancer effects of Adriamycin and Tamoxifen, two commonly used cancer drugs.[146] However, it goes ignored by cancer doctors even though it's known to help chemotherapy!

While Desferal, an iron-chelating cancer drug, has a modest effect because of its poor ability to get inside tumor cells and remove iron, IP6 is found in every cell in the body and is essential for life. By virtue of its ubiquitous presence in living

---

[143] Deliliers GL, British J Haematology 117: 577—87, 2002
[144] Fox CH, Complementary Therapy Med 10: 229—34, 2003
[145] Saied IT, Anticancer Research 18: 1479—84, 1998
[146] Tantivejkul K, Breast Cancer Research Treatment 79: 301—12, 2003

human cells, it is non-toxic.[147]

In 2001, Food and Drug Administration researchers reported that 8 of 12 chelating agents tested were mutagenic (caused gene mutations.) Among the four non-toxic chelators were IP6.[148]

The obvious choice among available iron chelators is inositol hexaphosphate (IP6.) IP6 meets all the requirements for a safe iron chelator to treat cancer. It penetrates inside cells. It is non-toxic, inexpensive, and very effective. It's just not a drug.

Dr. Paul Eggleton of Oxford University demonstrated the IP6 also assists our immune system in our battle against enemies by increasing the oxidizing agents within neutrophils to aid in destruction of cancer and disease.

Ip6 Summary:

- IP6 inhibits cell proliferation; helps stop cancer growth
- IP6 inhibits cell progression
- IP6 inhibits metastasis by interfering with CTC (circulating tumor cell) adhesion, migration, and invasion (it inhibits MMP-9 secretion)
- IP6 induces apoptosis in many cancer cell lines
- IP6 inhibits Angiogenesis (new blood vessel growth to cancer) by:
  o Inhibiting growth and differentiation of endothelial cells
  o Inhibits secretion of VEGF (vascular endothelial growth factor)
  o Blocking fibroblast growth factor

---

[147] Richardson DR, Critical review Oncology Hematology 42: 267—81, 2002
[148] Whittaker P, Environmental and Molecular Mutagenesis 38: 347—56, 2001

What We Use
IP-6

> shop.ConnersClinic.com/ip6

Note: IP-6 is also an excellent chelator to help pull toxins and heavy metals out of the body!

Artemisia

Artemisia annua is an herbal shrub that grows in hot, arid climates. It has been long touted as beneficial for malaria. The 2015 Nobel Prize in Physiology and Medicine was awarded to Professor Youyou Tu for her key contributions to the discovery of the key component of the plant, artemisinin. Artemisinin has saved millions of lives and represents one of the significant contributions of China to global health.

Recently, several published case reports and pilot phase I/II trials indicate clinical anticancer activity of these compounds.

The cellular response of Artemisinin and its derivatives towards cancer cells include oxidative stress response by reactive oxygen species and nitric oxide, DNA damage and repair, various cell death modes (apoptosis, autophagy, ferroptosis, necrosis, necroptosis, oncosis), inhibition of angiogenesis and tumor-related signal transduction pathways.

Artemisia is definitely one of my favorites for cancer as well as Lyme and other infections.

What We Use
Artemisinin Solo

> shop.ConnersClinic.com/artemisinin-solo

CHAPTER 5 – NUTRACEUTICALS

Artemisinin

shop.ConnersClinic.com/artemisinin

Vitamin D3

I hesitated about listing Vitamin D as a cancer "killer" as we tend to test for and place everyone on Vitamin D with K2 (MK7 form only), A, and E. I believe that you should add *all* of the fat-soluble vitamins together as they have a synergistic benefit to the body.

When we test for Vitamin D3 levels, I like to see our patients' blood levels between 60–150 nanograms/milliliter even though levels of 20 to 50 ng/mL is considered adequate for healthy people.

Two forms of Vitamin D can be measured in the blood: 25-hydroxyvitamin D and 1,25-dihydroxyvitamin D. The 25-hydroxyvitamin D is the major form found in the blood and is the relatively inactive precursor to the active hormone, 1,25-dihydroxyvitamin D. Because of its long half-life and higher concentration, 25-hydroxyvitamin D is commonly measured to assess and monitor Vitamin D status in individuals and is the one I speak of when looking at healthy levels.

What We Use

Vitamin D

shop.ConnersClinic.com/vitamin-d

Hormone Balancers

When we attempt to support hormonally driven cancer patients, we typically aren't trying to block estrogen

345

production like most drugs do; we would rather support healthy, normal elimination of estrogens through proper metabolism. However, some people may over-express estrogen in a state of "hyper-aromatization" and do well on nutrients such as Chrysin, Quercetin, Naringenin, Resveratrol, Apigenin, Genistein, Grape Seed Extract, and Oleuropein, all-natural slowing agents of aromatase.

Generally, our desire is to support healthy metabolism by supporting the cytochrome P-450 pathways (we also look at these genes.) Compounds found in vegetables such as cabbage, Brussels sprouts, and broccoli, from the Brassica plant family are essential for this (I3C and DIM are found in these foods.) Glutathione S-transferase is also upregulated by the sulfur constituents in cruciferous vegetables so make sure you look at and support genetic defects in the Transsulfuration pathway.

Other nutrients that support healthy estrogen balance may include Norway spruce lignan extract **and** Hops extract. Plant lignans are phytonutrients commonly found in small amounts in unrefined whole grains, seeds, nuts, vegetables, berries, and beverages, such as tea (green tea) and coffee. The friendly bacteria in our intestines convert plant lignans into the "human" lignans called enterodiol and enterolactone. Aromatic-PN is a concentrated, naturally occurring plant lignan called 7-hydroxymatairesinol, which is derived from the Norway spruce (Picea abies.) In humans, 7-hydroxymatairesinol is a direct metabolic precursor of enterolactone.

Enterolactone is a phytoestrogen that binds to estrogen receptors and has both weak estrogenic and weak antiestrogenic effects. The latter accounts for much of its cell-protective capacity. Additionally, in vitro work has demonstrated that enterolactone affects aromatase and the biosynthesis of estrogen and has strong free radical scavenging and antioxidant properties.

The protective effect of lignans and enterolactone on tissues, including those of the prostate and breast, is encouraging. At the same time, the estrogenicity of HMR and enterolactone, although milder than estradiol, offers promising applications for women with menopausal concerns. For instance, in a randomized, single-blind, parallel group pilot study, 20 menopausal women taking 50mg/d of hydroxymatairesinol for eight weeks experienced half as many hot flashes as compared to pretreatment. Furthermore, high serum enterolactone has repeatedly been associated with cardiovascular health.

Specific Nutrients

Sulforaphane

Sulforaphane (SFN) is an isothiocyanate found in cruciferous vegetables and is especially high in broccoli and broccoli sprouts as well as other cruciferous vegetables. Recent studies suggest that SFN offers protection against tumor development during the "post-initiation" phase and mechanisms for suppression effects of SFN, including cell cycle arrest and apoptosis induction.

Other studies show data that suggests sulforaphane inhibits cell growth, activates apoptosis, inhibits HDAC activity, and decreases the expression of key proteins involved in breast cancer proliferation in human breast cancer cells.

We've found it to be beneficial in many hormone-driven cancers.

See more info here:

ConnersClinic.com/broccoli-extract

ConnersClinic.com/nrf2

What We Use

Sulfora-Xym

shop.ConnersClinic.com/sulforaxym

DIM

Indole-3-carbinol (I3C) is an essential nutrient found in *Brassica* vegetables, such as broccoli, cauliflower, and collard greens. Diindolylmethane (DIM) is the digestion derivative of indole-3-carbinol via condensation formed in the acidic environment of the stomach. If you are going to use I3C as a nutritional supplement (and you may want to consider it after reading this), take DIM. DIM has long been studied for its anti-carcinogenic effects and its ability to bind and rid the body of "bad" estrogens. These so-called "bad" estrogens are both made in the body as intermediate metabolites and consumed through estrogen exposure in drinking water and estrogen disruptors such as plastics. The latter are termed xenoestrogens, as they are toxins from environmental sources.

DIM's history for cancer prevention and therapy[149] began when a mouse study showed its promising results in tobacco smoke, carcinogen-induced, lung adenocarcinoma. DIM was found to have "lung cancer preventive effects" that are mediated via modulation of the receptor tyrosine kinase/PI3K/Akt-signaling pathway.[150] DIM demonstrated "exceptional anti-cancer effects against hormone responsive

---

[149] Kim YS, Milner JA. Targets for indole-3-carbinol in cancer prevention. J Nutr Biochem. 2005;16(2):65–73. [PubMed]
[150] Qian X, Melkamu T, Upadhyaya P, Kassie F. Indole-3-carbinol inhibited tobacco smoke carcinogen-induced lung adenocarcinoma in A/J mice when administered during the post-initiation or progression phase of lung tumorigenesis. Cancer Lett. 2011 [PMC free article] [PubMed]

cancers like breast, prostate and ovarian cancers."[151] In a recent study, it was concluded that DIM rather than I3C was the active agent in cell culture studies destroying cancer.[152]

DIM transduces signaling via aryl hydrocarbon (Ah) receptor, NF-κB/Wnt/Akt/mTOR pathways, to help inhibit growth. These pathways are typically up regulated in cancer patients, yet DIM may help block many of these avenues.

DIM was also found to induce cell cycle arrest, helping slow replication of cancer cells. It also helps modulate key CYP enzymes in the liver, aiding important detoxification channels. DIM was found to alter angiogenesis, the lay-down of new vessels that cancers rely on for continued growth. It decreases cell invasion, metastasis and epigenetic behavior of cancer cells as well.[153]

DIM was found to induce Nrf2-mediated, intercellular detoxification (GSTm2, UGT1A1, and NQO1) and antioxidant (HO-1 and SOD1) genes. These pathways are our essential detoxification pathways inside every cell. Think of them as the cellular garbage service that gets rid of the poisons that would otherwise wreak havoc. Individuals with genetic defects on Nrf2, Glutathione, and SOD genes have an even greater need to support such cellular garbage service.

DIM has also shown synergistic benefits with isothiocyanates, and sulforaphane, the nutrients found in cruciferous

---

[151] Acharya A, Das I, Singh S, Saha T. Chemopreventive properties of indole-3-carbinol, diindolylmethane and other constituents of cardamom against carcinogenesis. Recent Pat Food Nutr Agric. 2010;2(2):166–177. [PubMed]

[152] Bradlow HL, Zeligs MA. Diindolylmethane (DIM) spontaneously forms from indole-3-carbinol (I3C) during cell culture experiments. In Vivo. 2010;24(4):387–391. [PubMed]

[153] Banerjee S, Kong D, Wang Z, Bao B, Hillman GG, Sarkar FH. Attenuation of multi-targeted proliferation-linked signaling by 3,3′ - diindolylmethane (DIM): From bench to clinic. Mutat Res. 2011[PMC free article] [PubMed]

vegetables that have been found to have such wonderful benefits for patients with cancer.[154]

Overall, DIM showed anti-cancer properties, especially in hormonally driven tumors. DIM is currently in clinical trials for various other forms of cancers, however given its benefits to boost other natural therapies, it may be a good add for all cancer patients.

What We Use

Clear DIM

shop.ConnersClinic.com/clear-DIM

I3C

Indole-3-carbinol (I3C) is a naturally occurring compound found in numerous cruciferous vegetables, such as broccoli, cauliflower, kale and cabbage. Following ingestion of I3C, the body converts it to several different metabolites, one of which is diindolylmethane (DIM.) Both of these compounds, as well as many other I3C metabolites, have been shown to impact metabolic shifts and cellular activities for improved health outcomes. I3C has also been shown to temper estrogen signals by competing for binding sites and inhibiting the activity of estrogen receptors.6-15 A study published in the *Journal of Nutrition* unveiled evidence that I3C supports healthy cellular function related to estrogen metabolism.

---

[154] Saw CL, Cintron M, Wu TY, Guo Y, Huang Y, Jeong WS, Kong AN. Pharmacodynamics of dietary phytochemical indoles I3C and DIM: Induction of Nrf2-mediated phase II drug metabolizing and antioxidant genes and synergism with isothiocyanates. Biopharm Drug Dispos. 2011;32(5):289–300.[PMC free article] [PubMed]

What We Use

CDG EstroDIM

shop.ConnersClinic.com/cdg-estroDIM

Norway Spruce Lignan

Conners Clinic Originals Estro Clear delivers a unique, proprietary blend of 8-prenylnaringenin (8-PN) from hops and plant-lignan extract at clinically relevant levels. Research suggests lignans and 8-PN can support the body's natural process of healthy aromatase activity and exert phytoestrogen (e.g. enterolactone) and antioxidant activity. This all-natural formula may support cardiovascular, bone, breast, and prostate health and help relieve normal menopausal discomforts.

What We Use

Estro Clear

shop.ConnersClinic.com/estro-clear

Fermented Soy

It is helpful to understand that most cancers with a hormonal component increase the gene expression of the estrogen receptors-alpha (ER-a) on cells. This is the receptor site, or "docking port" where estrogens attach to enter through the cell membrane to get into the cell. The gene expressions of ER-a and estrogen receptor-beta (ER-b) in healthy 20-year-old females and the gene expressions in postmenopausal women can be very different. Postmenopausal women can have increased ER-a sites and decreased ER-b sites in their cells.

I know this sounds confusing, but it is very important to understand. These two different receptors on the cell membrane (ER-a and ER-b) work very different from each other; where the ER-a is a true estrogen receptor, ER-b is not.

As women age and move towards perimenopause, ovarian secretion of estrogen slowly decreases, and adrenal secretion of estrogen should take up the slack. Here lies a major problem: women entering perimenopause with adrenal insufficiency and hypothalamus-pituitary axis lesions are exposed to have extreme fluctuations in estrogen levels that lead to the problem of having an increase in the amount of ER-a sites on their cell membranes with a concurrent decrease the other receptor site called ER-b (Estrogen receptor beta.) To further the problem, the greater the exposure to xenoestrogens the greater the disparity between the numbers of ER-a and ER-b occurs. This is neither normal nor healthy for several reasons and worse when it comes to leading to cancer because the ER-b sites function to stimulate apoptosis. When you down-regulate receptor sites for apoptosis, bad things happen!

I know this all sounds mighty confusing but stick with me for a minute. Research has shown that fermented soy phytoestrogens (fermented soy products) reduce the ER-a sites in these patients; that's **good**! Reducing ER-a on the cells and upregulating your ER-b sites reduces your cancer risks of all types and allows your Th1 (immune killer cells) system to kill cancer cells! Remember that I said there are *good* phytoestrogens and *bad* phytoestrogens? Fermented soy is a *good* phytoestrogen.

In summary, cells have two different named estrogen receptor sites, ER-a and ER-b. ER-a receptor sites are the ones that receive and process estrogens. If these sites are upregulated and increased in number, estrogen toxicity begins and the risk of cancer in both men and women increases dramatically. The ER-b sites (good guys) are actually sites where another hormone, 3-beta adiol (adiol), attaches which then upregulates immunity and kills cancer; you do not want this site downregulated, which is what happens in HRT and exogenous exposure of xenoestrogens. Compounds that occupy the ER-b receptor site are anti-estrogenic, regulate immunity and kill cancer cells. Compounds that go to the ER-a site are carcinogenic, estrogenic, and involved with increased cancer risks.

We need to understand that fermented soy phytoestrogens are not estrogens, nor do they act like estrogens. Fermentation improves bioavailability and eliminates undesirable compounds found in non-fermented soy.

I said all the above to introduce Haelan 951 and SanoGastril, fermented soy products that upregulate the ER-b (good guys) and down-regulate ER-a (the bad guys.) These are great products and should be considered by **all** patients with **any** hormonal involvement with their cancer breast cancer, ovarian, uterine, prostate and others!

What We Use

Sano-Gastril

shop.ConnersClinic.com/sano-gastril

Haelan 951

Haelan951.com

For Men

Blocking Testosterone and IL-6

Many oncologists that treat prostate cancer patients insist on using androgen-deprivation therapy (ADT) that blocks male hormone production and release. The theory that testosterone increases the growth of prostate cancer is based on the androgen receptor on cancer cells and its high-affinity binding of dihydrotestosterone (derived from testosterone) which can block this receptor.

The general positive response many prostate cancer patients have after beginning ADT reflects a dependence on androgen in tumor cell proliferation, at least in early stage disease. However, studies have shown that subsequent to androgen deprivation therapy, prostate cancers can recur and progress to a terminal stage despite reduced circulating testosterone.

There is research that shows that a specific androgen receptor, AR 3, is activated by testosterone stimulating normal prostate growth. In prostate cancer, it is thought that testosterone over-effects these receptors in a sense. Somehow the receptors become hyper-reactant to testosterone causing excess growth. This is called AR 3 overexpression. It is thought that certain genes (TIF2 and SRC1) can become expressed which then contribute the AR 3 overexpression.

Reducing testosterone with castration or ADT has proven to help early stage prostate cancer but researchers are still puzzled as to the mechanism of cancer return and re-growth in many patients. Using Lupron or another brand of ADT can dramatically reduce PSA levels and even greatly slow growth for a period of time. Then the cancer tends to reappear with a vengeance. How can we address this?

It has been known that elevated interleukin-6 (IL-6), a major mediator of the inflammatory response, has been implicated in androgen receptor (AR 3) activation, cellular growth and differentiation. Since IL-6 plays an important role in the development and progression of prostate cancer, is there a natural way to reduce these levels and slow the expression of the TIF2 and SRC1 genes?

Enter two natural products: Andrographis and EGCg. The traditional Chinese and Indian medicinal plant *Andrographis paniculata*, as well as EGCg, an active catechin from Green Tea have been shown to inhibit IL-6 expression and suppress IL-

6–mediated signals.

Furthermore, andrographis inhibits cell viability and induces apoptotic cell death in both androgen-stimulated and castration-resistant human prostate cancer cells without causing significant toxicity to normal immortalized prostate epithelial cells.

What We Use

Vira Clear: for Andrographis

shop.ConnersClinic.com/vira-clear

Teavigo: for EGCg

shop.ConnersClinic.com/teavigo

Saw Palmetto

Saw palmetto is an herb used to treat the symptoms of benign prostatic hyperplasia (BPH.) In vitro studies have found that saw palmetto inhibits growth of prostatic cancer cells and may induce apoptosis. Other studies revealed that Saw Palmetto down-regulated IL-6 as well as androgen receptor (AR 3.)

It has also been shown to reduce Cox-2 expression, an inflammatory marker associated with an increased incidence of prostate cancer so use can also be preventative.

What We Use

Prostate Health

shop.ConnersClinic.com/prostate-health

Prostate Supreme

shop.ConnersClinic.com/prostate-supreme

Chrysin

Chrysin is a natural flavone commonly found in honey that has been shown to be an antioxidant agent. Studies have shown it to have an antiproliferative effect on prostate cancer cells inducing apoptosis is several cell lines.

Another study revealed that Chrysin inhibited insulin-induced expression of HIF-1α by reducing its stability. I talk about HIF-1α in my *Cancer Genes* book because it closely relates to many cancer's ability to utilize lactic acid from glucose as a fuel source. Inhibition of HIF-1α by chrysin also may inhibit vascular endothelial growth factor (VEGF) expression thereby reducing the vasculization of tumors.

What We Use

FemGuard + Balance

shop.ConnersClinic.com/femguard

Prostate Health

shop.ConnersClinic.com/prostate-health

Prostate Supreme

shop.ConnersClinic.com/prostate-supreme

Sano-Gastril

shop.ConnersClinic.com/sano-gastril

Haelan 951

Haelan951.com

Minerals

Selenium

Selenium has been an interest to cancer patients since a study by Clark et al. (1996) that showed supplementation with selenized brewer's yeast was capable of decreasing the overall cancer morbidity and mortality by nearly 50%. It was a double blind, randomized, placebo-controlled trial involving 1312 patients (mostly men) who were recruited initially because of a history of basal cell or squamous cell carcinoma.

Adding selenium to one's diet seems appropriate. Brazil nuts, fish, most meat, eggs and rice have selenium. We recommend green drink products to most patients that also have added selenium, or we use selenium with iodine.

What We Use

Selenium + Iodine

shop.ConnersClinic.com/selenium-iodine

Iodine

Iodine is essential for thyroid function as it is a component of the thyroid hormone, but iodine is also essential for many cancers, especially breast cancer. Also, animal experiments have demonstrated a clear increase in incidence of thyroid epithelial cell carcinomas after prolonged iodine deficiency.

What We Use

Selenium + Iodine

shop.ConnersClinic.com/selenium-iodine

Magnesium

Magnesium is an essential mineral for just about every metabolic process in the body. Adding magnesium to one's protocol can have multiple benefits. We use magnesium to improve bowel habits, as it will loosen the stools. Our Magna Clear has TRAACS/ALBION brand (double bonded to an amino acid as in nature) of magnesium malate, citrate and lysinate to help calm the brain, feed the tissues and help with stools.

What We Use

MagnaClear

shop.ConnersClinic.com/magna-clear

Zinc

Zinc is an essential mineral for cancer patients as its ratio with copper is all-important. Copper is essential for growth and therefore added to many multi-mineral and multi-vitamin complexes. However, we do **not** want to add copper to a cancer patient's protocol!!

Several studies have shown that plasma copper concentrations are increased in various carcinomas. While copper stimulates growth, zinc acts as a cellular growth protector, including growth of neoplastic cells, and its deficiency was demonstrated to be involved in several stages of malignant transformation. Studies have shown a significant increase in the mean total serum Cu levels and the serum Cu/Zn ratio in all patient groups with cancer compared to a control group.

Measuring the copper to zinc ratio (Cu/Zn) can be helpful; we want that ratio to be as low as possible, meaning that we want to **lower** copper levels and **elevate** zinc levels. So, you don't need to run the lab test, just **stop** any supplements that have copper and start taking zinc!

What We Use

Clear Multi Min

shop.ConnersClinic.com/clear-multi-min

Reacted Zinc

shop.ConnersClinic.com/reacted-zinc

Dr. Conners Zinc/DMSO Topical Spray

shop.ConnersClinic.com/zinc-dmso

Benagene

Brain cancers, like aggressive glioblastoma, have been difficult to treat. A recent study has given us clues as to why they can continue to grow even with aggressive chemotherapy. It appears that the cancer cells plug into the brain's neuronal network and receive impulses that stimulate tumor growth. These impulses, which are transmitted via synaptic connections, may also explain how brain tumors spread so quickly.

The good news is that it also may give us a way to hinder growth through blocking this connection.

This discovery that cancer cells, like brain tissue, may be electrically/neurologically active was reported by scientists from Heidelberg University Hospital and the German Cancer Research Center. In the paper "Glutamatergic synaptic input to glioma cells drives brain tumor progression" that appeared in *Nature*, these scientists noted that previous research had already established that glioblastoma cells connect with one another rather like neurons. This finding has been extended in the new research, which argues that tumor cells not only interconnect like neurons, they also interconnect *with* neurons.

Even more intriguingly, "the interconnections are active. We report a direct communication channel between neurons and glioma cells in different disease models and human tumors: functional bona fide chemical synapses between presynaptic neurons and postsynaptic glioma cells," the authors of the *Nature* article wrote. "These neurogliomal synapses show a typical synaptic ultrastructure, are located on tumor microtubes, and produce postsynaptic currents that are mediated by **glutamate receptors of the AMPA subtype.**"

This discovery may be our key: **glutamate receptors of the AMPA subtype.** Glutamate is a neurotransmitter that can effectively be reduced through diet and specific nutrients. Decreasing the available glutamate may help decrease the communication signaling and help reduce cancer growth.

"We were able to show that signal transmission from neurons to tumor cells does, in fact, work like stimulating synapses between the neurons themselves," noted Thomas Kuner, a corresponding author of the current study and director of the department of functional neuroanatomy at Heidelberg University's Institute for Anatomy and Cell Biology.

The current study also explored the relationship between tumor-neuron signaling and tumor growth: "Glioma-cell-specific genetic perturbation of AMPA receptors reduces calcium-related invasiveness of tumor-microtube-positive tumor cells and glioma growth. Invasion and growth are also reduced by anesthesia and the AMPA receptor antagonist perampanel, respectively."

Using dietary approaches such as caloric restriction, time-restricted eating, and reducing animal protein consumption may prove beneficial for some tumors. Also consider glutamate reducing nutrients like oxaloacetate (Benagene) and Glutamate Scavenger.

360

What We Use

Benagene

> shop.ConnersClinic.com/benagene

Glutamate Scavenger 2

> shop.ConnersClinic.com/glutamate-scavenger

Dandelion Root

Dandelion root extracts (DRE) have long been a favorite in alternate circles to aide in liver detoxification, increase cellular health, and help with cancer. A recent study[155] demonstrated that DRE has the potential to induce apoptosis (help cancer cells die) and autophagy (clean up the trash around a cancer) in human pancreatic cancer cells with no significant effect on noncancerous cells. So, it leaves normal cells alone and helps kill cancer cells!

What We Use

Dandelion Root

> shop.ConnersClinic.com/dandelion-root

Homeopathic Remedies

The main principle of Homeopathy is stated as "let likes cure likes," *similia similibus curentur*. While the concept of "like curing like" dates back to the Greek Father of Medicine, Hippocrates (460-377 B.C.), it was German physician Dr. C.

155

https://journals.lww.com/pancreasjournal/Abstract/2012/10000/Selective_Induction_of_Apoptosis_and_Autophagy.8.aspx

F. Samuel Hahnemann (1755-1843) who first codified this principle into a system of medicine.

The second principle is that of "minimal dose." Typically, a homeopathic remedy, if taken to a biochemistry laboratory, would show no traces of the particular component in the remedy. Homeopathic remedies are thought to contain only the frequency of the component that then stimulate the body to make an appropriate response to such a frequency. This is where homeopathy has received the greatest amount of backlash from the medical community.

For the most part, homeopathic remedies are given in a liquid dropper or pellet form that are administered orally under the tongue. There are some general rules for best practices outlined below.

There are numerous classical homeopathic remedies for cancer. We create homeopathic remedies based on the needs of the patient. Here are some examples:

- **Remedy made from Cancer Biopsy slides**: Under the homeopathic understanding that "likes cure likes" a homeopath of a patient's cancer biopsy may be beneficial to help stimulate an immune reaction to the cancer.

- **Remedy to help detoxify**: Using a homeopath for mercury, for example, may be able to help a person detoxify mercury. The same is true to help detoxify radiation for X-Rays or CT Scans, radiation from radiation therapy, Gadolinium from MRIs, and other toxins as well.

Cayenne Pepper

Capsaicin is an ingredient in chili peppers that is found in many OTC topical pain relievers. It is available as a cream, ointment, stick, pad, gel, liquid, or lotion and marketed under many brand names including Zostrix, Icy Hot Arthritis Therapy, Capsagel, and Arthricare.

Capsaicin is actually an irritant to humans, producing a burning sensation in any tissue it touches which is one reason why it works. When you eat chili peppers (or take a tincture) it produces saliva and irritates any tissue it comes in contact with. This fires an immediate immune response (Th1) that is extremely helpful in cancer patients. Topically, it also interferes with substance P, a chemical involved in transmitting pain impulses to the brain. Make sure to wash hands thoroughly after applying a topical capsaicin to other areas of the body and never touch your eyes after handling either the topical or the real peppers. (Believe me, I know!)

Even with regular use of a topical capsaicin product, it may take some time to feel the benefits from arthritis pain. *Make sure not to use it on broken skin, or if you've had previous allergic reactions to capsaicin or hot peppers.*

The American Institute for Cancer Research noted in its February 2007 newsletter that capsaicin has shown some promise in the fight against cancer. The nonprofit organization reports that one 2006 study showed that capsaicin was capable of killing 80% of prostate cancer cells in laboratory mice. A second study that shortly followed showed that orally administered capsaicin reduced pancreatic tumors in mice by about 50% compared with mice that had a normal diet. Some research indicates that capsaicin might help fight cancer cells by disrupting the mitochondria that supply energy to the cancer.

Dr. Schultz has long been touting the benefits of peppers as a cancer cure. Recently, a Nottingham University study showed that the family of molecules to which capsaicin belongs, the vanilloids, bind to proteins in the cancer cell mitochondria to trigger apoptosis, or cell death, without harming surrounding healthy cells.

Lead researcher Dr. Timothy Bates said: "As these compounds attack the very heart of the tumor cells, we believe that we have in effect discovered a fundamental 'Achilles heel' for all cancers. The biochemistry of the mitochondria in cancer cells is very different from that in normal cells. This is an innate selective vulnerability of cancer cells." He said a dose of capsaicin that could cause a cancer cell to enter apoptosis, would not have the same effect on a normal cell.

Other authors believe that capsaicin can actually promote cancer in healthy people. I disagree based on physiology:

- Capsaicin is a strong Th1 stimulant and therefore shows great promise in cancer care, as nearly every cancer will be Th2 dominant at the cancer site

- But, because capsaicin is a strong Th1 stimulant, those individuals that are Th1 dominant autoimmune already may **not** benefit from use. It may actually make them worse! (Hence the opposing data)

- Because capsaicin also decreases mitochondrial function and thereby decreases cancer cell metabolism (a good thing), it may not be beneficial for those with adrenal fatigue and chronic fatigue syndromes.

What We Use

Cayenne

shop.ConnersClinic.com/cayenne

GcMAF

The following information must be understood in the context that GcMAF, in its original form, does **not** currently exist/is **not** currently available. There are sources (overseas) that claim to have GcMAF, but I question the authenticity. Proceed with caution.

I've stated before that should intracellular failsafe procedures that ensure cell death collapse, it is the function of your immune system to destroy rapidly replicating cells. How does the immunes system do this? It takes a strong Th1 system; the predominant part of an immune response that kills invaders to attack a growing cancer mass. One type of cell in this Th1 response is called a macrophage. In the destruction of cancer, the macrophage attaches to a binding receptor on a cancer cell and then activates to destroy the cell. With many types of cancer, an enzyme created by the growing cancer can halt this activation process. This is not good as it renders the immune response null and void.

A protein molecule circulating in the blood called Gc protein (also called Vitamin D binding protein) is abundant in healthy individuals and aids in the destruction of pathogens and cancer cells. It is a glyco-protein, meaning that it has specific sugars attached to it that form something like a key. Found in human blood serum, Gc protein becomes the molecular switch to activate macrophages when it is converted to its active form called Gc-macrophage-activating-factor (Gc-MAF/GcMAF.) Gc protein is normally activated by conversion to GcMAF with the help of the B and T cells (white blood cells in the immune response.) Unfortunately, cancer cells get smarter over time and begin to secrete an enzyme known as alpha-N-acetylgalactosaminidase (also called Nagalase) that completely blocks conversion of Gc protein to GcMAF, preventing the "last ditch" macrophage protection against cancer. This is the way cancer cells escape detection and destruction: they disengage the immune system's ability to kill the cancer. This also leaves cancer patients prone to infections and many then succumb to pneumonia or other infections, stuck in a Th2 dominant state.

I must also remind you that a suppressed immune system (from radiation or chemotherapy) leaves a similar result. Without a healthy immune response, a growing cancer is left on its own, unrestricted. This is why I'll say it again:

You cannot kill cancer with chemotherapy, radiation and surgery alone! You **must** do other immune stimulating therapies and search for the cause!

Understanding the above phenomenon, there is another promising way to stimulate the activation of a macrophage through the use of a nutrient called GcMAF. Taking GcMAF injections directly activates the macrophage response, thereby sharply stimulating a Th1 reaction that *turns on* macrophages.

Researchers testing GcMAF stated it, "works 100% of the time to eradicate cancer completely, and cancer does not recur even years later." (This was stated based on the tested group of patients; nothing works 100% for everyone) The weekly injection of GcMAF, a harmless glyco-protein, activates the immune system, which can then kill the growing cancer. Studies among breast cancer and colon cancer patients produced complete remissions lasting 4 and 7 years respectively. This glyco-protein "cure" is totally without side effect, but currently goes unused and is completely ignored by cancer doctors. Why? Maybe it is because there is little money to be made in selling it. For less than $2,000 a cancer patient can obtain an adequate amount of GcMAC.

The once-weekly injection of just 100 nanograms (billionths of a gram) can activate macrophages and allow the immune system to pursue cancer cells with vigor, sufficient to produce total long-term cures in humans. But remember, there is not one drug, medicine, herb, or nutraceutical that works for everyone. Everyone's body is unique.

I spoke to Dr. Nobuto Yamamoto, director of the Division of Cancer Immunology and Molecular Biology at Socrates Institute for Therapeutic Immunology, Philadelphia, Pennsylvania. He told me that GcMAF is "the most potent macrophage activating factor discovered, yet oncologists ignore the research." As I discussed a patient with him, he laughed at the treating oncologist's demand for the patient to continue chemotherapy: "they don't even know what they are doing," he said, as he then pointed me to research data published in peer-reviewed Cancer journals from as far back as 1996 and as recent as 2008 that proved the benefits of GcMAF.

Unfortunately, there is simply too much money in chemotherapy!

How do you know if GcMAF will work for your cancer? There are a few ways to tell. A specialized medical lab test measuring Nagalase enzyme levels will reveal either normal (low) levels, indicating that GcMAF is not going to be your first choice, or abnormal (high), indicating GcMAF may be a perfect complement to help stimulate Th1 macrophage responses. One can also utilize kinesiology to easily test if GcMAF will potentially help a patient with cancer or measure other markers through blood.

Once a sufficient number of activated macrophages are produced, another GcMAF injection is not needed for at least a week because macrophages have a half-life of about six days. The studies revealed that after 16-22 weekly doses of GcMAF, the amount of Nagalase enzyme fell to levels found in healthy people, which serves as evidence tumors have been completely eliminated. "The treatment was fool-proof, it worked in 100% of 16 breast cancer patients (tested) and there were no recurrent tumors over a period of 4 years."[156]

---

[156] January issue of the International Journal of Cancer. [International Journal Cancer.2008 January15; 122(2):461-7]

In my conversations with Dr. Yamamoto, he kept telling me that he has always been "neutral" in the traditional vs. alternative cancer fight. He repeated that he just wished doctors would look at the facts. He and colleagues stated in an article published in Cancer Immunology Immunotherapy, "Gc-MAF therapy totally abolished tumors in 8 colon cancer patients who had already undergone surgery but still exhibited circulating cancer cells (possible metastases)." After 32-50 weekly injections, "all (the tested) colorectal cancer patients exhibited healthy control levels of the serum Nagalase activity, indicating eradication of metastatic tumor cells," said researchers. "An effect that lasted 7 years with no indication of cancer recurrence either by enzyme activity or CT scans." [157]

Though Dr. Yamamoto first described this immuno-therapy in 1993,[158] there are very few clinics utilizing the therapy.

In an animal experiment published in 2003, researchers in Germany, Japan, and the United States collaborated to successfully demonstrate that after they had injected macrophage activating factor (GcMAF) into tumor-bearing mice, it totally eradicated tumors. [159] In 1997 Dr. Yamamoto injected GcMAF protein into tumor-bearing mice, with the same startling results. A single enzyme injection doubled the survival of these mice and just four enzyme injections increased survival by 6-fold. [160] In 1996 Dr. Yamamoto reported that all 52 cancer patients he had studied carried elevated blood plasma levels of the immune inactivating alpha-N-acetylgalactosaminidase enzyme (Nagalase), whereas healthy humans had very low levels of this enzyme.[161]

---

[157] Cancer Immunology, Immunotherapy Volume 57, Number 7/July 2008

[158] The Journal of Immunology, 1993 151 (5); 2794-2802]

[159] Neoplasia 2003 January; 5(1): 32–40

[160] Cancer Research 1997 Jun 1; 57(11):2187-92

[161] Cancer Research 1996 Jun 15; 56(12):2827-31

In the early 1990s, Dr. Yamamoto first described how the human immune system is disengaged by enzymes secreted from cancer cells, even filing a patent on the proposed therapy.[162]

Activated Gc protein has been used in humans at much higher doses without side effect. This Gc macrophage activating factor (GcMAF) has been shown to be effective against a variety of cancers including breast, prostate, stomach, liver, lung, uterus, ovary, brain, skin, head/neck cancer, and leukemia. Although GcMAF is also called Vitamin D binding protein, the activation of macrophages does not require Vitamin D (though many cancer patients are deficient.)

GcMAF is a naturally made molecule and is not patentable (hence the reason why drug companies have ignored the data), though its manufacturing process is patent protected. One could argue that if an effective treatment for cancer would come into common practice, the income stream from health-insurance plans for treatment would collapse the medical monopoly in America. The National Cancer Institute estimates cancer care in the U.S. costs $100,000 to over a million dollars per year, per patient, and produces only marginal improvements in survival.[163]

The AMAS Test is another alternative to Nagalase Testing and is easier to obtain here in the United States. Its promoters state that the AMAS test is useful both as a screening test for early cancer and for monitoring cancer therapies. AMAS is elevated when cancer is present and goes down below baseline when cancer is undetected. They say it is over 99% accurate (when done twice) and can be used instead of Nagalase to find and follow cancers.

---

[162] US Patent 5326749, July 1994; Cancer Research 1996 June 15; 56: 2827-31
[163] Targeted Oncology 2007 April, 2 (2); 113-19

The AMAS test measures a naturally occurring antibody present in blood serum accurately detecting early cancer of all types. It will show positive if any type of cancer exists with greater than 95% accuracy; repeat testing greater than 99% accurate; false positive and false negative rates less than 1%. AMAS results will help monitor treatment choice as well because the numbers will decrease with successful cancer treatment; normal levels in successfully treated cancer patients indicate absence of malignancy. I cannot promote the AMAS test personally though as I do not have experience using it and cannot find much data supporting it. That doesn't mean that it is not valid; I would consider utilizing any newer test alongside current acceptable testing. It isn't an expensive test and is sure worth the expense.

Unfortunately, at the time of the most recent update of this book, GcMAF is **no longer available** for whatever reason (you can only guess.)

Hoxsey Therapy

Currently, this herbal approach to cancer therapy, involving an internal tonic, a topical salve, and a topical powder, can be obtained in its original form from Mexico. For decades it was a thriving cancer therapy in the U.S. It was the first widely used non-toxic cancer approach, but was so heavily opposed by the American Medical Association that it was finally forced out of the United States in the 1950's. Melanomas and lymphomas are considered the best responders to this herbal approach.

Hoxsey Therapy is a mixture of herbs and was first marketed as a purported cure for cancer in the 1920s by Harry Hoxsey (a former coal miner and insurance salesman), and Norman Baker (a radio personality.) Hoxsey claimed that he traced the treatment to his great-grandfather, who observed a horse with a tumor on its leg cure itself by grazing upon wild plants growing in the meadow. John Hoxsey gathered these herbs and mixed them with old home remedies used for cancer. Among the claims made in his book, he purports his therapy aims to restore "physiological normalcy" to a disturbed metabolism throughout the body, with emphasis on purgation, to help carry away wastes from the tumors he believed his herbal mixtures caused to necrotize.

Over time, people sought out Hoxsey for the treatment of their cancer and he opened 17 clinics, all of which would eventually be closed by the FDA. Dogged in many states by legal trouble for practicing medicine without a license (he wasn't a doctor), Hoxsey frequently shut down his clinics and reopened them in new locations. In 1936, Hoxsey opened a clinic in Texas which became one of the largest privately-owned cancer centers in the world. At one point in the 1950s, Hoxsey's gross annual income reached $1.5 million from the treatment of 8,000 patients. No one can doubt the success he had in treating cancer patients, and he won the respect of several heavy critics after successfully treating their family members, but Hoxsey made some critical errors, and his ego was his downfall. He claimed to "cure cancer" and stuck to his statements of "cure" despite what the AMA and FDA did to shut him up. He may have "cured" many cancer patients, but **no one** can claim a "cure" regardless of how a patient responds. Ego and pride are the downfall of many.

The truth: due to the herbs used, the Hoxsey formula is a great detoxification tool, which we make good use of with many of our patients. You do not need to go to Mexico to utilize Hoxsey protocols.

What We Use

Hoxsey-Like Supplement

shop.ConnersClinic.com/hoxsey

Parent Essential Fatty Acids (DPAs, ALAs, EPAs & DHAs)

Essential fatty acids have undergone extensive studies with cancer and their potential anti-inflammatory effects on the body. In a recent study out of Finland, Jyrki Virtanen, from the University of Eastern Finland, analyzed blood levels of omega-3 fatty acids, as well as C-reactive protein (CRP, a marker of inflammation,) in Finnish men, ages 42 to 60 years. Results showed that if omega-3 levels increased, CRP levels decreased. Specifically, docosapentanoic acid (DPA) and docosahexanoic acid (DHA) increase significantly, whereas no change in levels of eicosapentaenoic acid (EPA) or alpha-linolenic acid (ALA) were observed. The authors of the study concluded: "Serum (omega-3 polyunsaturated fatty acids) and especially the long-chain (omega-3 polyunsaturated fatty acids) concentration, a marker of fish or fish oil consumption, were inversely associated with serum (C-reactive protein) in men."

Essential fatty acids are a great anti-inflammatory fat that everyone needs to consume. How much is enough? First understand that farm-raised salmon and other fish are **not** a good source of Omega-3s. Do **not** buy fish that are farm-raised; these are fed prepared fish foods and not natural. To get EFAs from food, eat cold water, ocean caught fish that are products of their natural environment. There are also arguments on whether it is best to take supplements of fish oil or use Parent oils (which are cold pressed seed oils; I list the source we use below.) Either way, you must spend the money and purchase a good brand that ensures little to no contaminants and has a reputation for quality.

Because omega-3 fatty acids are in shortest supply in the typical American diet and have been so imbalanced in most people for decades, I often recommend you obtain EFAs from a **Parent** source. This means the oils are from unadulterated sources that are from sources that contain the "parents" of both Omega-3 and Omega-6. These "parent essential oils" (PEOs) are Linoleic Acid and Linolenic Acid. This is one of the simplest, safest, yet most effective steps you can take to quell chronic inflammation in your body. I also recommend that everyone include a small handful of raw nuts and seeds in your diet daily, especially walnuts, which are good sources of PEOs.

It is important to have the proper ratio of omega-3 and omega-6 in the diet and to let the body make them through using PEOs. We know that Omega-3 fatty acids help reduce inflammation, and most omega-6 fatty acids tend to promote inflammation which, from the outside looking in, isn't good. However, there **must** be a proper balance between an inflammatory "attack" response and the anti-inflammatory "clean-up." Everything in life is about balance!

Prof. Brian Peskin is a world-leading scientist specializing in parent EFAs (termed PEOs) and their direct relationship to both cancer and cardiovascular disease. He currently spends time advancing the scientific understanding of the role of essential fatty acids in the body's metabolic pathways, and has developed a means for alleviating cancer's prime cause, as postulated by Nobel Prize-winner Otto Warburg, M.D., Ph.D., by increasing cellular oxygenation (*The Hidden Story of Cancer*.)[164] From an immune standpoint, there is a fundamental cancer/heart disease connection whereby the same physiologic solution helps solve both conditions.

Dr. Peskin's protocol, termed "the Peskin Protocol," will lead to a new understanding of how to better care for patients with both cancer and heart disease. The basis for Peskin's current work, grounded in physiology, can be found in his seminal work and peer-reviewed medical journal articles. Clinical physicians throughout the world have validated Prof. Peskin's EFA recommendations. In the most exciting development to

[164] Pinnacle-Press.com

373

date, Dr. Peskin's theoretical conclusions were recently and completely validated in a physiological experiment by precise instrumentation capable of measuring arterial compliance. This experiment (IOWA experiment) provided the first conclusive clinical proof and validation of Prof. Peskin's theory. Peskin pharmaceuticals have a patent pending on the medicament that embodies this development.

What is a Parent Essential Oil (PEO)?

There are really only two essential fatty acids, LA (parent omega-6) and ALA (parent omega-3.) They **must** come from food. To work properly, they **cannot** be heated, chemically processed, and **must** be organically raised to guarantee full physiologic functionality.

The typical American diet tends to contain 15-30 times more omega-6 fatty acids than omega-3 fatty acids; and they are all adulterated! A 1:1 ratio of parent omega-3 : parent omega-6 would be perfect, but not very practical if you think you are getting them from your current food sources.

The Mediterranean-type diets have a healthier balance between omega-3 and omega-6 fatty acids. I prefer even a stricter Paleo type diet for most people, eliminating grains, "bad" carbohydrates, grain-fed meats, and obtaining most of your nutrition from your vegetables, juicing, and stone fruits. Many studies have shown that people who follow this diet are less likely to develop heart disease and have a much greater chance of surviving cancer.

People who follow an anti-inflammatory diet tend to have higher HDL or "good" cholesterol levels, which help promote heart health. Inuit Eskimos, who get high amounts of omega-3 fatty acids from eating fatty fish (and even blubber), also tend to have increased HDL cholesterol and decreased triglycerides (fats in the blood.) Yes, they eat fat and are healthier, have less fat in their blood and liver, and have less cancer! Finally, walnuts (which are rich in alpha linolenic acid or ANA, which converts to omega-3s in the body) have been reported to lower total cholesterol and triglycerides in people with high cholesterol levels.

Most clinical studies examining parent omega-3 : parent omega-6 fatty acid supplements for autoimmune disorders have focused on rheumatoid arthritis (RA), an autoimmune disease that causes inflammation in the joints. A number of small studies have found that it helps reduce symptoms of RA, including joint pain and morning stiffness by reducing the acute inflammation.

Eating foods rich in PEOs seems to reduce the risk of colorectal cancer according to research and observance. For example, Eskimos, who tend to have a high fat diet as described above, but end up eating high amounts of PEOs, have a low rate of colorectal cancer. Animal studies and laboratory studies have found that omega-3 fatty acids prevent worsening of colon cancer as well. Preliminary studies suggest that taking PEOs daily may help slow the progression of colon cancer in people with early stages of the disease. Although not all experts agree, women who eat foods rich in PEOs over many years may be less likely to develop breast cancer.

Population based studies of groups of men suggest that a "good" fat diet including PEOs help prevent the development of prostate cancer. The biggest thing to remember about good oils and cancer is the anti-inflammatory benefits. Remember, rapidly reproducing cells (cancer) give off a large amount of acidic waste that form an inflammatory "slime" layer around the growing mass that protects it and prevents your immune system from killing it. Anything one can do to decrease this "slime" layer will have benefits in allowing your body to kill the cancer cells.

PEOs and Cancer

In his book *The Hidden Story of Cancer*, Dr. Peskin details the molecular biochemistry of why cancer develops and shows that no "genetic cause" will ever be found to the majority of cancers. Remember that cancer is not a foreign invader but is rather a primitive defense mechanism for survival in a very unhealthy environment. Medical research understood that cancer comes from within our own bodies, but they viewed our bodies' cells as being somehow genetically programmed to "turn against themselves." "This is where they make their mistake: The body is not turning on itself; instead, it is struggling to survive in the only way it can," writes Peskin. Cancer cells survive by making energy using fermentation.

Most cancers are not, and have never been, genetic in origin. What is correct is that the cancerous tissue is surrounded by unhealthy, oxygen-deprived tissue that has allowed the uncontrolled growth to take place. However, it gets worse. Many tissues are oxygen deprived along with the cancerous ones; it is **not** a local problem, it is a systemic problem. Homer Macapintac, M.D., chair and professor of nuclear medicine at The University of Texas M.D. Anderson Cancer Center stated this truth: "Breast cancer is not a local problem. It is a systemic (whole body) disease."

One **major** reason that our tissue becomes oxygen deficient and more acidic is simple: by eating adulterated oils and fats from the food processing industry and from your supermarket's cooking oil section! These adulterated oils have a long shelf-life but have lost their oxygenation ability. They started out containing the functional, vitally needed oxygen-transferring PEOs, but they were ruined by processing and refining. Your body can't make them on its own; they **must** come from food. We are giving ourselves cancer by eating common, everyday processed foods! Trans fats are only the tip of the iceberg of the methods used by food processors to obtain long shelf-life and ruin the oxygenation capability of fats.

PEOs work like tiny magnets drawing oxygen into all cells, tissues, and vital organs.

Dietary Sources

Plant and nut oils are the primary dietary source of PEOs. ALA is found in flaxseeds, flaxseed oil, canola (rapeseed) oil, soybeans, soybean oil (but do **not** take canola oil or soy products with cancer!!), pumpkin seeds, pumpkin seed oil, purslane, perilla seed oil, walnuts, and walnut oil.

Taking a supplement is really necessary unless you eat a perfect diet. I often use (each patient is different, I test them) Dr. Peskin's Protocol now with PEOs. Some of our non-cancer patients fare better with fish oils (see our book on this subject, *You're Crazy*, available as a free download at ConnersClinic.com/books) and recommend Premier Research Labs products. Premier Research Labs has Parent Essential Oils (PEOS) that are organically produced, cold-pressed seed oils containing "parent" omega-6 and "parent" omega-3. They are often better than fish oil supplements for those with cancer.

What We Use

Fatty Acid Liquescence

shop.ConnersClinic.com/FAL

Poly-MVA

Palladium Lipoic Acid Complex (PdLA) is the most active ingredient in a dietary supplement called Poly-MVA. In the palladium lipoic acid complex, the element palladium is covalently bound to the antioxidant alpha-lipoic acid, a potent "cancer killer." In addition to PdLA, the proprietary blend of Poly-MVA is formulated with minerals, vitamins, and amino acids such as molybdenum, rhodium, ruthenium, thiamine, riboflavin, cyanocobalamin, acetyl cysteine, and formyl methionine.[165] Dr. Merrill Garnett invented Poly-MVA. His inquiry and screening of thousands of organo-metallic compounds led to the discovery of the non-toxic supplement and found it to have potent chemotherapeutic properties.

Poly-MVA, is not merely a cocktail of different nutrients, it is *how* they are put together that makes them work differently. Alpha-lipoic acid (ALA) is a great nutrient by itself, working to help liver detox pathways and dozens of other metabolic functions, but there is really no free ALA or free palladium in Poly-MVA. They are bound together; that makes them function differently and *this* is what makes it a special product. This compound was synthesized by Dr. Garnett to create a "metallic bio-organic molecule" that demonstrates enhanced fat and water-solubility. Furthermore, it is prepared in a unique fashion, so it does not produce toxic products upon consumption. This is unlike many other chemotherapeutics, which break down, accumulate in tissue, and eventually become toxic.

Its unique properties appear to be the key to its physiological effectiveness. When glucose enters a cell, it is broken down under anaerobic conditions (absence of oxygen in glycolysis) into pyruvate. Pyruvate subsequently enters the mitochondria, and is quickly oxidized, in the presence of alpha-lipoic acid (ALA), to acetyl-CoA so that it can enter the Citric Acid Cycle and produce even more energy. In aerobic respiration, acetyl-CoA is then channeled into the Krebs/Citric Acid Cycle to create the reduced forms of nicotinamide adenine dinucleotide (NADH) and flavin adenine dinucleotide (FADH2.) NADH and FADH2 donate their electrons to the electron transport chain to make the high energy molecule ATP. This is how

---

[165] Garnett 1995, 1997, 1998

378

your body makes energy.

Recent studies in India[166] have demonstrated Palladium Lipoic Acid Complex's ability to facilitate aerobic metabolism, which is responsible for ATP production in healthy cells. The energy needs of the body are supplied by splitting ATP into adenosine diphosphate (ADP) and a free phosphate (Griffin et al. 2006.) Studies have demonstrated that Poly-MVA provides electrons to DNA, via the mitochondria.

Let's simplify: Poly-MVA helps energy production by providing electrons to speed up production. Whenever anything increases electrons to your body, it increases pH as well. That's all good!

Electrons are lost in normal cells as a result of oxidative damage from radiation and chemotherapy;[167] that's **bad** and exactly how poisons work. Poly-MVA electron transfer provides an additional energy source to normal cells that increases pH and overall health. However, cancer cells are metabolically challenged, and function in a hypoxic (without oxygen) environment. Since there is less oxygen and more free electrons in the cancer cell, generation of free radicals occurs at the tumor mitochondrial membrane.[168] This activates apoptosis by facilitating the release of cytochrome C from the inner mitochondrial membrane, allowing the formation of an apoptotic complex in the cytoplasm. This complex results in the subsequent activation of enzymes that destroy the malignant cells. At significantly higher concentrations of Poly-MVA, necrosis becomes apparent in the malignant cell. Given that normal cells are richly oxygenated, Poly-MVA is non-toxic to them and they actually benefit from the energy

---

[166] Sudheesh et al., 2009
[167] Garnett and Garnett 1996
[168] Antonawich et al. 2004

boost.[169]

So, Poly-MVA appears to be a "selective" metabolic modulator as it increases the apoptotic function of cancer cells (helps them undergo normal cell death) and helps normal cells thrive. But, like every "cancer killer" discussed, it just doesn't work on everyone. Sometimes (most of the time) a combination of diet, Th1 stimulators, and specific "killers" are necessary.

What We Use
Poly MVA

shop.ConnersClinic.com/poly-mva

Protocel

This unique liquid formula is one of the easiest and least expensive alternative approaches to cancer, yet may be one of the most successful. Protocel is non-toxic and because it is so easy to use it is often ideal for administering to small children or the elderly with cancer. It was developed by a chemist to interfere with the anaerobic (without oxygen) function of cancer cells. The fact that cancer cells obtain their energy primarily through anaerobic means (glycolysis) was proven in the 1930s and 1940s by two-time Nobel Prize-winner Otto Warburg. Since all healthy cells in the body use aerobic functioning, Protocel leaves healthy cells unharmed. In 1990, the National Cancer Institute tested this formula (under its previous name of Cancell®), and the results showed it to work better than chemotherapy on a large variety of cancer cells lines. A great book to help understand Protocel is *Outsmart Your Cancer*; the only source in print to present the history, theory,

---

[169] Antonawich et. al 2006

and correct usage of Protocel, and it also presents 16 inspiring testimonials from cancer patients who used it successfully to fight their cancer.

What We Use
Protocel 23

shop.ConnersClinic.com/protocel-23

Protocel 50

shop.ConnersClinic.com/protocel-50

Budwig Diet

Flaxseed oil and cottage cheese, combined in the right way, is the mainstay of this dietary approach to cancer. Developed by the brilliant German biochemist, Dr. Johanna Budwig, it has been used very successfully by thousands of cancer patients. Dr. Budwig was one of Germany's top biochemists as well oas ne of the best cancer researchers throughout all of Europe. She was born in 1908 and seven times she was nominated for the Nobel Prize. Dr. Budwig claimed to have had over a 90% success rate with her diet and protocol with all kinds of cancer patients over a 50-year period. This approach is based on the fact that flaxseed oil is one of the highest sources of omega-3 and omega-6 fatty acids, and cottage cheese is one of the highest sources of sulfur-based proteins. Taken together, the fatty acids bind to the sulfur-based proteins, which results in optimum transport of the fatty acids to cancer cells.

The underlying concept is that the omega-3 and omega-6 fatty acids repair the damaged cell walls and chemical communication of the cancer cells to the point where they normalize. Dietary restrictions and extra supplementation are also recommended. People with many different types of cancer have responded well to this method, but prostate cancer appears to show a particularly good response to this approach.

Instructions from The Budwig Center

Generally, each tablespoon of Flaxseed Oil (FO) is blended with 2 or more tablespoons of low-fat organic Cottage Cheese (CC) or quark.

Note: *Whenever Tablespoons are mentioned it is the standard US tablespoon which is the equivalent of the British "dessert" spoon (the Budwig Center is in Spain).*

1 US Tablespoon (T) = 15ml

1 British Tablespoon = 18ml

16 Tablespoons = 1 cup

4 Tablespoons = 1/4 cup

Directions

- To make the Budwig Muesli, blend 3 Tablespoons (British dessert spoons) of flaxseed oil (FO) with 6 Tablespoons **low-fat** (**less than 2%**) Quark or Cottage Cheese (CC) with a hand-held immersion electric blender for **up to a minute**. If the mixture is too thick and/or the oil does not disappear you may need to add 2 or 3 Tablespoons of milk (goat milk would be the best option.) Do not add water or juices when blending FO with CC or quark. The mixture should be like rich whipped cream with no separated oil. Remember you must mix **only** the FO and CC and nothing else at first. Always use organic food products when possible.

- Now once the FO and CC are well mixed, grind 2 Tablespoons of whole flaxseeds and add to the mixture. Please note that freshly ground flaxseeds must be used within 20 minutes after being ground or they will become rancid. *Therefore, do not grind up flaxseeds ahead of time and store.*

- Next mix in (by hand or with the blender) 1 teaspoon of honey (*raw non-pasteurized is recommended.*)

- (Optional) For variety, you may add other ingredients such as sugar free apple sauce, cinnamon, vanilla, lemon juice, chopped almonds, hazelnuts, walnuts, cashews (no peanuts), pine kernels, rosehip-marrow. For people who find the Budwig Muesli hard to take, these added foods will make the mixture more palatable. Some of our patients have even added a pinch of Celtic sea salt and others put in a pinch of cayenne pepper for a change.

- (Optional) Dr. Harvey Diamond, who wrote a book on the importance of "food combining," and other experts recommend not mixing fruit with other foods (*they say to eat fruit on its own on an empty stomach and wait 10 minutes before eating other foods.*) If, however, you do not have any digestion problems, you may want to add various fruits, especially berries (fresh or frozen.) No more than 1 cup of fruit should be added.

- (Optional) Add ground up ***Apricot kernels*** (no more than 6 kernels per day.) Or you may decide to eat these apricot kernels on their own

Nausea

Some people get nausea from the ground flaxseeds. Counter this by taking a small bowl of papaya immediately afterwards. Also put a lot of papaya into the morning muesli; it may be there is a special enzyme in the papaya that quells the nausea.

The Basic Rule with the Budwig diet is: *"if God made it then it's fine, and try to eat it in the same form that God made it."*

Here are some foods that many are not sure of, but they are accepted on the Budwig diet:

- Sweeteners: Stevia, raw non-pasteurized honey, dates, figs, berry and fruit juices serve

- Herbs in their natural form (pure, nothing added)

- All nuts (raw, unroasted) are fine (***except peanuts***)

- All seeds are good; sunflower seeds are very complete and filling

- Raw, unprocessed cocoa, shredded (unsweetened coconut), and rose hip puree

- A cup of black tea is accepted (coffee beans are toxic and not recommended)

- Any flour is permissible as long as it's 100% whole grain. Corn is generally believed by the group to be an exception because of mold/fungus and genetic manipulation

- 2 or 3 slices of health food store pickles (no preservatives, read the label!)

- Freezing cottage cheese/quark as well as fruits and vegetables is okay

- ***Very Important***: The flaxseed oil must always be kept in the refrigerator. It will keep for 12 months in the freezer. Arrange to purchase as direct as possible from a manufacturer (like Barlean's, cold pressed) and when it arrives put it right away in the refrigerator

- Drink only distilled water or reverse osmosis water

- *No* hydrogenated oils, *no* trans-fats, (cold pressed sunflower seed oil is a better choice than olive oil)

- *No* animal fats, *no* pork (pigs are the cleaners of the earth and their meat is loaded with toxins. Ham, bacon, sausages, etc. should be avoided)

- *No* seafood (lobsters, clams, shrimp, and all fish with a hard shell are cleaners of the sea and are loaded with toxins)

- White, regular pasta is eliminated, as is white bread, (gluten-free pasta and bread is a better choice than wheat as many cancer patients have an intolerance to wheat, whole rye, oat, multigrain bread is good. Corn is very discouraged because of mold and genetic modification issues)

- *No* ice cream or dairy products (other than the cottage cheese and some cheese)

- *No* cane sugar, white sugar, molasses, maple syrup, Xylitol, preservatives

- *No* processed foods (*no* store-bought pastries), make your own with our recipes

- *No* soy products (unless fermented or used for 2 or 3 weeks at the beginning if you cannot tolerate the cottage cheese)

- Avoid pesticides and chemicals, even those in household products & cosmetics. Good old vinegar, as well as baking soda, are excellent household cleaners (look on the internet for more info)

- **No** microwave, **no** Teflon or aluminum cooking ware or aluminum foil. We recommend, and provide during your stay at Budwig Center, enamel cooking ware. Stainless steel, ceramic, cast iron, glass and corning cookingwear are fine.

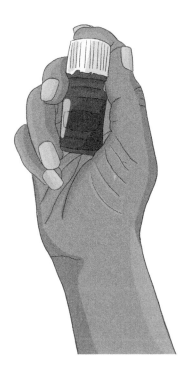

Essential Oils

There are numerous essential oils that have been shown, with peer-reviewed studies, that they can be beneficial for cancer. While we don't use the same treatment for every patient, there are several oils that we almost always use for patients with cancer. We also synergistically link oils with specific nutraceuticals (vitamins, herbs.)

We do a lot of testing to find out what each patient needs because everybody is different. No one should simply stick to one out-of-the-box protocol that they read online or that a friend shared with them. When we look at detox pathways, we always use genetic testing because there are specific genes that are real drivers for specific pathways. If a person has defects on those pathways, they're going to have a difficult time detoxifying.

More information: ConnersClinic.com/essential-oils-cancer

What We Most Often Use

Sacred Frankincense

shop.ConnersClinic.com/sacred-frankincense

Frankincense

shop.ConnersClinic.com/frankincense

Copaiba

shop.ConnersClinic.com/copaiba

Lemongrass

shop.ConnersClinic.com/lemongrass

Myrrh

shop.ConnersClinic.com/myrrh

Oregano Oil

shop.ConnersClinic.com/oregano-vitality

High Dose Melatonin

Melatonin could be an excellent candidate for the prevention and treatment of several cancers, such as breast cancer, prostate cancer, gastric cancer, and colorectal cancer. Melatonin is a hormone synthesized and secreted by the pineal gland in the brain to help us fall asleep.

Data from several clinical trials and multiple experimental studies performed both in vivo and in vitro have documented that the pineal hormone inhibits endocrine-dependent mammary tumors. However, hundreds of recent reports demonstrate an anticancer effect of the pineal hormone on many other kinds of cancers.

When we say, "High-Dose Melatonin" we mean taking 20-60mg before bed. Normal dose for someone using it to help induce sleep would be 3mg before bed.

What We Use

Melatonin 20mg

shop.ConnersClinic.com/melatonin

Green Tea Extract: EGCg

I write about EGCg elsewhere because it simply does so many things. Green tea (*Camelia sinensis*) is an abundant source of antioxidants; notably, epigallocatechin gallate (EGCg), the most potent reducer of IL-6, a powerful pro-inflammatory cytokine. Previous studies have suggested that supplements of green tea extract may confer a variety of cardiovascular and cancer protective effects.

More recently, Nagi B. Kumar, from the H. Lee Moffitt Cancer Center & Research Institute (Florida, United States), and colleagues enrolled 97 men who had premalignant prostate lesions or high-grade intraepithelial neoplasia. Tracking for changes in high-grade prostatic intraepithelial neoplasia (HGPIN) and/or atypical small acinar proliferation (ASAP), study participants were randomly assigned to receive either a supplement containing green tea extract (400mg EGCg), or placebo, for one year.

The researchers observed that the men who received the green tea supplement experienced reduced combined rates of HGPIN/ASAP, as well as decreased levels of Prostate Specific Antigen (PSA.) The study authors report that, "Daily intake of a standardized, decaffeinated catechin mixture containing 400mg EGCg per day for 1 year accumulated in plasma and was well tolerated but did not reduce the likelihood of PCa in men with baseline [high-grade prostatic intraepithelial neoplasia] or [atypical small acinar proliferation]."

EGCg may cause apoptosis in oral cancer cells while leaving normal cells alone, according to researchers at Penn State. Previous studies had shown that EGCg destroyed oral cancer cells without harming healthy ones, but researchers did not understand the mechanism of action behind this. This study, published online in *Molecular Nutrition and Food Research*, demonstrates that EGCg may trigger apoptosis in the mitochondria, leading to cell death.

The researchers determined that the protein known as sirtuin 3 is critical to the process. Sirtuin 3 plays an essential role in antioxidant activity and in mitochondrial function in many tissues throughout the body. They conclude that EGCg's potential ability to selectively regulate the activity of sirtuin 3 (to turn it off in cancer cells and to turn it on in normal cells) is a key factor and may be relevant to many kinds of cancers.

EGCg is also a powerful assistant in the fight against bone loss. Both Primary Osteoporosis and bone loss due to pathological reasons (cancer) involves elevated IL-6 levels. Clear EGCg may be a beneficial nutrient to anyone's protocol should bone loss exist.

Important

Most Green Tea from China is heavily contaminated (this includes supplements!!) We ***only*** use very reputable companies (now using a de-caffeinated EGCg that is spot-checked for heavy metals and pesticides) that run labs on ***every*** batch!

What We Use

Teavigo

shop.ConnersClinic.com/teavigo

Fenbendazole

Fenbendazole, an over-the-counter drug used often to treat rodent pinworm infections in dogs, is fast becoming a success in many late-stage cancers in humans. One study revealed, when testing cancer cell lines against the off-label drug, "the group supplemented with both vitamins and fenbendazole exhibited significant inhibition of tumor growth." Another study suggested, "it caused mitochondrial translocation of p53 and effectively inhibited glucose uptake, expression of *GLUT* transporters as well as hexokinase (*HK II*), a key glycolytic enzyme that most cancer cells thrive on." While I've discovered positive studies, there are others that show no benefits of Fenbendazole, so we must take a balanced approach.

There are numerous anecdotal testimonies of people in very late-stage cancers going into full remission (with documentation) by adding Fenbendazole into their protocol, but I realize these are most often dismissed with a casual eye-roll by the pompous establishment. I'm willing to try anything that may help as long as it doesn't cause harm; and I tend to believe most cancer patients would feel similarly.

How Would I Take It?

If someone wanted to give Fenbendazole a try, I would suggest the following protocol: (***Note***: the Fenbendazole is taken for three straight days and then four days ***off***, e.g. only 3 days in a given week. The other nutritional products are taken daily.)

1. Fenbendazole (shop.connersclinic.com or directly from Amazon): Get the Panacur-C brand (Canine Dewormer); it comes in a white and yellow box with three, 1-gram packets of the products. One box of three packets will last a week since you take ***one*** packet per day for three straight days and then take ***four days off***. Example: Take the Fenbendazole on Monday, Tuesday, and Wednesday ***only*** of each week. Do ***not*** follow the weight-dependent dosing (for dogs) that is given on the back of the packaging! It may be best to place the powdered substance directly in one's mouth and chase it down with a flavored drink such as cranberry juice. It doesn't dissolve well in any liquids. Others may try to mix it into a smoothie or something. It can be taken as a single dose in the morning, with or without food.

2. Apop-E, a specific Vitamin E (with the delta and gamma tocotrienal components): take 1/day always (even on your "days off.") **Note**: more on this particular Vitamin E and cancer can be found here: shop.ConnersClinic.com/apop-e

3. Curcu Clear, the current best source of Curcumin: take 2/day always (even on your "days off.") It can be found here: shop.ConnersClinic.com/curcu-clear

4. Evolv Entourage2 CBD, the current best quality CBD: take 1/2 dropper full (1ml), per day always (even on your "days off.") It can be found here: shop.ConnersClinic.com/evolv-entourage

How Long Should I Give This a Try?

I like to be reasonable in my approach, but if the above protocol is working (talk to your Oncologist), continue it indefinitely. If there is no change after a few months (meaning the cancer continues to progress), or if you experience any ill-effects, this protocol may not be your best choice.

As always, we are providing this information for just that: information. Speak to your doctor about proceeding.

Black Seed Oil

For many centuries, seeds of Nigella sativa (black cumin), have been used as a spice in Middle Eastern and Mediterranean cuisine. These small black seeds contain over 100 chemical compounds, with many more still unidentified. Black cumin seeds are a rich source of amino acids, phytosterols, omega-6 and omega-9 essential fatty acids, proteins, and Vitamins B1, B2 and B3. They also contain calcium, folic acid, iron, copper, zinc and phosphorous.

As studies have shown, black cumin seed oil is a potent antibacterial, anti-fungal, antiviral, and anti-parasitic oil. Traditionally, the seeds have been used medicinally for: asthma, hypertension, diabetes, inflammation, cough, bronchitis, headache, eczema, fever, dizziness, and gastrointestinal disturbances. The literature and studies regarding the biological activities of black cumin seeds is extensive, supporting that this oil could be beneficial for the management of epilepsy, autoimmune disorders, skin irritation and disorders, kidney stone prevention, chronic fatigue, and much more.

Rich in heart-healthy omega-6 and omega-9 fatty acids and phytosterols, *Andreas Black Cumin Seed Oil* may help prevent cardiovascular disease. It may be beneficial for enhancing immune functions, lowering cholesterol.

Due to the process used to press *Andreas Black Cumin Seed Oil*, the nutrient-coded fibers naturally remain in the oil, enhancing the flavor and aiding delivery of the full benefits of the seeds.

Black cumin seed oil is a potent ***anti-cancer, antibacterial, antifungal, antiviral, and anti-parasitic oil***.

What We Use

Black Cumin Seed Oil

shop.ConnersClinic.com/black-cumin-seed-oil

Delta Tocotrienols

Is Vitamin E good for Cancer? If so, is there a difference between the different options out there? What is Tocopherol and Tocotrienol? I answered these questions in this episode of Conners Clinic Live: ConnersClinic.com/vitamin-e

Vitamin E has actually 8 main components, four inner tocotrienols and four outer tocopherols. Vitamin E has long been heralded for its antioxidant properties. Antioxidants are generally believed to inhibit the development of cardiovascular disease and cancer by neutralizing free radical damage.

Tocotrienol derivatives did not attract much attention from researchers until the late 1980s, when their cholesterol-lowering potential[170] and anticancer effects were described.[171]

Tocotrienol has been shown to reduce the transcription factor NF-κB, which is closely connected to the process of tumorigenesis (growth.) A mouse model study of human pancreatic cancer, oral administration of tocotrienol inhibited tumor growth and enhanced the antitumor properties of gemcitabine by inhibiting NF-κB (Kunnumakkara et al. 2010).

What We Use

Apop-E

shop.ConnersClinic.com/apop-e

Rauwolfia Vomitoria

Mirko Beljanski, PhD (1923-1998), was a French molecular biologist who worked for over 40 years studying DNA replication and transcription. Born in the former Yugoslavia, he worked his way from a small village with no resources to become a researcher at the Pasteur Institute in Paris, France,

---

[170] Qureshi et al. 1986
[171] Kato et al. 1985; Sundram et al. 1989

one of the top research institutions in the world.

At the time of his untimely death in 1998, he left behind a legacy of fearless innovation as well as an impressive body of work including two books, 133 articles published in peer-reviewed scientific journals, and numerous patents. One of his primary ambitions was to find a natural chemical that would aide cancer patients.

He found that a selective extract from the bark of the roots of ***Rauwolfia vomitoria***, an African tree, traditionally used as a regulator of the digestive and the hormonal system, also helped slow cell replication in Pancreatic and Ovarian cancer patients. A 2013 study[172] showed, "Rau decreased cell growth in all 3 tested ovarian cancer cell lines dose dependently and completely inhibited formation of colonies in soft agar. Apoptosis was induced in a time- and dose-dependent manner and was the predominant form of Rau-induced cell death."

Another 2018 study on Pancreatic Cancer revealed, "The poor treatment outcomes of pancreatic cancer are linked to an enrichment of cancer stem cells (CSCs) in these tumors, which are resistant to chemotherapy and promote metastasis and tumor recurrence. The present study investigated an extract from the root of the medicinal plant Rauwolfia vomitoria (Rau) for its activity against pancreatic CSCs. In vitro tumor spheroid formation and CSC markers were tested, and in vivo tumorigenicity was evaluated in nude mice. Rau ***inhibited the overall proliferation of human pancreatic cancer cell lines*** with a 50% inhibitory concentration (IC50) ranging between 125 and 325µg/ml, and showed limited cytotoxicity towards normal epithelial cells. The pancreatic CSC population, identified using cell surface markers or a tumor spheroid formation assay, was ***significantly reduced***, with

---

[172] Antitumor Activities of Rauwolfia vomitoria Extract and Potentiation of Carboplatin Effects Against Ovarian Cancer, Curr Ther Res Clin Exp. 2013 Dec; 75: 8–14. doi: 10.1016/j.curtheres.2013.04.001

an IC50 value of ~100µg/ml treatment for 48 h and ~27µg/ml for long-term tumor spheroid formation. The levels of CSC-related gene Nanog and nuclear β-catenin were decreased, suggesting suppression of the Wnt/β-catenin signaling pathway. In vivo, 20mg/kg of Rau administered five times per week by oral gavage significantly reduced the tumorigenicity of PANC-1 cells in immunocompromised mice. Taken together, these data showed that Rau preferentially inhibited pancreatic cancer stem cells. Further investigation is warranted to examine the potential of Rau as a novel treatment for pancreatic cancer."[173]

What We Use

OnKobel-Pro

shop.ConnersClinic.com/onkobel-pro

Laminine

Laminine is the only natural source of Fibroblast Growth Factor or FGF. The role of FGF is to "reprogram" stem cells in the body of an adult so that they can begin repairing damaged areas in your body. This process may enable easier tissue repair and healing; thus, the body gets to recover faster from a vast range of problems.

The human body has amazing regenerative abilities already but Laminine can speed things up and enhance the process. Poor diet, chronic stress, a sedentary lifestyle, and even genetic factors can make it much more difficult to heal.

FGF and amino acids work together to help the body recover

---

[173] Inhibition of pancreatic cancer stem cells by Rauwolfia vomitoria extract. Dong R1, Chen P1, Chen Q1. Oncol Rep. 2018 Dec;40(6):3144-3154. doi: 10.3892/or.2018.6713. Epub 2018 Sep 18

from such detrimental influences and start healing fast once again. New technology has facilitated the extraction of both FGF and essential amino acids, which has resulted in more powerful and beneficial supplements.

The name of the supplement is derived from laminins: proteins that have high molecular weight. The laminins play an incredibly important role in the human body: they lay the foundation of the basal lamina, the network of proteins that affect and stimulate the establishment of tissues and organs.

The combination of Fibroblast Growth Factor and essential proteins is the most distinctive characteristic of Laminine. Fibroblast Growth Factor sends signals, indicating that stem cells and amino acids have to be used for the regeneration of damaged tissues or organs.

The supplement is 100% natural. It gives the body essential amino acids, trace minerals, and other nutrients that play a role in human health. The formula is enriched further through the addition of antioxidants that protect the cells against the damage caused by free radicals. Thus, Laminine gives the body everything that it needs to keep systems functioning properly and to repair damaged tissues.

What We Use

Laminine

shop.ConnersClinic.com/laminine

Vitamin C: IV and Liposomal

Vitamin C is a potent water-soluble antioxidant, and even in small amounts can protect us from damage by free radicals. It is vital to immune function and is an essential cofactor in many enzymatic reactions in the body. It is truly our most universal antioxidant.

Intravenous administration of Vitamin C has been shown to decrease oxidative stress and, in some instances, improve physiological function in adult humans. Oral Vitamin C administration is typically less effective than intravenous, due in part to inferior Vitamin C bioavailability. The purpose of a recent study was to determine the efficacy of oral delivery of Vitamin C encapsulated in liposomes (Liposomal C.) On 4 separate, randomly ordered occasions, 11 men and women were administered an oral placebo, or 4g of Vitamin C via oral, oral liposomal, or intravenous delivery. The data indicate that oral delivery of 4g of Liposomal Vitamin C produces circulating concentrations of Vitamin C that are greater than encapsulated oral (non-liposomal) but less than intravenous administration.

So, while Liposomal C is a much better choice that regular Vitamin C, intravenous C gives even a higher concentration in the blood. However, IV Vitamin C can cause damage to the veins and just isn't for everyone. This is where Liposomal shines; it is easy on the stomach and highly absorbable.

Liposomal C is about 5x as potent as regular oral *or* intravenous Vitamin C. Three teaspoons per day (3750mg/day) is nearly equivalent to 10,000mg/day IV, which has advantages in that you can take it every day. There are 60 teaspoons/bottle.

Liposomal Vitamin C is a vegetarian product that provides 3 forms of Vitamin C. Liposomal encapsulation of ingredients represents a new delivery system that appears to offer important advantages over existing methods of delivery. The liposome has hydrophilic and hydrophobic sides offering a fat and water portion, which allows Vitamin C to be absorbed through the fat and water-soluble pathways for optimal utilization by the body. Each 8-ounce bottle provides 48 servings. Each serving provides 1250mg of Vitamin C. Liposomal C is especially beneficial for patients who have had gastric bypass surgery or who have general gastro-intestinal dysfunction.

What We Use

Liposomal C

shop.ConnersClinic.com/liposomal-c

Astaxanthin

Astaxanthin, classified as a type of carotenoid, is a form of microalgae that gives the red color to salmon, lobster, and crab, and the pink color to the feathers of flamingos.

It has been found to inhibit cell growth in a dose- and time-dependent manner by arresting cell cycle progression and by promoting apoptosis. One study investigated the effects of astaxanthin on the antitumor effector activity of natural killer (NK) cells suppressed by stress in mice in order to define the immunological significance of astaxanthin and found that it increased natural killer cell activity.

While astaxanthin also is a great help in supporting the PON1 detoxification pathway, thereby helping most cancer patients indirectly, it is proving to be an excellent choice for helping kill cancer directly.

What We Use

PON1 Assist

shop.ConnersClinic.com/pon1

Alpha-Lipoic Acid

Alpha-lipoic acid (ALA) is a unique, vitamin-like antioxidant that can combat radiation sickness, repair damaged livers, treat diabetes and diabetes-related conditions (polyneuropathy) and protect against oxidative processes.

Unlike normal cells, tumor cells tend to survive in a redox environment where the elevated reactive oxygen species contribute to enhance cell proliferation (growth) and to suppress apoptosis. Alpha-lipoic acid, a naturally occurring reactive oxygen species scavenger, has been shown to possess anticancer activity due to its ability to suppress proliferation and to induce apoptosis in different cancer cell lines.

One study showed evidence that ALA can effectively induce apoptosis in human colon cancer cells. Other studies support its use in the ancillary treatment of many diseases, such as diabetes, cardiovascular, neurodegenerative, autoimmune diseases, cancer, and AIDS.

The studies on this nutrient are abundant; it helps too many pathways to be left out of nearly any nutritional regimen. Free radical damage can promote the activity of a particular cell protein called NF kappa B. (NF-kB.) NF-kB works to promote inflammation and genetic changes that have been linked with the development of cancer. Studies at the University of California at Berkley have found that when cells are bathed in ALA, NF-kB is inhibited thus preventing cell mutations from replicating. Researchers believe that this has significant implications in inhibiting the formation of cancerous tumors.

What We Use

BerberClear

shop.ConnersClinic.com/berber-clear

Garlic

The benefits of garlic are great for many conditions and can be a strong Th1 stimulant, but the studies in cancer patients are not as positive. Garlic is not a "main player" in my book regarding cancer treatment which works synergistically with other nutrients listed here and bears mentioning. Many studies have shown that organic ingredients of garlic are effective in inhibiting or preventing cancer development, which I believe is a function of Th2 suppression.

What We Use

Allicidin

shop.ConnersClinic.com/allicidin

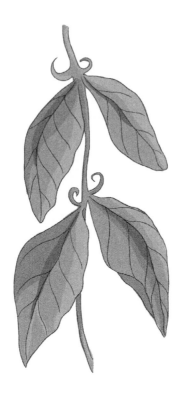

Cat's Claw

Cat's Claw (*Uncaria tomentosa, Uncaria guianensis, Una de Gato, Samento, Saventaro*) is an herb traditionally used by the Asháninka Indians of Peru. The tribe recognized two different types of this plant (one was used therapeutically, the other was rarely used.) This difference has been verified phytochemically and two chemotypes have been identified: the preferred chemotype contains predominantly only pentacyclic oxindole alkaloids (POAs) speciophylline, mitraphylline, pteropodine, isomitraphylline and isopteropodine; the other chemotype, which was never used, contains predominantly the tetracyclic oxindole alkaloids (TOAs) rhynchophylline and

402

isorhynchophylline in addition to the POAs. The preference for the POA chemotype Cat's Claw has been backed up by scientific research even though there has been more than enough puff made about TOAs, we still must point out that all Cat's Claw contains some. I like to use a product that utilizes the synergistic benefits of Cat's Claw with a few other herbs. Coriolus, Green Tea and Olive Leaf extract blend well with Cat's Claw.

Cat's Claw acts as an immune stimulant; it aids the Th1 response. It also has some anti-inflammatory actions as well and is therefore a great benefit to a bio-toxin generated autoimmune disorder in the brain. Because of its anti-inflammatory benefits, it can help brain issues like depression, anxiety, ADD/ADHD and the like.

Cat's Claw is particularly beneficial in treating Lyme disease. Lyme just may be the most misdiagnosed problem in America leading to many autoimmune disorders. Doctors are inclined to rule out Lyme disease based on the negative result of a laboratory test that are just plain poor! Since there has been no reliable laboratory test for Lyme, most clinicians are ill-equipped to diagnose chronic Lyme disease and I have had scores of patients that were refused treatment of acute Lyme due to a false negative test. These are the patients who have suffered needlessly for years, hopelessly lost in the maze of the health care system, looking for answers and enduring the skepticism of practitioners inexperienced with autoimmune disease.

What has been needed for years has been a better Lyme test or some other objective measure to persuade practitioners to consider the diagnosis of Chronic Lyme disease.

Recently, researchers Dr. Raphael Stricker and Dr. Edward Winger discovered that Chronic Lyme patients exhibit a decrease in a specific marker called CD57+. White blood cells (a.k.a. eukocytes) are the components of blood that help the body fight infections and other diseases. White blood cells are categorized as either granulocytes or mononuclear leukocytes. Mononuclear leukocytes are further sub-grouped into monocytes and lymphocytes.

The main lymphocyte sub-types are B-cells, T-cells, and natural killer (NK) cells. B-cells (part of the Th2 response) make antibodies after the T-cells in the Th1 response fail to destroy the antigen in "round one." T-cells and NK cells are the initial cellular aggressors in the immune system and are the sub-group that the CD57 markers are a piece of.

CD markers are a part of the chemical slurry making up an immune response. CD, which stands for "cluster designation," is a glycoprotein molecule on the cell surface that acts as an identifying marker. Cells have thousands of different identifying markers, or CDs, expressed on their surfaces, and about 200 or so have been recognized and named so far.

Natural Killer cells have their own specific surface markers; the predominant NK cell marker is CD56. The percentage of CD56 NK cells is often measured in patients with chronic diseases as a marker of immune status, e.g., the lower the CD56 level, the weaker that particular portion of the immune system. With Chronic Lyme disease, Dr. Raphael Stricker and Dr. Edward Winger discovered, CD57 NK cells are lower than individuals that are healthy and lower than patients suffering from other chronic, autoimmune disorders. This makes measuring CD57 counts a great marker for these chronic patients who often think they are going crazy. Believe it or not, these chronic and often hidden disorders like Chronic Lyme can be responsible for lowering the Th1 response enough to "set-up" cancer!

The reason I bore you with the details is that Cat's Claw has been shown to be a tremendous help to increase CD57 values.

Who knows what other diseases may be helped with increased CD57 markers? Unfortunately, Lyme disease can be an underlining "cause" of immune dysfunction that can lead to cancer.

What We Use

Cat's Claw

shop.ConnersClinic.com/cats-claw

Arginine

Brain cancer, especially the most prevalent form known as glioblastoma, can be devastating, with a dismal prognosis (medically speaking) for this particular tumor. Many cancers develop and progress due to a decreased immune function, allowing single cancer cells to reproduce and metastasize to different organs in the body. Th1 lymphocytes and cytokines (the "killer" side of the immune system composed of different types of white blood cell neutrophils and specialized chemicals) are responsible for destroying aberrant tumor cells before they have the opportunity to develop. This is what is known as normal cell death; cells divide, the old cell dies, aided in part by the "killer cells" that your body uses to clean of possible cancer growth. Normally, immune response declines as we age, in large part due to excess sugar consumption (our poor diets accelerate this process), systemic inflammation (chronic, even sub-clinical autoimmune disorders) and poor cellular oxygenation (made worse by sedentary lifestyles.) Researchers publishing in the journal *Clinical Cancer Research* have found that natural arginine (an amino acid) supplementation may reactivate cancer-fighting T-cells in glioblastoma patients, allowing reactivation of the immune system to fight cancer progression.

Cool, now what do we need to learn from this information? Eat foods that contain higher amounts of arginine like nuts, seeds, beans, and fish. These are all things we encourage cancer patients to consume; this is part of our cancer-regimen "snack food." Raw peanuts, almonds, walnuts, and hazelnuts are great brain snack food that increase arginine levels (as well as good fat levels) and decreases inflammation. Tuna, salmon, and eggs all have high arginine levels. Neutrophils, a type of white blood cell necessary in this immune attack on cancer cells, are an ancient and nonspecific cell that neutralizes invading bacteria and viruses. Neutrophils are a part of the Th1 response to provide a powerful immune response to knock out pathogens. Low-grade and often sub-clinical autoimmune disorders as well as general obesity, sedentary lifestyles, and individuals living with poor diet and lifestyle choices all develop chronic, systemic inflammation.

Chronic inflammation suppresses Neutrophils and other Th1 cytokines (the cancer killer side of the immune system) and they become desensitized to the persistent, systemic inflammation and act less responsive to disease-causing agents. Cancer cells thrive in an inflamed cellular environment and, if left unchecked, lead to the destruction of healthy tissue and unchecked tumor formation. Neutrophils stop the immune response by secreting an enzyme called arginase. Researchers have found that patients with glioblastoma (as well as other cancers) do not exhibit the normal neutrophil-mediated immune response and cancer cells grow and spread unabated.

Again, cancer tends to be a Th1-suppressed disorder!

Scientists from the University of Colorado Cancer Center found that Th1 cells are critically dependent on arginine for activation and function. They were able to determine that the lack of arginine suppresses the "killer side" of the immune system. The researchers concluded that "persistent arginase production from neutrophils suppresses the immune system and keeps cancers from becoming immune targets."

Arginine is a well-researched, natural compound (an amino acid) largely associated with helping lower blood pressure and improves both cardiovascular and brain health. The result of past research demonstrates that arginine is a precursor to the production of friendly nitric oxide (eNOS) and supports blood vessel relaxation to effectively lower out of range blood pressure readings in at-risk individuals. Cancer prevention can now be added to the list of chronic conditions that benefit from regular arginine supplementation and it is **always** best to get your nutrients from your **food**.

Eat more **raw** seeds, nuts, almonds, walnuts, ocean-caught cold-water fish, and organic eggs. Decrease inflammatory foods like red meat, dairy, sugar, and grains. Be conscious of what you eat and even your temperament. Forgive and forget; do what is right.

What We Use

L-Arginine

shop.ConnersClinic.com/l-arginine

Echinacea

A recent study by McGill University, Montreal, Quebec, Canada revealed startling good news regarding Echinacea and cancer. They induced leukemia in mice and treated them with the herb to study if Echinacea would increase Natural Killer Cells (NKCs.) Remember, NKCs are part of the first line of defense against disease and cancers. The concept that herbal compounds could enhance NKCs has recently gained considerable attention and indeed, excellent reviews on the roles of NKCs in tumor combat and the role of such compounds in modifying antitumor responses, have been provided by leading researchers.

So, they induced leukemia in mice via injection of a dose of leukemia cells known to consistently result in death 3.5 weeks later and on the same day as leukemia induction, Echinacea was added to their diet. A "Control Group" of leukemia-injected mice also consumed a regular diet with **no** Echinacea added. The results were most encouraging. NKC numbers by 9 days after tumor onset were "very significantly elevated over control." Three months after leukemia onset (long after all control, those mice with **no** Echinacea, leukemic mice had died) NKCs were recorded at more than *twice* the numbers present in normal mice of identical age, strain and gender. That is: the mice with leukemia that were given Echinacea had ***twice*** the NKCs then normal mice!!

Furthermore, the study reports, "all the other hemopoietic (blood cell) and immune cell lineages in both bone marrow and spleen in these long-term, Echinacea-consuming, originally leukemic mice were indistinguishable from the corresponding populations of cells in normal mice. Life span analysis indicated that not only had Echinacea extended life span but also the survival advantage provided to leukemic mice by consuming Echinacea daily was statistically significant. One-third of all Echinacea-consuming mice that survived until 3 months after leukemia onset went on to live a full-life. We believe that further manipulation of Echinacea dose/frequency/duration regimens could allow many more if not the other full two-thirds to go on to live a full life."

Echinacea mediates its antineoplastic (cancer killing) activity via the immune system and has no influence on the tumor cells themselves (it stimulates the NKC activity.) By stimulating the first line of defense, e.g. NKCs, which are so effective in detecting and killing tumor cells immediately upon detection, the value of Echinacea can be readily seen.

What We Use

Rapid Immune Boost

shop.ConnersClinic.com/rapid-immune-boost

Andrographis

Several cellular processes and targets modulated by andrographis have been identified in human cancer and immune cells. It inhibits the in vitro proliferation of different tumor cell lines, representing various types of cancers.

I wrote about Andrographis when discussing prostate cancer as well. Coupled with EGCg from Green Tea extract (our Teavigo product), it makes a great combo for many cancers.

What We Use

ViraClear

shop.ConnersClinic.com/vira-clear

Astragalus

Astragalus, an ancient immune booster, has been used for centuries to heal the sick. A growing amount of detailed German and American research has confirmed the herb's powers and identified an important potential role in cancer treatment.

For example:

- Researchers from the University of Texas, Houston, have reported that cancer patients receiving Astragalus have twice the survival rate of those only receiving placebos.

- Astragalus is often used in conjunction with other herbs. In a 1994 Italian study (Morazzoni, Bombardelli) breast cancer patients were given a combination of Iigustrum and Astragalus. Patients given this mix showed a decline in mortality from 50% to 10%.

- In another study of patients with advanced non-small-cell lung cancer all undergoing chemotherapy, the group taking the dual herb mix showed an average life span increase of 130%.

- Astragalus doesn't merely enhance interferon levels; there is strong scientific evidence that it benefits liver function (often impaired in the cancer sufferer.) In China, Astragalus is widely used in the treatment of hepatitis. It seems to reduce toxin levels significantly, boost interferon levels and inhibit viral protein expression whilst having little or no effect on normal DNA. (Zhang 1995, Fan 1996)

The FDA is currently considering it or approval as an anti-cancer agent, although you shouldn't hold your breath, as they have never given approval to an herb in their history! Again, that which cannot be patented cannot be profitable.

Remember what I said earlier, most studies on alternatives must be "in conjunction with" standard chemo, radiation and surgery in order to get study approval. In keeping, studies show that Astragalus improves the effectiveness of Radio- and Chemotherapy (or maybe it works **despite** the chemo?!)

One extremely important conclusion from several US studies is that Astragalus seems to help the immune system differentiate between healthy cells and foreign cells, thereby boosting the body's total "cancer fighting system." One effect of this is the added benefit of improving the effectiveness of radiotherapy and chemotherapy treatments.

- In Chinese hospitals, Astragalus is now routinely used to help people recover from the negative effects of radiotherapy and chemotherapy.

- MD Anderson Cancer Center (Texas) researchers reported that cancer patients undergoing radiotherapy had twice the survival rates if they took Astragalus during the treatment.

- In the West, some herbalists routinely provide chemotherapy and radiotherapy patients with Astragalus, and apart from boosting the immune system (which of course both orthodox treatments damage) it also seems to stop the spread of malignant cancer cells to secondary healthy tissues.

What We Use

Astragalus Complex

shop.ConnersClinic.com/astragalus

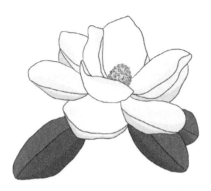

Magnolia

Magnolia (*magnolol, honokiol*) has long been used as an anti-inflammatory agent and now shows promise in blocking a pathway for cancer growth.

A laboratory led by Jack Arbiser, MD, PhD, at Emory University School of Medicine, has been studying the compound honokiol, found in Japanese and Chinese herbal medicines, since discovering its ability to inhibit tumor growth in mice in 2003. "Knowing more about how honokiol works will tell us what kinds of cancer to go after," says Arbiser, who is an associate professor of dermatology. "We found that it is particularly potent against tumors with activated Ras." Ras refers to a family of genes whose mutation stimulates the growth of several types of cancers. Although the Ras family is mutated in about one third of human cancers, medicinal chemists have considered it an intractable target.

"Honokiol's properties could make it useful in combination with other antitumor drugs, because blocking Ras activation would prevent tumors from escaping the effects of these drugs," Arbiser says. "Honokiol could be effective as a way to

412

make tumors more sensitive to traditional chemotherapy," he says. Again, studies for Magnolia center around improving chemotherapy benefits in order to get approval of the study by the FDA.

One of the effects of Ras is to drive pumps that remove chemotherapy drugs from cancer cells. In breast cancer cell lines with activations in Ras family genes, honokiol appears to prevent Ras from turning on an enzyme called phospholipase D. It also has similar effects in lung and bladder cancer cells in the laboratory. Phospholipase D provides what have come to be known as "survival signals" in cancer cells, allowing them to stay alive when ordinary cells would die.

Understanding the physiology, one might conclude that the effect of Magnolia may be that it stops cancer cells from extruding waste and forces them to self-destruct.

Researchers at the University of Pittsburgh wanted to learn how effectively Magnolia kills cancer cells, and how and why it triggers cancer cell death. When they treated several different types of human prostate cancer cells with magnolol (the magnolia compound) for 24 hours, they found that the compound both decreased the number of cancer cells, and changed their shape in a way that suggested the cells were undergoing apoptosis (cell death.) The treatment worked on many different types of prostate cancer cells, regardless of their invasiveness. The higher the dose of magnolol, the more significant the damage it caused to cancer cells (that's called "dose dependant.") Meanwhile, magnolol treatment did not appear to harm healthy prostate cells.

The researchers then took their investigation a step further, looking at the pathways by which magnolol affected prostate cancer cells. "It is very important to understand how magnolol acts as an anticancer agent," says lead author Yong Lee, PhD, Professor in the Department of Surgery and Pharmacology at the University of Pittsburgh. "If we understand the mechanisms of killing (pathways, model of death, etc.), we can improve the efficacy of the drug and avoid side effects."

Dr. Lee's team discovered that magnolol alters the activity of various proteins that are involved in the apoptosis process, in order to promote cancer cell death. It also inhibits growth factor receptors that are typically produced in larger-than-normal amounts by cancer cells to help those cells survive. "Its ability to destroy cancer cells without harming healthy cells makes magnolol a promising treatment strategy. Although this study focused on prostate cancer, the treatment may also be useful for other types of cancers," Dr. Lee says.

What We Use

CortiClear

shop.ConnersClinic.com/corticlear

Tranquinol

shop.ConnersClinic.com/tranquinol

Dr. Conners Medicinal Mushroom Blend

shop.ConnersClinic.com/medicinal-mushrooms

Chlorella

Chlorella is a single-celled freshwater algae that has been used for centuries to promote healing and detoxification. It contains Vitamin C and carotenoids, both of which are antioxidants that block the action of free radicals (unstable molecules that can damage cells.) Chlorella is also reported to contain high concentrations of iron and B-complex Vitamins. It is widely used in Japan for a variety of health conditions, but again, there are not many scientific studies to support its effectiveness for preventing or treating cancer or any other disease in humans.

According to the American Cancer Society's (ACS) website, "Chlorella is promoted as an herbal remedy for a wide range of conditions. Proponents claim it kills several types of cancer, fights bacterial and viral infections, enhances the immune system, increases the growth of 'friendly' germs in the digestive tract, lowers blood pressure and cholesterol levels, and promotes healing of intestinal ulcers, diverticulosis, and Crohn's disease. It is said to 'cleanse' the blood, digestive system, and the liver. Chlorella supporters also say that it helps the body eliminate mold and process more oxygen. Supporters state that chlorella supplements increase the level of albumin in the body. Albumin is a protein normally present in the bloodstream, and promoters claim it protects against diseases such as cancer, diabetes, arthritis, AIDS, pancreatitis, cirrhosis, hepatitis, anemia, and multiple sclerosis. Chlorella is said to prevent cancer through its ability to cleanse the body of toxins and heavy metals. Some websites describe it as the perfect food, saying that it regulates blood sugar, kills cancer cells, strengthens the immune system, and even reverses the aging cycle."

I highly recommend Chlorella as I believe it is a great support for detoxification and overall liver support. The ACS website adds this disclaimer: "Available scientific evidence does not support these claims. Because of this, the U.S. Food and Drug Administration (FDA) has warned the proprietors of at least one website to stop making unproven statements about chlorella's benefits." Oh brother, pharmaceutical companies can claim anything they want while they get paid up to $15,000 per chemo treatment yet a nutritional product made by God and sold for less than $50 for a month's supply needs to be stifled for making "false claims." Give me a break!

415

What We Use

Chlora-Xym

shop.ConnersClinic.com/chlora-xym

Japanese Knotweed

Though Japanese Knotweed (*Polygonum cuspidatum, Chinese knotweed, Hu Zhang, Kojo, Itadori, Hojang*) can act as a great Th1 stimulator and must be tested in individual patients, it can work well to modulate the immune response. Studies have revealed anti-parasitic, antibacterial, antifungal, anticancer properties as well as central nervous system calming properties. It also protects the body against endotoxin damage from "die-off" of bio-toxins killed through other sources. Other studies have shown it to be anti-inflammatory and may be extremely useful in calming Th17 inflammation in the brain as it crosses the blood-brain barrier readily.

Some bio-toxins (living organisms invading the body) can release compounds called matrix metalloproteinases (MMPs, of which there are several different types) that destroy our body's tissue. Many anti-inflammatories that I highly recommend in this group have shown to help clear the body of these MMPs, but only one (Japanese knotweed) has proven to block several types of MMP production. It also contains Resveratrol, by itself a Th2 stimulant, but in combination with the whole herb, it acts to inhibit MMP levels as well. Other research has shown that it inhibits arachidonic acid metabolites that force the COX inflammatory pathways as well as iNOS (the "bad" nitric oxide that causes inflammation in the brain.) It has also been proven to interfere with nuclear factor-kappaB, a chemical linked to inflammation, autoimmune disorders and cancer. It helps regulate normal cell death (apoptosis) where that has been altered (in cancer), and just modulates the immune response, especially in the

416

brain and spinal cord.

Knotweed has also show to increase circulation to the small vessels of the eye, ear, joints, heart, and skin. I test all Cancer, Lyme, Hepatitis C, and other bio-toxic patients on knotweed. It can also work well for acute infections.

What We Use

AdrenaVen

shop.ConnersClinic.com/adrenaven

Tranquinol

shop.ConnersClinic.com/tranquinol

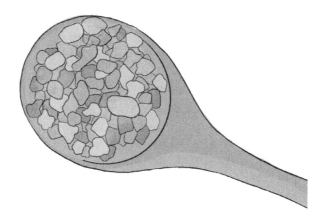

Boswellia

Boswellia Serrata is an extract of Indian frankincense. It has long been a favorite of mine to help decrease inflammation in

417

the gut and brain, and now studies are coming out that are proving its effectiveness in cancer. The most promising study came from Streffer et al, who investigated the use of a Boswellia preparation in 12 patients with cerebral edema and demonstrated a clinical or radiological response in 8 of 12 patients. Boeker and Winking had similar results in a small prospective study. In a systematic review, Ernst found 7 controlled clinical trials investigating the anti-inflammatory effects of Boswellia. These studies were related to the treatment of asthma, rheumatoid arthritis, Crohn disease, collagenous colitis, and osteoarthritis.

Another study showed almost unbelievable benefits of Boswellia on patients with brain tumors; notorious for mobility due to chronic inflammation. They conducted a randomized, placebo-controlled, double-blind study to investigate the efficacy of Boswellia on cerebral edema in patients irradiated for brain tumors.

The results were astonishing: "Compared with baseline and if measured immediately after the end of radiotherapy and BS/placebo treatment, a reduction of cerebral edema of >75% was found in 60% of patients receiving BS and in 26% of patients receiving placebo ($P = .023.$) These findings may be based on an additional antitumor effect."

For them to even document the "anti-tumor effect" was exciting and a bit risky for them to report.

I realize that many people have brain inflammation from a variety of sources. Think about adding Boswellia to your protocol and see if you notice any changes in brain fog, memory, headaches, and such. Let me know what your results are!

Links to studies referenced: ConnersClinic.com/boswellia

What We Use

Clear Inflam

shop.ConnersClinic.com/clear-inflam

Vitamin B12

Vitamin B12 is often an essential for those with cancer. While I would not consider it a "cancer killer" by any means, one problem with long-term cancer patients is often anemia. There are multiple different types of anemia and "anemia of chronic disease" may be the most common with cancer. Another common anemia is "B12 deficient anemia" due to intestinal wall damage and absorption issues. Adding a good form of B12 is a good idea, but which one should you take?

There are four types of B12 (cobalamin) currently available. Cyanocobalamin is commonly used in less expensive supplements and is what I consider to be a synthetic, very poor source; do *not* use. Methylcobalamine is the most common form of B12 and may be the best for *non*-cancer patients as long as they take lower doses to start. It donates its methyl-group to aide in methylation, but this form is *not* recommended for cancer patients as excess methyl-groups can *turn off* tumor suppressor genes and interferes with some chemotherapy drugs.

We recommend either hydroxocobalamin or adenosyl cobalamin as better choices for cancer patients because they are non-methylated.

What We Use

Adenosyl-Cobalamin B12 Assist

shop.ConnersClinic.com/ab-b12

Pro Hydroxo-Cobalamin

shop.ConnersClinic.com/pro-hc

Vitamin B

Sufficient B vitamins prepare the body to counteract the toxic effects of pesticides, environmental toxins, and stressors. B Vitamins are also imperative for healthy red blood cells, energy metabolism, oxygen transport, nerve function, DNA production, and much more.

We recommend non-methylated, whole-food B Vitamins for our cancer patients to prevent genetic triggers which could disrupt the optimal function of tumor suppressor genes.

What We Use

B Specific Naturally

shop.ConnersClinic.com/b-specific

Probiotics

The benefits of probiotics for gut health are widely known. However, many people aren't aware of the importance of cycling probiotic brands and bacterial strains to introduce the widest array of healthy bacteria into our microbiome as possible.

We carry numerous brands of probiotics, both shelf-stable varieties (non-refrigerated) and those needing to be kept in a refrigerator. Meaning, whether a cancer patient is staying home or traveling abroad, they'll have access to high-end probiotics.

What We Use

Clear Pro 100

shop.ConnersClinic.com/clear-pro-100

Biome-Xym

shop.ConnersClinic.com/biome-xym

Pain & Inflammation Relief

Battling pain can become one of the greatest threats to cancer patients' successful healing journey. An additional threat is the horrific side effects associated with extended prescription opioid and NSAID use. We want our patients to pursue as many natural, pain-reducing routes as possible to help minimize their dependence on intense (and sometimes dangerous) pharmaceutical interventions.

Finding a "natural" pain relieving formulation is difficult. Most are based in decreasing inflammation. The hemp-based products (THC and CBD) are probably the most powerful, but you would need to check your local legislation.

What We Use

Curcu Clear

shop.ConnersClinic.com/curcu-clear

421

Evolv Limitless

shop.ConnersClinic.com/evolv-limitless

Clear Inflam

shop.ConnersClinic.com/clear-inflam

Kannaway Gold Premium CBD Paste

shop.ConnersClinic.com/cbd-gold-premium

Kannaway Pure CBD Caps

shop.ConnersClinic.com/pure-cbd-caps

Kannaway Premium CBD Caps

shop.ConnersClinic.com/premium-cbd-caps

Kannaway Premium CBD Oil

shop.ConnersClinic.com/premium-cbd-oil

Kannaway K-Salve CBD Salve

shop.ConnersClinic.com/k-salve-cbd

Evolv Entourage 2 CBD Liquid Dropper

shop.ConnersClinic.com/entourage

Evolv Ease CBD Salve

shop.ConnersClinic.com/evolve-ease

More info on pain relief: ConnersClinic.com/pain-relief

Chrysin

Chrysin is a natural flavone that I discussed when writing about prostate cancer. Other benefits of this nutrient show that it inhibits aromatization. Aromatase is an enzyme responsible for a key step in the biosynthesis of estrogens from androgens. The aromatase enzyme can be found in many tissues in the body and even found in some cancer tissues. It is an important factor in sexual development. Some bodybuilders taking steroids also take Chrysin to prevent excess testosterone conversion into estrogens, which can cause gynecomastia (men developing breasts.) Chrysin, along with several of the Medicinal Mushrooms, have been shown to be extremely effective in reducing aromatization, helping those with all types of cancer.

What We Use

FemGuard + Balance

shop.ConnersClinic.com/femguard

Anxiety Support: Calming the "Bunny Brain"

Rabbits are prey. Their cute, little, ever-wiggling noses, giant fluffy ears and large eyes are all designed for their protection with heightened senses always looking for the next attack. Their nervous systems are tipped in a constant sympathetic dominance that leads to quickly accelerated blood pressure, ease of escape, and continual worry. We are not rabbits.

However, our "bunny brain," as I like to call it, can bend

towards getting stuck in a similar scenario. This may be more appropriately termed post-traumatic stress disorder, anxiety disorder, or some form of obsessive-compulsive issue, but it's all relatively the same. Whether it was a past experience that left us in a state of helplessness to danger or a current condition that steals our control, we can easily get trapped feeling like we are defenseless bunny rabbits surrounded by a hundred hungry wolves.

Our bunny brain can get stuck on high alert long after the predators have gone. Neurologically, we call this being in a state of sympathetic dominance. Our sympathetic nervous system is part of our autonomic nervous response, responsible for "fight, flight, or freeze" largely protective, survival reactions. It's counterpart, the parasympathetic system, is calming, healing, detoxifying, and resting. They are polar opposites and are supposed to be in balance, for the most part, in a resting, non-emergency, situation.

The problem comes in when our brain gets stuck thinking that wolves surround us. The ramped-up sympathetics can lead to high blood pressure, blood sugar control issues, and even cancer. Even worse, when someone is diagnosed with such disease, it can lead to greater morbidity as the diagnosis itself increases sympathetic tone.

Surrender your past or current issues to God. If you are not a believer, I have no other help for my first point. Life is full of predator situations where we are the helpless prey, whether we like it or not. This is a simple fact of the fallen world we live in. All will experience the inevitable struggles of life and trying to overcome without knowledge of and dependence on our Creator is impossible.

Keep your mind occupied. I like to stay busy, both mind and body. I am constantly listening to books and good sermons and lectures that help me grow in faith and knowledge to help others. I have a difficult time sitting still, even on vacation, and

I see this as a good thing. It helps me keep my bunny brain from activating.

Always be asking better questions. The worst things I see my patients do is ask, "Why is this happening to me?" Instead ask questions like, "What am I supposed to learn for this?" "How can I help others through what I am going through?" "How can I be a blessing to someone today?"

Stay in the present. When we focus on the possibility of a bleak future, our bunny brain is in full swing. Focus on today; take one day or one hour at a time. This brings us back to the good questions to ask: ask them in the present tense. Instead of, "When I get better, I want to help others," think, "How can I help someone **today**." There is always someone you can encourage **now** whether it is your spouse or the barista at your local coffee shop. Who can you bless today? It is the gentle word of encouragement, the "thank you" and unexpected compliment that adds love to life.

Become a giver instead of a taker. Those who see themselves as victims often become needy takers that suck the life out of everyone around them. Be introspective enough to recognize that we all can slip into this position from time to time. Fight against it. Be a giver even if you can only give kindness right now. You pour out what is inside of you; so, if people bump into you and you get drenched with anger and pity and bitterness, you had better look inside and make some changes.

Ask for assistance. Accountability is a necessary tool of change. We need others who love us enough to tell us the truth. I thank God for my wife who is secure enough in our relationship to speak truth into me when I need a slap. Surround yourself with those who will "sharpen your iron" and be slow to take offense.

Pray for hope and the joy that comes along with future grace. God has, in His sovereignty, planned all you are experiencing to draw you closer to Him and the future grace He has for you in eternity. See everything as a molding and shaping and your bunny brain will calm down.

Supplements That Can Be of *Great* Assistance

Decreasing Glutamates

While glutamine may provide a direct fuel source for growing cancer, it also converts to glutamate, which is an excitatory neurotransmitter. Glutamine is an amino acid found in animal protein and in many supplements aimed at healing the gut. We ***never*** recommend a cancer patient to be taking glutamine (usually found as L-Glutamine) because of its potential to ***increase*** cancer growth and its conversion to glutamate, which can cause sleep issues and anxiety.

What We Use to Lower Glutamates

Glutamate Scavenger 2

> shop.ConnersClinic.com/glutamate-scavenger

Benagene

> shop.ConnersClinic.com/benagene

More on Glutamates: ConnersClinic.com/glutamine

Add Adaptogens

An adaptogen (or Adaptogenic herb) is an herb that has been shown to improve the body's ability to adapt to stress, whether it's a hectic schedule, heat or cold, noise, high altitudes, or any number of other stressors, typically by helping balance the Pituitary, Adrenal, and Thyroid glands. This elite class of herbs imparts strength, energy, stamina, endurance, and improve mental clarity.

What We Use

Adapto Clear

shop.ConnersClinic.com/adapto-clear

Adaptogen-R3

shop.ConnersClinic.com/adaptogen

Corti Clear

shop.ConnersClinic.com/corti-clear

More on Adaptogens: ConnersClinic.com/stress

Improve Sleep and Increase Exercise

There are numerous studies that show that increasing the quality and quantity of our sleep as well as increasing our exercise can greatly improve our anxiety.

What We Use

Insomnitol

shop.ConnersClinic.com/insomnitol

Tranquinol

shop.ConnersClinic.com/tranquinol

Modified Citrus Pectin

I discussed Modified Citrus Pectin (MCP) when I addressed ways to limit metastasis. But, regular doses of regular citrus pectin support digestive health since the molecules are too large to enter the circulation; meaning benefits are restricted to the GI tract alone. PectaSol-C, our MCP solves this limitation with an advanced modification process that reduces the size and structure of the pectin. This allows PectaSol-C to absorb into the circulation and deliver total-body benefits related to cellular health, immunity and more.

Supports Healthy Cells & Blocks Galectin-3

Over the last decade, scientists and researchers have shown that cellular, cardiovascular, and other critical areas of health are significantly affected by elevated levels of "rogue protein" galectin-3. Therefore, finding a way to maintain healthy galectin-3 levels is of utmost importance in supporting wellness and longevity. Modified Citrus Pectin is the most-researched galectin-3 blocker, and PectaSol-C is the most-researched modified citrus pectin, delivering unparalleled support for numerous areas of health through its ability to successfully bind and block excess galectin-3.

What We Use

PectaSol-C MCP

shop.ConnersClinic.com/pectasol-c

Vitamin B6

The most **common** reason for B6 deficiency in our patients is **chemotherapy drug use**. People who have a history of taking birth control pills, hormone replacement, or antibiotics, or those who have been on diuretics or bronchodilators have a good chance they have suboptimal levels, or what we call a functional deficiency of B6.

Vitamin B6 is also a key link in the utilization of Essential Fatty Acids (EFAs), particularly the conversion of ALA to EPA and DHA.

The classic symptoms of gross Vitamin B6 deficiencies include seizures, mental retardation, and anemia. However, there is a whole host of functional deficiencies. A deficiency in B6 can cause pain and inflammation, numbness, Heberden's nodules, trigger finger, joint stiffness, carpal tunnel syndrome, sensitivity to bright lights, tingling of extremities (neuropathy), sore tongue, depression, hypochlorhydria, fissures/cracks in the tongue, burning sensation in the mouth, history of birth problems like spontaneous abortions or fetal abnormalities to name a few.

Vitamin B6 also acts in many genetic pathways as an essential cofactor and subclinical deficiencies can lead to numerous issues. Again, the most common sign for the need of Vitamin B6 is peripheral neuropathy following chemotherapy.

What We Use

B Specific Naturally

shop.ConnersClinic.com/b-specific

B6/B1 Zinc

shop.ConnersClinic.com/b6-b1

Antihistamines

Our body has two distinct methods of clearing things that could bring it harm: our immune system kills living toxins (bacteria, virus, parasites...) and our detoxification pathways clear non-living toxins (chemicals, heavy metals, drugs....) We have one other system that sits somewhere in the middle between the immune and the detoxification systems that helps with both: the mast cells.

Mast cells make a chemical called histamine, which has numerous, distinct, beneficial roles. As part of the immune response, histamine doesn't kill bad guys itself. It draws fluid to tissues by rendering capillaries more permeable making it easier for immune killer cells to "ride the waves" to a nasty bacterium to destroy. Histamine's immune and detoxification connection runs deep as its functions vary depending on tissue site and specific receptors on the outside of cells to which it binds.

In the brain, histamine can keep us awake, is involved in our reflex reaction to pain, temperature changes, vibration, and hormone balance. It affects our appetite, helps control gastric secretions helping balance blood pH, and serves as a gatekeeper for neurotransmitters that balance mood, concentration, and focus. This makes sense if you think about it: if exposed to an infection, a chemical irritant, something that stimulates pain, or a dangerous vibration felt in the legs or feet, you would need to wake the brain to increase circulation, and flee such harm, buffer the blood to maintain life, and alert us to possible threat.

Histamine so serves in "flight or fight" mechanism to ensure life. Its role in the periphery demonstrates this as well. If histamine attaches to one receptor (there exists 4 main histamine receptors, H1, H2, H3, and H4 with different functions) it is vasoconstrictive, enabling quick movement of blood to extremities to fuel muscles for a quick "getaway." Attaching to a different receptor, histamine dilates small vessels and constricts the bronchial tubes as an immediate protective "freeze" mode. It enhances a hypersensitivity to harmful stimuli creating its most known response: the histamine rash and itch. This would serve to keep us safe from poisonous fauna and teach us that those berries are possibly not edible.

However, histamine, when created in excess, over a period of time, will create an environment of chronic inflammation, disturbing cell-to-cell communication and thereby changing its function. Cell function is dependent on their interaction with the environment. If we think of individual cells as people, an organ could be equivalent to a crowded stadium gathered to observe a football game. Communication to your friend seated next to you may be relatively easy during slow play and more challenging when the home team is guarding the one-yard line. The roar lifts, chants of "de-fence" try to drown out the opposing quarterback's play call, and you can barely hear yourself think as you stand, scream, cheer, and cover your ears. A touchdown is scored, and silence calms the saddened crowd. All sit. Equilibrium ensues.

If we could liken this scenario to cells in the milieu of the body with thousands upon thousands of conversations taking place, sodas being ordered from barkers selling cold beer and peanuts, opposing fans arguing, people shuffling between rows and hundreds of other activities, we would need to envision a million stadiums with hundreds of millions of observers to understand the complexity of the human body. Think of how difficult it is communicate when the opposing team has the ball at the one-yard line and this is similar to a cell receiving correct information in the chaos of chronic inflammation.

When histamine levels increase both within and between the cells, causing fluid to accumulate, our body responds with an intricate system to remove the water and regain equilibrium. It signals a special gene called the HNMT gene to make an enzyme that quickly drops histamine levels and fluids decrease accordingly. The crowd sits during a lull in the game. So it is, when we are exposed to allergens, histamine is released, bringing a washing of fluid, the HNMT gene makes its histamine-degrading enzyme, and tissues are cleansed, the cells are bathed, and balance is achieved. This cycle of the histamine cleanse helps us get rid of things that we eat and breath that are not beneficial.

Histamine's relationship with the stress response brings a bit of clarity on how the system can go wrong. In its protective role in the "flight, fight or freeze" response, histamine is released with an uptick of the sympathetic nervous system (SNS.) The SNS controls adrenal output and cortisol release. When we perceive danger, SNS stimulation protection raises blood pressure, shunts blood to extremities, and dilates pupils enabling us to best survive the assault. All functions considered non-essential to survival are suppressed. Our brain conserves energy. One need not reproduce when chased by a tiger; shut that down. A tiger is going to eat me; who cares if I die from mercury poisoning in ten years, shut down detoxification! I'm soon to be food to a predator, stop all wasted energy on digestion, immune function, and fighting chronic disease.

By now you're probably understanding how the modern, chronic predators of running a business, raising a family, stressful, abusive relationships, paying the bills and filling out tax forms can influence cell communication and our ability to fight disease. One could argue that modern society has created its own tigers and even rewards the increased productivity gained by the chase. The downfalls of such a system is evidenced in the rise of chronic disease, including cancer.

Higher histamine levels together with its stimulation of the H4 cell receptors have been reported in many different tumors including melanoma, colon, pancreatic, and breast cancer. Moreover, histamine content increased unequivocally in other human cancer types such as ovarian, cervical and endometrial carcinoma in comparison with their adjoining normal tissues suggesting the participation of histamine in carcinogenesis.

Histamine's story worsened when recent studies noted that most malignant cell lines express their own histamine-synthesizing enzyme, L-histidine decarboxylase (HDC) and contain high concentrations of endogenous histamine that can be released to the spaces between the cells.

Why would a cancer cell want to create commotion and disturb communication between itself and the body? One might theorize that histamine may regulate diverse biological responses related to tumor growth. Growing cancers require angiogenesis, cell invasion, migration, differentiation, stunted apoptosis and modulation of the immune response, indicating that histamine may be a crucial mediator in cancer development and progression. Many cancers have even revealed a much higher concentration of histamine receptors on their cell membranes, further suggesting that histamine stimulates proliferation.

Researchers in Finland, Sweden, and Switzerland have shown how the most aggressive form of brain cancer, glioblastoma, can be stopped in its tracks by an antihistamine drug that triggers a form of cell death caused by leaky lysosomes. Though this was a mouse study as most initial studies are, it is very promising. Headed by Pirjo Laakkonen, PhD, at the University of Helsinki, the studies demonstrated an association between the fatty acid binding protein: mammary-derived growth inhibitor (MDGI) and poorer prognosis in patients.

MDGI shuttles fatty acids into cells where they, among other things, become integral components of lysosomal membranes. Lysosomes are little organelles inside our cells that contain numerous digestive enzymes that remove waste and recycle worn-out cellular parts to help keep a cell alive. Healthy lysosomal membranes enclose these enzymes and release them inside the cell only when necessary. If we could destabilize these membranes, we could spill the content of the lysosomes (the digestive enzymes) into the cell and essentially stimulate apoptosis (cell death).

The study focused on Glioblastoma, one of the most aggressive brain cancers we face. The team's studies found that blocking the MDGI gene (thereby **not** allowing fatty acids into the cell as readily) in glioblastoma cell lines disrupted fatty acid transport into cells and their incorporation into lysosomal membranes, which compromised lysosomal membrane composition and integrity, resulting in lysosomal membrane permeabilization (LMP.) LMP is an intracellular cell death pathway triggered when the lysosome contents leak into the cell. The team's subsequent studies in cell lines and in live mice found that treatment with the anti-histamine Clemastine (Dayhist, Dayhist Allergy, and Allergy Relief), an older type of antihistamine that can cross the blood-brain barrier, effectively mirrored the effects of MDGI, triggering LMP and causing glioblastoma cell death, without harming healthy cells.

In non-brain tumors where crossing the blood-brain barrier is not an issue, theory may admit that any antihistamine, drug or natural histamine blockers, may illicit the same response in many tumors. Should all cancer patients go on antihistamine medications or histamine blocking nutrients? That remains to be answered with more studies, but this looks very promising!

Through further experiments the investigators showed that MDGI was essential to glioma cell survival. Glioma cells engineered to overexpress MDGI also grew more aggressively and invasively than non-engineered tumor cells following implantation into experimental mice. Conversely, silencing the MDGI gene dramatically reduced the viability of patient-derived glioma cells and blocked cell proliferation. Human glioblastoma cells lacking MDGI were also unable to form tumors when transplanted into mice. "These results demonstrate a dose-dependent effect of MDGI silencing on glioblastoma cell growth and viability."

A Few Ideas We Are Beginning to Implement at Conners Clinic

- The use of DAO enzyme both orally and as a rectal suppository. DAO is the specific enzyme made by the HNMT gene in the tissues as well as the ABP gene in the gut cavity. The problem with oral dosing has been its failure to be absorbed and enact any benefit to the tissues. Genetic aberrations (SNPs) or defects (mutations) may result in a lesser ability to produce such enzyme, a decreased capacity to clear histamine and a tendency to histamine related disorders including (possibly) cancer.

- The DAO enzyme requires flavin adenine dinucleotide (FAD) as its cofactor and FAD requires the B Vitamin riboflavin (B2) for its synthesis. So, adding a whole-food source of B2 may also be in order.

- A novel use of Rife frequencies in an attempt to regain the normal synchronicity of over-productive mast and basophil cells.

- Use of relatively higher dose, unique enzymes (beta glucanase, chitinase, xylanase, alpha galactosidase, phytase, astrazyme, serratiopeptidase, peptidases, and proteases) orally to aide in the reduction of histamine stimulating antigens in the digestive tract, break biofilms (histamine-responsible) surrounding the cancer, and help bond to receptor sites on the cancer.

435

- Coupling nutritional therapies with Sauna Therapy which has been shown to decrease mast cell activation.

- Stimulation of parasympathetic receptors to reduce sympathetic dominance and lower histamine release.

- Employing the Fasting Mimicking Diet (FMD) as well as Time Restricted Eating (TRE).

- Cognitive, mindful meditation and prayer.

- A deeper look at genetic pathways gives us other clues to assist DAO production. The HNMT and ADH genes require supplemental zinc, Vitamin C, magnesium, and thiamine.

- Quercetin, a natural compound found in apples, onions, and capers is a wonderful natural histamine reducer. Unfortunately, it is poorly absorbed (about 1%) so use as a suppository may prove more beneficial.

- Holy Basil, Milk Thistle, and EGCg (from green tea extract), Aloe, Bromelain, Stinging Nettle, Pine Bark Extract, Marshmallow Root, Bitter Orange, and Licorice can be helpful as may Ellagic acid found in raspberries, strawberries, walnuts, mango kernel, and pomegranate.

See Study Links:

ConnersClinic.com/histamines

ConnersClinic.com/histamine-and-cancer

What We Use

HistaClear DAO Enzyme

shop.ConnersClinic.com/hista-clear

Histamine Scavenger

shop.ConnersClinic.com/histamine-scavenger

Natural Clear Hist

shop.ConnersClinic.com/clear-hist

Burdock Root

The common burdock weed (that I hate as it grows wild in the fields near my house and is a source of annoying burrs matted in dog's fur) is also a medicinal herb of considerable reputation. Called *gobo* in Japan, burdock root is said to be a food that provides deep strengthening to the immune system. In ancient China and India, herbalists used it in the treatment of respiratory infections, abscesses, joint pain, and cancer. European physicians of the Middle Ages and later used it to treat cancerous tumors, skin conditions, venereal disease, and bladder and kidney problems.

Burdock was a primary ingredient in the famous Hoxsey cancer treatment. Other herbs in his formula included red clover, poke, prickly ash, bloodroot, and barberry. Burdock is also found in the famous herbal cancer remedy Essiac.

We use burdock quite frequently as it is in our Black Salve Bloodroot (which I take), our Essiac, our Hoxsey, and several other formulas.

What We Use

Black Salve Bloodroot

shop.ConnersClinic.com/black-salve-bloodroot

Essiac Extract

shop.ConnersClinic.com/essiac

Hoxsey-like Liquid

shop.ConnersClinic.com/hoxsey

Graviola (Soursop)

Graviola comes from a tree in the rain forests of Africa, South America, and Southeast Asia. It is a common food there. It is commonly known as custard apple, cherimoya, guanabana, soursop, and Brazilian paw paw. The active ingredient is a type of plant compound (phytochemical) called annonaceous acetogenins. People use graviola pulp in juices, smoothies, and ice cream.

There are laboratory studies that show that graviola extracts can kill some types of liver and breast cancer cells that are resistant to some chemotherapy drugs. A more recent study showed that graviola pulp extract has an effect on prostate cancer cells in mice.

Modern science still discounts any benefits of graviola, as it does to anything else they can't patent, but we have found it very beneficial when coupled in our formulas giving us the belief there is a synergistic effect among herbs.

What We Use

Black Salve Bloodroot

shop.ConnersClinic.com/black-salve-bloodroot

Glucosamine, Chondroitin and MSM

A study published in *International Journal of Cancer* suggests that taking glucosamine and chondroitin as dietary supplements may help reduce the risk of developing colorectal cancer. The current study led by E. D. Kantor from Fred Hutchinson Cancer Research Center in Seattle, WA, USA and colleagues shows that men and women using a combination of glucosamine and chondroitin for more than three years had a 45% reduced risk of colorectal cancer, compared with those who did not take the supplements.

An early study in which participants were followed for a shorter period already observed the association between use of glucosamine and chondroitin and reduced risk of colorectal cancer. For the current study, the researchers analyzed more data from an additional 2-year follow-up and found men and women reporting use of glucosamine and chondroitin on more than four days a week for more than three years were 45% less likely to be diagnosed with colorectal cancer, compared with non-users.

The researchers added, "There is great need to identify safe and effective cancer preventive strategies, suggesting that glucosamine and chondroitin may merit further attention as a potential chemo preventive agent." ***Glucosamine and chondroitin*** as dietary supplements have been commonly used for joint pain and osteoarthritis because they have anti-inflammatory properties. Many forms of cancer are believed

439

to be associated with inflammation and it is hypothesized that glucosamine and chondroitin may reduce risk of CRC through an anti-inflammatory mechanism.

See study links: ConnersClinic.com/g-and-c

What We Use

Glucosamine Sulfate/Chondroitin Sulfate MSM

shop.ConnersClinic.com/g-c

Fasting Mimicking Diet

Pre-clinical and clinical studies have proven that ***periodic fasting***, done for several consecutive days, is a very powerful intervention that our bodies learned to naturally cope with by protecting and rejuvenating itself. These two factors are both anti-aging measures that offer additional health benefits. Our 5-Day ProLon Fasting Mimicking Diet has been clinically tested and found to promote beneficial effects in a wide variety of conditions ranging from excess weight and fasting blood glucose, to growth factors associated with DNA damage and aging.

A recent randomized, controlled trial of 100 subjects, of which 71 completed 3 cycles of **ProLon** either in a randomized phase (N=39) or after being crossed over from a control diet group to the Fasting Mimicking Diet group (N=32.) Control subjects continued their normal diet. ProLon participants consumed the fasting mimicking diet (FMD) for 5 consecutive days per month for 3 months. Measurements were performed prior to the diet and during the recovery period after the 3rd cycle.

IGF-1 levels decreased, which is significant for cancer patients, and one of the main reasons we suggest this diet. Studies have shown that cancer patients with higher IGF-1 level don't fare as well as those able to keep their IGF-1 lower. Diet is typically considered the main contributing factor to keeping this under control.

The ProLon clinical trials protocol included three consecutive cycles of ProLon (5-day only per month over three consecutive months.) This is what we typically recommend. If a patient is not overweight and eats and exercises well, we suggest the product 1-2 times a year.

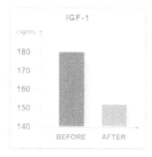

IGF-1, marker associated with increased mortality and DNA damage in human cells, was reduced by 14%.

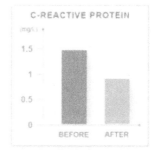

C-reactive protein (CRP) levels decreased from 1.5 mg/L to 1.0 mg/L after participants had resumed their normal diet for 5-8 days after cycle 3.

More on FMD: ConnersClinic.com/fmd

441

What We Use

Prolon FMD

shop.ConnersClinic.com/prolon-fmd

Tooth and Gum Oil

Infections of the teeth and gums are highly prevalent, often leading to tooth extractions but much more frequent than most would think. Most infections are subclinical, meaning they produce little or no symptoms and can be very difficult to detect since they are not seen on x-ray. The disease and associated symptom pattern initiated from subclinical dental infections are commonly displayed elsewhere in the body including headaches, infections of the throat, tonsils, breasts, lymph nodes and even cancer. Missing teeth can thus be considered as proxy for chronic dental infections, caries or periodontitis.

A recent study followed-up a cohort for 24 years investigating the association between missing teeth and the incidence of cancer with the hypothesis that dental chronic inflammation links to cancer.

Conclusion: In periodontally healthy subjects extracted molars, proxy for past dental infections, seemed to predict cancer risk in the studied age group; hence supporting a role of chronic dental infection/inflammation in carcinogenesis.

Another study revealed that an infection from a common type of mouth bacteria can contribute to colorectal cancer. The bacteria, called *Fusobacterium nucleatum*, can attach to colon cells and trigger a sequence of changes that can lead to colon cancer, according to the team at Case Western Reserve University School of Dental Medicine.

Swollen gums, halitosis, and cavities are serious concerns, but may be insignificant problems compared to greater dangers of subclinical tooth infection: hepatitis, cancer, heart disease, and more. Bacteria in the mouth can multiply in damaged teeth and migrate throughout the body, causing significant damage, especially in teeth that have had root canals performed, leaving them to be virtual hotels for bacteria with no blood supply to carry immune cells to mitigate their livelihood.

Bacteria Flourish in the Mouth and Teeth

Damaged teeth and root canal teeth are ideal environments for bacterial growth. The dentin of each tooth contains microscopic tubules that enter its pulp and nerve, which are hospitable to "bad" anaerobic bacteria. Root canals are especially susceptible because immune cells cannot enter the dead tooth to destroy the bacteria. Mold, fungus, bacteria, and viruses that infect the tooth can move into the bloodstream at a constant rate. The following are early signs that a root canal may be leaking bacteria into the blood:

- Periodontitis
- Halitosis
- Soreness and bleeding
- Gum or cheek inflammation

Our special Tooth and Gum oil was designed to help your body kill any periodontal infections that can destroy your health. This oil was created to simply add a drop onto your finger and rub (apply) gently over your gums, both top and bottom, inside and out. It is a proprietary blend of Black Cumin Oil and Oregano Oil. It may "sting" a bit for a short time and doesn't necessarily taste great, but it works.

What We Use

Tooth and Gum Oil

shop.ConnersClinic.com/tooth-gum-oil

Superoxide Dismutase (SOD)

Superoxide, a free radical that is supposed to be reduced through the SOD genes, may play a huge roll in the survival of a cancer cell as it blocks a major apoptotic pathway. I've created a helpful video on this subject here: ConnersClinic.com/SOD

What We Use

Pro SOD/Catalase

shop.ConnersClinic.com/pro-sod

OncoClear: Avemar Fermented Wheat Germ

There can be many health benefits from foods are derived from wheat germ. However, with the advent of gluten sensitivities, wheat germ has fallen from grace. The molecular composition of different wheat germ containing products greatly differ as shown by normal-phase HPLC-mass spectrometry analysis; thus, experimental data obtained by one of them is not necessarily true for the other.

Avemar is a nontoxic wheat germ extract registered as a special nutriment for cancer patients in Hungary. It shows potent anticancer activity on cell lines by deeply interfering with glucose metabolism and affecting expressions of several

444

kinases. In in vivo experimental models, Avemar is also effective by enhancing the activity of the immune system such as stimulating Natural Killer cell (NK cell) activity, enhancing tumor necrosis factor secretion of the macrophages. It has also been shown to increase ICAM 1 molecule expression on the vascular endothelial cells which helps stimulate an immune response. All of these lead to apoptosis of tumor cells.

There is a wide range of biological activity with Avemar. Since there are numerous experimental data and the clinical benefit repeatedly confirmed, Avemar can be a potent and well researched food supplement available for cancer patients.

What We Use

Dr. Conners' Onco Clear

shop.ConnersClinic.com/onco-clear

Galangal Root Powder

Galangal root powder (*Alpinia officinarum*) is a traditional oriental spice often used in folk medicine. Galangin, the active flavonol, exerted anticancer effects on several cancers, including melanoma, hepatoma, and colon cancer cells. Apoptotic pathways in cancer cells might be activated by prolonged stress on an organelle in the cell's cytoplasm called the endoplasmic reticulum. Studies have shown that galangin induced endoplasmic reticulum stress in hepatocellular carcinoma cells. In addition, galangin also induced autophagy in hepatocellular carcinoma cells, via activating the TGF-β receptor/Smad pathway which can also help fight cancer.

We use a raw, powdered galangal root that can be added to a smoothie or even used by itself in hot water as a tea. It has a ginger-like taste that is quite pleasant.

What We Use

Galangal Root Powder

shop.ConnersClinic.com/galangal-root-powder

Suppressing RAS Oncogenes

The family of proteins known as "Ras" and "Raf" play a central role in the regulation of cell growth; and in cancer, they suppress, or slow growth. They fulfill this fundamental role by integrating the regulatory signals that govern the cell cycle and proliferation, something grossly out of balance in a growing tumor. This means that Ras oncogenes help *turn on* normal cell death.

Defects in the Ras-Raf pathway can result in uncontrolled cancerous growth. Mutant Ras genes were among the first oncogenes identified for their ability to transform cells into a cancerous phenotype (e.g. a cell observably altered because of distorted gene expression.) Mutations in one of three genes (H, N, or K-Ras) encoding Ras proteins are associated with upregulated (increasing) cell proliferation (growth) and are found in an estimated 30-40% of all human cancers. The highest incidences of Ras mutations are found in cancers of the pancreas (80%), colon (50%), thyroid (50%), lung (40%), liver (30%), melanoma (30%), and myeloid leukemia (30%.)

The differences between oncogenes and normal genes can be slight. The mutant protein that an oncogene ultimately creates may differ from the healthy version by only a single amino acid, but this subtle variation can radically alter the protein's functionality. Remember, proteins are just a long chain of amino acids; one seemingly small change changes everything. The Ras-Raf pathway is used by human cells to transmit signals from the cell surface (the membrane) to the cell nucleus.

Such signals direct cells to divide, differentiate, or even undergo programmed cell death (apoptosis), therefore the **signals are important**.

A Ras gene usually behaves as a relay switch within the signal pathway that instructs the cell to divide. In response to stimuli transmitted to the cell from outside, cell-signaling pathways are *turned on*. In the absence of stimulus, the Ras protein remains in the *off* position. A mutated Ras protein gene behaves like a switch stuck on the *on* position, continuously misinforming the cell, instructing it to divide when the cycle should be *turned off*. So, the question is: How do you turn this switch *off*?

A number of natural substances impact the activity of Ras oncogenes. For example, limonene is a substance found in the essential oils of citrus products. Curcumin also inhibits RAS, and causes cell death in breast cancer cells expressing RAS mutations.

Japanese researchers examined the effects of Vitamin E on the presence of K-Ras mutations in mice with lung cancer. Prior to treatment with Vitamin E, K-Ras mutations were present in 64% of the mice. After treatment with Vitamin E, only 18% of the mice expressed K-Ras mutations .[174] Vitamin E decreased levels of H-Ras proteins in cultured melanoma cells.[175]

Researchers at Rutgers University investigated the ability of different green tea polyphenols to inhibit H-Ras oncogenes. The Rutgers team found that all the major polyphenols contained in green tea except epicatechin showed strong inhibition of cell growth.[176] Investigators at Texas A&M University also found that essential oils decreased colonic Ras

---

[174] Yano et al. 1997
[175] Prasad et al. 1990
[176] Chung et al. 1999

membrane localization and reduced tumor formation in rats. In view of the central role of oncogenic Ras in the development of colon cancer, the finding that essential fatty acids modulate Ras activation could explain why good omegas protect against colon cancer.

What We Use
Curcu Clear

shop.ConnersClinic.com/curcu-clear

Apop-E

shop.ConnersClinic.com/apop-e

Fatty Acid Liquescence

shop.ConnersClinic.com/FAL

Gut Health and Cancer

Surprise, surprise, what we've been saying for years is now being verified by "real science": the gut plays a huge part in cancer. Top scientists at Roche Holding AG and AstraZeneca Plc are sizing up potential allies in the fight against cancer: the trillions of bacteria that live in the human body.

"Five years ago, if you had asked me about bacteria in your gut playing an important role in your systemic immune response, I probably would have laughed it off," Daniel Chen, head of cancer immunotherapy research at Roche's Genentech division, said in a phone interview. "Most of us immunologists now believe that there really is an important interaction there."

Two recent studies published in the journal *Science* have intrigued Chen and others who are developing medicines called immunotherapies that stimulate the body's ability to fight tumors.

Our Gut Check Protocol

Remove Foods That Cause Damage

- Food sensitivities such as gluten, corn, soy, and dairy cause inflammation in the gut that damages cells and allows passage of toxins across the gut wall.

- Testing for toxins is essential and ***complete removal*** is absolutely necessary!

Begin a Course of Prebiotics

Prebiotics feed the intestinal cells, which increases the healthy mucus layer that is necessary for your microbiota to grow and live.

- SunFiber, SunSpectrum, and SBI Protect are the best products as they are a source of indigestible fiber and gut healing nutrients. This is essential for your gut to create butyrate, the desired food for intestinal cells that then enable them to create the mucus necessary for the perfect home for your flora.

- These foods eaten every day feed your gut cells:
    o Raw dandelion greens
    o Raw garlic
    o Raw onions, leeks and the onion family
    o Raw asparagus
    o Green bananas
    o Chicory (often used in coffee substitutes)

Begin Taking Oral Probiotics

We recommend rotating different brands and strains based upon your need/condition.

Probiotic Enemas

See ConnersClinic.com/pro-enema

Begin Fecal Microbiota Transplantation (FMT) Therapy

What We Use

SunFiber

shop.ConnersClinic.com/sunfiber

SunSpectrum

shop.ConnersClinic.com/sunspectrum

Clear SBI Protect

shop.ConnersClinic.com/clear-sbi-protect

Clear Pro 100

shop.ConnersClinic.com/clear-pro-100

Enema Kit

shop.ConnersClinic.com/enema-kit

Compounds That Slow Glycolysis

As a young scientist in the 1920's, Otto Heinrich Warburg described an elevated rate of glycolysis occurring in cancer cells, even in the presence of atmospheric oxygen (the Warburg effect) that earned him a Nobel Prize. Glycolysis is the metabolic pathway where cells take glucose to produce energy for cell function and replication.

The alternative cancer world has long seen this fact as a therapeutic strategy to help block cancer's fuel source. Here contains some of the latest scientific data that support various natural compounds effect on glycolysis to inhibit the Warburg effect.

Hypoxia inducible factor-1 (HIF-1) is one of the key transcription factors that play major roles in tumor glycolysis and could directly trigger the Warburg effect. Thus, how to inhibit HIF-1-dependent, Warburg effect, to assist the cancer therapy is becoming a hot issue in cancer research. While the pharmaceutical industry scrambles to produce a patentable drug, research is backing natural substances that we can use now.

Here are a few details about HIF-1. It up regulates the glucose transporters (GLUT) that increase the amount of glucose getting into the cell, a bad thing for those with cancer as it fuels the fire. It induces the expression of glycolytic enzymes, such as hexokinase, pyruvate kinase, and lactate dehydrogenase, so glucose is more readily used as an energy source. If there exist natural compounds to help regulate these glycolysis-signaling pathways, we may help more people with cancer.

First let's explore nutrients that may regulate the glucose transporters that are related to glycolysis. Many natural compounds affect expression of glucose transporters (especially GLUT1 and GLUT4) indirectly. Flavones, polyphenols, and alkaloids are interesting bioactive anticancer molecules isolated from plants, as several of them have been repeatedly reported to control glucose transporter activity in different cancer cell models.

Flavones are plant-derived compounds that are commonly consumed in the diet as flavonoids. These are present in fruits, vegetables, tea, red wine, dark chocolate, and herbs such as ginkgo biloba, and milk thistle. Polyphenols give fruits, berries, and vegetables their vibrant colors, and contribute to the bitterness, astringency, flavor, and aroma. They are found in a wide variety of foods, herbs, berries, fruits, and spices.

These compounds have various names (*Fisetin, myricetin, quercetin, apigenin, genistein, cyanidin, daidzein, hesperetin, naringenin,* and *catechin*) with distinct properties. As a matter of fact, comparative studies indicated that these compounds do not exhibit the same mode of action as they bind different domains of GLUT1 to slow glucose transmission. Genistein (an isoflavone found in soy) binds the transporter on the external face whereas quercetin (a flavonoid found in many fruits and vegetables) interacts with the internal face. It's as if they play different positions on the team's defensive line, blocking the opposition at alternate angles.

Numerous research articles have been written on the benefits of each of these, but it may be the synergy between them, as they are naturally found in food sources that really make them winners. Together, they are well-known inhibitors of glucose uptake in human cells making them beneficial for cancer patients but also diabetics and just about any other inflammatory disorder.

There are also genetic mutations that influence aerobic glycolysis that curcumin (the active form of the Indian spice turmeric) has proven to reverse. Another natural isoflavinoid, 4-O-methyl alpinumisoflavone, isolated from the tropical rainforest tree, Lonchocarpus glabrescens, could inhibit HIF-1 activation and hypoxic induction of HIF-1 target genes (CDKN1A, GLUT-1, and vascular endothelial growth factor (VEGF)).

Also, long chained fatty acid derivatives extracted from Graviola have recently shown multiple anticancer activities on pancreatic cancer cell models. Torres et al. highlighted the ability of this compound to inhibit glucose uptake, and it has strong ability to reduce the expression levels of GLUT1 and GLUT4, HKII, and LDH-A pathways, making it a great player against most cancers.

I believe that getting your nutrition from your food is the best approach to care whenever possible. We can get plenty of GLUT blocking players from organic vegetables, fruits, herbs and spices. It is best to eat them as near to the way God made them, organic, fresh, and whole. While juicing has advantages in predigesting, it removes some of its value. Maybe blending is a better option. Other nutrients mentioned, like Curcumin and Graviola, might better be consumed a supplement. You can get CurcuClear at shop.ConnersClinic.com/curcu-clear

While the alternative cancer world has long seen this fact as a therapeutic strategy, current research is giving us multiple avenues to support cancer patients naturally. Let's explore the latest scientific data that support various natural compounds effect on glycolysis to inhibit the Warburg effect.

Hexokinase (HK) is an enzyme found in all cells that aides the processing of glucose thereby increasing a fuel source for cancer. Ionidamine, a HK inhibitor, has become new drug that interferes with mitochondrial functions, thereby inhibiting cellular oxygen consumption and energy metabolism in both normal and cancerous cells. Some natural compounds have been described as promoting the detachment of HK from mitochondria without any nasty side effects.

Prosapogenin A, a saponin from Chinese herb Veratrum nigrum (black false hellebore or Li Lu in Chinese herbalism), could inhibit cell growth and promote cell apoptosis. Methyl jasmonate, a plant stress hormone produced by many plants including rosemary, olive, and ginger, inhibits HK, triggering apoptosis in cancer cells.

Another enzyme, pyruvate kinase, is specifically expressed in cancer cells and plays an important role in the metabolism and replication. Oleanolic acid, a triterpene found in numerous herbs (*Bearberry, Heather, Reishi, Chinese Elder, Olive Leaf Extract,* etc.) is an anti-tumor compound that suppresses aerobic glycolysis in cancer cells and targets numerous other pathways that stimulate cell death.

Another novel therapeutic target in inhibiting cancer aerobic glycolysis is to slow the function of another enzyme, LDH-A. As an important factor in NAD regeneration, LDH-A was found to be overexpressed in various types of cancer including renal, breast, gastric, and nasopharyngeal cancer. Inhibition of LDH-A might lead to an energy production blockade in cancer cells.

EGCg from Green tea extract (we use Teavigo)nhas been recently shown to have LDH-A inhibiting activity. But other natural compounds, such as furanodiene and maslinic acid (found in curcumin, ginger, and olive oil derivatives) could increase the LDH release in cancer cells by inducing cancer cell injury.

Grab your Teavigo at shop.ConnersClinic.com/teavigo

Study Links

ConnersClinic.com/glycolysis-1

ConnersClinic.com/glycolysis-2

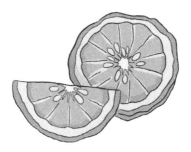

Bergamot

Acetyl-CoA, an important compound for cellular energy production, is the precursor for the synthesis of fatty acids, energy production, and cholesterol. Both glucose (sugar) and glutamine (amino acids) can contribute to the body's generation of acetyl-CoA. Acetate has recently been shown to be yet another source of acetyl-CoA for many different cancer types, including breast, prostate, liver, primary glioblastomas and brain metastases. Some of these cancerous tissues incorporate acetate into fatty acids to support the cancer's veracious need for structural elements in growth, whereas others have been shown to use acetate to fuel the TCA (Krebs energy) cycle that feed its need for energy.[177]

Therefore, acetate might become a crucial nutritional source in poorly vascularized regions of tumors. The acetyl-CoA generated from glucose, glutamine or acetate (or potentially other nutritional sources) supplies the cholesterol and fatty acids synthesis demand of cancer cell growth.

There has been a hypothesis that cancer patients treated with

---

[177] Comerford et al., 2014; Kamphorst et al., 2014; Mashimo et al., 2014; Schug et al., 2015

statins could be associated with a reduced incidence of cancer. This has stimulated some research on the use of statins for cancer prevention.[178] However, to date, clinical trials designed to specifically test cancer prevention by statin treatment have not been conclusive[179] and the other negative effects of statins (liver damage, decreased function of liver detoxification pathways, and CoQ10 depletion) seem to be too great a risk to take for cancer patients especially since liver metastasis is so common.

A novel approach to naturally hindering the same pathway without any of the side-effects may be in the use Bergamot Bioactive Polyphenolic Fractions (BPFs.) BPFs contains a powerful and unique array of cholesterol-balancing and cardio-protective polyphenolic flavonoids that act similarly to statins. Emerging clinical research has demonstrated that BPFs help maintain healthy total cholesterol (TC), high density lipoprotein (HDL), low density lipoprotein (LDL), very low-density lipoprotein (VLDL) and triglyceride (TRI) levels naturally.

Bergamot (*Citrus bergamia*) is a citrus plant that grows almost exclusively in the narrow coastal Calabria region in southern Italy. The local population quickly discovered bergamot juice could be used to help support healthy cholesterol levels and optimize cardiovascular wellness.

Bergamot's health benefits derive from its unique profile of phenolic compounds such as, neoeriocitrin, neohesperidin, naringin, rutin, neodesmin, rhoifolin and poncirin. Naringin has been shown to be beneficial in maintaining normal inflammatory balance, while neoeriocitrin and rutin have been found to exhibit a strong capacity to quench free radicals and maintain healthy LDL cholesterol levels. Also, bergamot is rich in brutieridine and melitidine, which have a unique

---

[178] Baandrup et al., 2015; Boudreau et al., 2010
[179] Bertagnolli et al., 2010; Cardwell et al., 2015

ability to dampen HMG-CoA reductase, and ***that*** is the key!

The tumor-promoting effects of enhanced fatty acid synthesis were first appreciated in the 1990s when fatty acid synthase (FASN) expression was identified as prognostic marker of aggressive breast cancers.[180]

The tendency of ovarian cancers to metastasize to the omentum has been shown to be driven by crosstalk between adipocytes (fat cells and accompanying fatty acids) and the ovarian cancer cells.[181] The uptake of fatty acids not only by the tumor cells but also the connective tissue cells necessary for building new cancer cells can affect continued tumor progression. In short, the more a cancer can efficiently make use of fatty acids, the poorer the prognosis.

Furthermore, cancers crave fatty acids and can activate adipose triglyceride lipase (a very specific enzyme that breaks down the body's fat) in the white adipose tissue and skeletal muscle to make use of such fatty acids for continued growth. This has been linked to cachexia, suggesting that inhibition of such lipases might help alleviate the devastating problems associated with it.[182]

Enter ***Bergamot***, one possible hero.

One study on Colorectal cancer (CRC) revealed evidence that citrus bergamia juice extracts (BJe) reduces CRC cell growth by multiple mechanisms. Another showed that bergamot even eradicated cancer stem cells!

---

[180] Kuhajda et al., 1994
[181] Nieman et al., 2011
[182] Das et al., 2011

Study Links

ConnersClinic.com/bergamot

What We Use
Bergamot BPF

shop.ConnersClinic.com/bergamot

Blocking Metastasis

Most cancers shed malignant cells called circulating tumor cells (CTCs) or cancer stem cells. These can be considered micro metastases that, thanks to your healthy immune system, usually fail to grow in their new locations. CTCs are doing just as they are named: they are circulating through the body looking for a place to set up a home and raise a family. This is the deadly metastasis that we all dread. What encourages a micro metastasis to become a clinically apparent macro metastasis? New data is encouraging for doctors like me:

Primary Cancers Release CTCs

CTCs are kept "at bay" by a healthy immune system. This, unfortunately, is the catch-22 of chemotherapy; as it may help destroy the primary cancer, it also destroys the patient's immune system allowing an increased risk for CTCs become a full-blown metastasis. Keeping a healthy immune system is paramount.

Primary Cancers Release Exosomes

Exosomes (membrane vesicles of endocytic origin that contain lipids, DNA, RNA, and proteins) are released by malignant cells, travel to the liver, and prepare it to foster growth of metastatic cells. A recent study showed that exosomes released by pancreatic ductal adenocarcinoma cells traveled to the liver and were "ingested" by Kupffer cells in the liver. The contents of the exosomes caused the Kupffer cells to elaborate various factors that fostered growth of micro metastases. In particular, exosomes, rich in macrophage migration inhibitory factor (MIF) were most likely to foster growth.

In lay person terms, primary cancers release chemicals (exosomes) that ***inhibit*** (through MIF) an immune attack on the primary cancer as well as the CTCs. Cancer is trying to survive, grow, and reproduce!

The next question should be: How do we stop, bind, and block, exosomes from inhibiting our immune system?

Here's what we have found:

- Use a Rife Machine!

- Using chelating agents such as modified citrus pectin (MCP), chlorella, NAC, cilantro, garlic, and ALA can help bind both CTCs and exosomes to rid them from your body.

- Decreasing inflammatory cytokines through green tea extract (EGCg), Boswellia, curcumin, quercetin, rutin, ginger, nettles, and rosemary can greatly decrease the risk of metastasis.

- Supporting liver detoxification pathways including diagnosing methylation defects is essential.

- Supporting a healthy immune system is a must!

Cachexia Support

Cachexia is a condition that relates to an excessive, uncontrollable loss of body weight, and occurs because a person's fat and muscle mass break down and burn as energy for a growing tumor. The term "Cachexia" comes from two Greek words: "Kakos" (bad), and "hexis" (condition.) Stopping the downward spiral has been difficult, as medications have not proven successful.

Take a look at my video on supporting Cachexia at ConnersClinic.com/cachexia

Nausea Support

Nausea is a common issue with those with cancer and something with which I've often struggled. There are several things you should address, from making sure your bowel habits are regular, adding digestive enzymes to your meals, and potentially increasing your frequency of coffee enemas.

Two products taken orally have been a great help for me: Not Now Nausea, an oral spray, and Digize, an essential oil. I use Digize taking just a few drops when nausea becomes annoying and have found it very helpful. I've also used Cinnamon essential oil with success.

Many of my patients have also found that Not Now Nausea worked well. Tempering nausea makes life much more pleasant and keeps you from losing too much weight.

What We Use

Digize

shop.ConnersClinic.com/digize

Not Now Nausea

shop.ConnersClinic.com/not-now-nausea

Liver Support

Milk Thistle

Milk Thistle extract has been used for many decades in the treatment of liver disorders and as a standard liver detoxification herb. Approximately 80% of this extract consists of silymarin and is believed to be responsible for most of the liver-protective activity of silymarin and Milk Thistle extract. Just within the last decade scientists have learned that silibinin has considerable potential for preventing and treating cancer; mainly through stimulating liver detox pathways.

Milk Thistle has also been shown to have growth inhibitory effects on a wide range of human cancer cell lines including cancers arising from the prostate, breast, colon, lung, liver, bladder, and cervix. It can suppress the proliferation of these cells, while at the same time increasing the rate at which they die. In addition, it can sensitize cancer cell lines to the killing effects of certain cytotoxic chemotherapeutic drugs. Thus, Milk Thistle may have potential both for retarding the growth and spread of cancer and for boosting the response of cancers to chemotherapy.

The mechanisms responsible for these effects have been studied most intensively in human prostate cancer cells. Also note that Milk Thistle, though it may retard the growth of cancers, does not influence the growth of healthy normal cells. The anti-proliferative effects of Milk Thistle on prostate cancer cells have been traced to decreased function of the epidermal growth factor receptor (EGF-R.) This is a key mediator of growth signals in prostate cancer and in many other types of cancer. Milk Thistle binds to this receptor and prevents it from interacting with hormones that activate it; some of which are produced by prostate cancers. Furthermore, Milk Thistle induces prostate cancer cells to make more of a compound, known as IGFBP-3, that binds to and inhibits the activity of insulin-like growth factor-1 (IGF-1), a key growth factor for many cancers.

Also, other studies have shown that Milk Thistle may suppress the NF-kappaB signaling pathway. This effect increases the sensitivity of cancers to certain chemotherapy drugs. The impact of orally administered Milk Thistle on the growth of human tumors in immune-deficient mice has been studied with three different types of tumors: prostate, lung, and ovarian. In each case, it has been found to have a substantial and dose-dependent suppressive effect on tumor growth in doses that had no apparent toxicity to treated animals.

Prior to using Milk Thistle, *please* review the detoxification pathways outlined in Section 4 of Chapter 2.

Important Note

Please understand that I cannot possibly list every beneficial nutrient in this book. Please don't write me with complaints; *but* please *do* write me if something not listed here has helped you. I am extremely open-minded and desire nothing but to help others. If you have knowledge that I don't have, I want to know about it!

I also am not so naïve to believe that this book and its contents will make everyone happy. We have those that hate the fact that "common people" like us are able to know as much as the "elite few" who control the purse strings of officials in the FDA and government. I look forward to the day "Dr." Stephen Barrett lists me on his "quackwatch" site; it would be a badge of honor!

There are just too many other beneficial nutrients to detail. Here are just a few more:

Lemon Balm (*Melissa officinalis*), Olive Leaf extract, Barley Grass, Wheat Grass, Kamut Grass, Oat Grass, Alfalfa Grass, Gynostemma Leaf, Ashitaba, Hydrilla, Verticillata, Spirulina, Dunaliella salina, Lycium fruit, Gynostemma Leaf Extract, Polygonum Multiflorum Extract, Tibetan Rhodiola Root Extract, Ashwaganda Root Extract, Asparagus Root Extract, Agaricus Mushroom Extract, Juicing (Brussels Sprouts, Cabbage, Carrot, Cauliflower, Celery, Cucumber, Green Bell Pepper, Kale, Onion, Spinach, Tomato), Amaranth Sprout, Azuki Sprout, Chia Seed Sprout, Flax Seed Sprout, Garbanzo Bean Sprout, Kidney Bean Sprout, Lentil Sprout, Millet Sprout, Pumpkin Sprout, Quinoa Sprout, Sesame Seed Sprout, Sunflower Seed Sprout; Garlic, Ginger, Kombu Extract, Bladderwrack, Grapestone, Sea Fern, Schizandra, Blueberry, Lycium, Cherry, Acerola Cherry, Papaya, Luohanguo, Bitter Melon, Rice Bran Solubles, Arabinogalactan, Apple Pectin, Guilin Sweetfruit, Pineapple Concentrate; Taking Probiotics such as Lactobacillus Acidophilus, Lactobacillus Delbreukii, Lactobacillus Bulgaricus, Lactobacillus Plantarum.

Things We Recommend You *Not* Take

Human Growth Hormone (HGH) and Growth Hormone Stimulators

HGH has been a big hype in the professional athletic world and nutritional companies have been selling HGH stimulators for years. HGH stimulates production of insulin-like growth factor 1 (IGF-1), a hormone that has growth-stimulating effects on a wide variety of tissues. It helps tissues grow, including bones and muscles.

In addition to increasing height in children and adolescents, growth hormone has many other effects on the body:

- Increases calcium retention, and strengthens and increases the mineralization of bone
- Increases muscle mass
- Promotes lipolysis (breakdown of fat)
- Increases protein synthesis
- Stimulates the growth of all internal organs excluding the brain
- Plays a role in homeostasis (normal balance of everything)
- Reduces liver uptake of glucose
- Promotes gluconeogenesis in the liver
- Contributes to the maintenance and function of pancreatic cells
- Stimulates the immune system

On paper, it seems that HGH would be great for cancer, but it's **not**! It has been shown to cause cancer cells to grow!! I have never promoted hormone therapy, and this is another reason why I take that stance. Simple: Don't artificially mess with hormones. Also, do **not** take the HGH stimulators if you have cancer!!

More on IGF-1

There have been recent studies that higher levels of IGF-1 can increase the risk of different cancers. I already stated above that taking HGH or HGH stimulators will increase IGF-1, but dietary considerations are important as well. IGF-1's primary action is mediated by binding to its specific receptor in the cell membrane, the Insulin-like growth factor 1 receptor (IGF1R), present on many cell types in many tissues. When IGF-1 docks into the IGF1R, it initiates intracellular signaling; IGF-1 is one of the most potent natural activators of the AKT signaling pathway, a stimulator of cell growth and proliferation. That's what it's supposed to do: stimulate ***growth***. ***But*** it also is an extremely potent inhibitor of programmed cell death (apoptosis).

So, higher levels of IGF-1 = decreased death of cells that are supposed to die. Increased IGF-1 = increased cancer growth!

What can you do about it?

- Don't take HGH or natural stimulators of HGH
- Watch your diet! Sugar stimulate IGF-1 production
- Stop/decrease bad carbohydrates other than sugar (see *Cancer Diet*)
- Reduce body fat (exercise)
- Get help for Metabolic Syndrome (talk to your doctor)

Should I Drink Alkaline Water?

The acid-alkaline balance is controlled by a powerful buffering system largely mediated by calcium channels. Much has been written about cancer and alkalization and it has become a popular belief that cancer cells cannot grow in an alkaline environment. Let's try to understand where this information came from and how we can separate fact from fiction; there will be much to benefit as far as health is concerned.

Fact: The pH of the body is important and needs to be maintained in a semi-neutral state to achieve homeostasis.

Fact: Diet does play an important role in maintaining a neutral pH

Fact: Poor diet, including the typical American diet, contribute to lowering tissue pH levels (create a greater acidity).

Fact: Increased acidity (lower pH levels) in the cells and extracellular spaces contributes to poorer cellular function and more sluggish removal of extracellular toxins.

Fact: Cancer cells do have an acidic "slime" layer that surrounds the growing mass.

Fiction: Cancer cannot grow in an alkaline environment. This is not true. The reason that cancer has an acidic layer that surrounds it is because the rapidly replicating cells are producing a vast amount of waste that cannot be cleared quickly enough by the lymphatic system. This acidic layer then protects the growing cells limiting the Th1 immune cytokines from making an assault. Dr. Tullio Simoncini, the Italian MD who was imprisoned for injecting sodium bicarbonate solution into cancer sites had some success in breaking down the acidic wall. There are just too many buffering systems to think that alkalization of the stomach can perform the same feat.

Fact: You have to understand physiology; pH of the blood will always be maintained at the expense of the tissue. A diet high in carbs, additives, flavorings, chemicals, excitotoxins, etc. tend to acidify the system, **not** because they are acidic themselves, but because of what the body needs to do to detoxify such garbage. Our bodies do not become alkaline because we drink alkaline water any more than we become acidic because we eat things that have a low pH. Sure, soda pop is acidifying to the system but **not** because it is acidic (it is), it is acidifying because of the increased (and overwhelming) pressure the accumulation of poor food choices has on the liver and cellular organelles.

How do we alkalize the tissue? Is that a goal? Yes and no. Our goal should be to detoxify and stop toxifying the body by getting back to the way we were meant to eat. Vegetables and whole fruit help to bring balance back to the system and are alkalizing to the tissue, **not** because they register higher on the pH scale (lemons are extremely acidic) but because of what they do **inside** us. They are filled with nutrients and enzymes that aide healing. Understand, I can destroy a carrot by growing it conventionally with fertilizers and pesticides, process it, blanch it, can it, and let it store on a grocers shelf for nine months and **think** I'm doing right by eating vegetables, but my carrot side dish may now be equally acidifying to my system as a can of soda. It is both the type and quality of food choices that either brings healing or destruction.

Live, raw, organic food is the best "alkalizer." This is why juicing (making your own homemade carrot, apple, celery juice, etc.) is the best. It is a pre-digested bundle of nutrition that alkalizes your tissue. It also carries an abundant number of enzymes that assist the breakdown of the acidic "slime" layer of cancer.

Fiction: What's wrong with alkaline water, doesn't that help? **No**, I am firmly against drinking alkaline water in an attempt to alkalize the tissue. First, it can contribute to the hypochlorhydria that has setup your ill health in the first place. Hypochlorhydria is probably the most common health problem in the modern world and is characterized as a decreased stomach acid production largely caused by the chemicals in food that have irritated the stomach's acid producing cells. Symptoms include increased gas, GERD, reflux, upset stomach, etc., and most people treat the symptoms with antacids (Prilosec, Tagamet or Rolaids.) These medications will relieve the symptoms but are exactly what **not** to do. People with a deceased stomach acid are not able to digest their food and it sits in the stomach longer, causing upset, fermentation of carbohydrates, and possible

467

regurgitating what little acid is there up through the esophagus causing reflux. Again, you can negate the symptoms by using antacids or you can fix the problem by adding digestive enzymes and HCl (in supplement form) to the diet with each meal until the stomach cells have healed enough to take over their responsibility.

There are several other reasons I do not recommend alkalizing your water but will comment on just one more. Several recent studies in *JAMA* have pointed out that subclinical, undiagnosed H. Pylori infections are far more common that otherwise thought. One study stated that nearly 50% of the world's population suffers from an undiagnosed H. Pylori infection. H. Pylori can be responsible for ulcers but can also infiltrate the epithelial tissue to cause autoimmune inflammation of the cardiovascular tissue and even sinusitis and Rosacea. Alkalizing a stomach that is meant to give the individual a first-line defense against pathogens, maintain a pH of about 1.5 to digest food, and quickly do its job to move bolus through the system seems counterproductive.

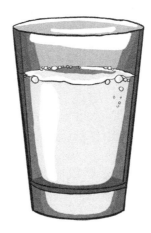

Water Purification

There is much to be said about toxins in our water, but let's just take a commonsense approach. If we are attempting to detoxify poisons in our body, it only makes sense to eliminate as many sources of toxic exposure as possible. Drinking water is one source.

Out of all the types of water purification, I like Reverse Osmosis (RO) filtration best. RO is a process in which dissolved inorganic solids (such as salts, heavy metals, etc.) are removed from a solution (water in this case.) This is accomplished by household water pressure pushing the tap water through a semi permeable membrane. The membrane (which is about as thick as cellophane) allows only the water to pass through, not the impurities or contaminates. These impurities and contaminates are flushed down the drain. Good RO systems remove most everything larger than .001 microns.

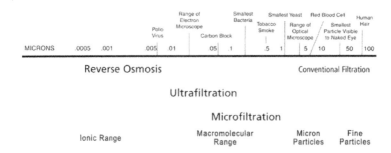

Though RO purification removes all "bad" things like heavy metals and contaminants, it also removes good minerals; so you must make sure you are taking a mineral supplement if you are drinking RO water. This is why some say that RO water is "dead" water. I agree. It's a pretty easy "fix" and the benefits of removing all the stuff that RO does far outweigh the negative of having to take a mineral supplement.

Like everything, not every RO unit is created equal. We use a unit produced by EcoWater Systems and it seems to be the best that I've researched. Just don't buy a super cheap one as the quality of the membrane equals the quality of filtered water at the opposite end.

Remarks

Regardless of what you choose about healthcare, I pray that you make wise, rational decisions based on facts (though often hidden) and not fear. You need to take responsibility and not hand it over to any practitioner, conventional or alternative. Get advice from many, weigh it all against their biases, and pray for peace about your decisions.

CHAPTER 6

Conclusion & Final Thoughts

"You gain strength, courage, and confidence by every experience in which you really stop to look fear in the face."

— Eleanor Roosevelt

Dealing with Specific Problems

Decreased Platelet Counts

Low blood platelet levels are called thrombocytopenia and can result in excessive bleeding when injury occurs. It is common with cancer patients, especially if they've done some chemotherapy or radiation as their body decreases production. Platelets are the tiny cells in your blood that function to take part in the clotting process. Each platelet contains granules that enhance the platelets' ability to stick to each other and the surface of a damaged blood vessel wall. An adequate number of platelets prevent hemorrhaging from a ruptured blood vessel. You can naturally increase your platelets to ensure the prevention of a leakage of red blood cells and lessen the chance of hemorrhage through diet.

Thrombocytopenia can also be a side effect of chemotherapy drugs that damage the bone marrow stem cells that normally produce platelets. The Phase I trial showed that Beljanski's

RNA fragments (now available as a nonprescription nutraceutical) could prevent thrombocytopenia by inducing the production of new platelets. Patients taking the RNA fragments had their platelet levels return to normal and chemotherapy treatments were completed without dose reductions, platelet transfusions, or suspensions. The RNA fragments protected platelet levels in patients with many different types of cancer who were taking many different anti-cancer drugs. Moreover, patients did not suffer any negative side effects as a result of taking the RNA fragments. The results suggest further studies aimed at establishing the RNA fragments as a standard component in all chemotherapies that cause significant platelet loss.

Cancer Treatment Centers of America® (CTCA) have completed a clinical trial on the Beljanski's formula of RNA fragments, which was conducted among cancer patients undergoing different chemotherapies. Thanks to the RNA fragments prepared according to Dr. Beljanski's proprietary process, the cancer patients all recovered a stronger immune system and managed to go through the end of their chemotherapy treatment without getting thrombocytopenia (a frequent and dangerous side effect of the chemotherapy drugs.)

Other things to consider to help increase platelet activity:

- Fresh fruits
- Green leafy vegetables
- Cod Liver or flax seed oil
- Tomatoes
- Berries
- Mushroom capsules
- Fresh garlic

As stated in our *Cancer Diet* section in Chapter 4:

- Avoid refined sugars, saturated fats, processed foods and grains and aerated (carbonated) beverages. These foods cause the platelets to fall.

- Stay away from all dairy products, alcohol, and food additives.

- Consume only healthy organic foods, fruits and vegetables. This helps to stimulate your internal mechanism, which increases your platelet count. Eat tomatoes and berries, which are loaded with vitamins and minerals with strong antioxidant properties that help you to increase your platelets. Add many green leafy vegetables to your daily diet. They tend to increase the hemoglobin level of blood, tackling the underlying cause of low levels of platelets. Red foods like tomatoes, cherries, watermelon, plums and berries are helpful.

- Wash all raw foods thoroughly to remove any parasites or viruses that could result in lowering your platelet counts. Parasitic antigens are the most common cause of low platelet counts. If you can get checked and treated for bio-toxin, parasitic, mycotoxin disorders, do so immediately.

- Strengthen your immune system using parent omegas (PEOs.) These oils will also reduce inflammation, improve your circulation and increase your ratio of high-density lipoprotein to low-density lipoprotein levels.

- Take a supplemental mushroom extract (not mushrooms.) Look for a capsule that has the extract of shitake, maitake and other mushroom varieties that help to balance out the immune system.

- Add plenty of fresh garlic and supplement your diet with vitamins and minerals such as Coenzyme Q10; selenium; zinc; melatonin; Vitamins A, B, D and E;

Omega-3; and iron supplements. These will enhance your immunity and ability to fight diseases.

- Papaya leaf powder or papaya leaf tea is a great natural platelet booster. The powder can be mixed into water, juice or any shake and the tea can be used in milder conditions.

Cachexia

Cachexia is the term we use for a "wasting disorder" seen in cancer patients when their body is literally eating up their muscles in order to produce glucose for the growing tumor.

"Cachexia is the wasting away of the cancer patient's body. The person is reduced to skin and bones, while the cancer continues growing vigorously. What is happening is that the cancer incompletely metabolizes glucose, turning it into lactic acid ... This lactic acid (if it reaches the bloodstream) travels to the liver where it is converted back into glucose by a procedure that consumes an enormous amount of the body's energy. This happens over and over again as the cancer grows and the rest of the body wastes away. Hydrazine Sulfate blocks a key enzyme in the liver that allows lactic acid to be converted into glucose."[183]

We read something interesting at the end of this quote: *"Hydrazine Sulfate blocks a key enzyme in the liver that allows lactic acid to be converted into glucose."* Hydrazine Sulfate was developed by Dr. Joseph Gold of Syracuse University. It helps metabolize excess lactic acid which causes an imbalance and extreme stress on the system. This imbalance causes the liver to expend enormous amounts of energy to convert the lactic acid back to glucose only to be reconverted back to lactic acid in cancer cell as it uses the glucose for energy. The body's expenditure of energy in this process eventually results in it wasting away and a "stealing" of muscle protein to keep up with the demand of glucose.

---

[183] http://www.alkalizeforhealth.net/cancerpain.htm

Here is another way of looking at this cycle:

"Cachexia: in a chronic infection/chronic disease, the patient's temperature rises, the CD4 count drops below the CD8 count, and the appetite wanes until the patient develops pathological anorexia. The body still needs nourishment, so it begins breaking down its fat stores, the process of glycogenesis, and also begins to break down proteins (muscles) to deliver these sugar precursors, the ones produced by glycogenesis, to the body. The metabolism of tumor/cancer cells is much less efficient than those of normal cells: normal cells metabolize aerobically, using oxygen, which is 15 times more efficient than cancer cells that metabolize anaerobically, through a process of fermentation. Fermentation, being less efficient, requires much more sugar than aerobically metabolizing cells. Additionally, the metabolism rate of a tumor is much higher than that of normal cells, so the amount of sugar needed is still greater. Eventually the patient dies trying to feed the tumor. Starvation is the major cause of death in cancer and AIDS patients."[184]

In short, when the person quits eating, the body starts to eat itself in order to feed the cancer cells.

Questions and Answers About Hydrazine Sulfate from The National Cancer Institute

What is Hydrazine Sulfate?

Hydrazine sulfate is a compound that has been studied as a treatment for cancer and for cancer-related anorexia (loss of appetite) and cachexia (loss of muscle mass and body weight.)

---

[184] http://www.mnwelldir.org/docs/cancer1/altthrpy2.htm

What is the History of the Discovery and use of Hydrazine Sulfate as a Complementary or Alternative Treatment for Cancer?

It has been known since the early 1900s that hydrazine compounds are toxic to animals and to humans. More than 400 hydrazine-related compounds have been tested for their ability to kill cancer cells. One of these compounds, procarbazine, has been used to treat Hodgkin's disease, melanoma, and lung cancer since the 1960s.

In view of procarbazine's anticancer activity, hydrazine sulfate (a compound similar to procarbazine) was studied for its effectiveness in fighting cancer beginning in the 1970s. Studies of hydrazine sulfate as a treatment for cancer-related cachexia also began during this time.

Hydrazine compounds have also been used to make rocket fuel, as herbicides (chemicals that kill plants), and as chemical agents in boiler and cooling-tower water systems. Many scientists consider hydrazine sulfate and other similar substances to be cancer-causing agents and are concerned about the safety of using these compounds.

What is the Theory Behind the Claim that Hydrazine Sulfate is Useful in Treating Cancer?

Two theories have been suggested to explain how hydrazine sulfate acts against cancer and cachexia:

1. Hydrazine sulfate may prevent the body from making sugar that cancer cells need to grow. It has been suggested that cachexia occurs because the cancer is using too much of the body's sugar, preventing healthy cells from getting what they need to live. This causes tissues to die and muscle to waste away, and the patient loses weight.

2. Hydrazine sulfate may block tumor necrosis factor-alpha (TNF-alpha.) This is a substance made by the body's white blood cells to fight infection and tissue damage. High levels of TNF-alpha have been found in cancer patients. These high levels of TNF-alpha may cause loss of appetite, tiredness, and the breakdown of muscle tissue. As muscle breaks down, it makes sugar that the cancer cells use to grow. Blocking the TNF-alpha might stop tumor growth and prevent cachexia.

How is Hydrazine Sulfate Administered?

Hydrazine sulfate is taken by mouth in pills or capsules. There is no standard dose or length of treatment time.

To read more on what the NCI has to say, go to their website.[185]

Bottom Line: Using hydrazine sulfate is an option if a patient is wasting away. I don't believe that it kills cancer cells or should be a part of a cancer regimen unless the patient is rapidly losing weight and dwindling away. Make sure you see your doctor and talk to them about this as there are some negative effects of hydrazine and it can interfere with some natural approaches as well. Overall, the ***best*** treatment for cachexia is the *Cancer Diet* with an increased amount of juicing.

If taking Hydrazine, you must avoid any foods that contains Tyramine, a monoamino from the amino acid Tyrosine that Hydrazine acts on by limiting its breakdown. Do not consume foods containing tyramine; most of these you shouldn't be consuming anyway:

• Aged, fermented, or pickled foods, such as most cheeses (except cottage cheese, cream cheese, and fresh

---

[185]

http://www.cancer.gov/cancertopics/pdq/cam/hydrazinesulfate/patient/Page2#Section_29

Mozzarella), lunch meats, hot dogs, yogurt, wines and beers

- Barley grass, which would exclude all barley supplements

- Dry and fermented sausage (bologna, salami, pepperoni, corned beef, and liver), pickled herring and salted dried fish, broad beans and pods (lima, fava beans, lentils, snow peas, and soybeans)

- Meat extracts, yeast extracts/brewer's yeast, beer and ale, red wine (chianti, burgundy, sherry, vermouth), sauerkraut

- Fruits such as oranges, tangerines, lemon, grapefruit, bananas, avocados, canned figs, raisins, red plums, raspberries, pineapples

- Cultured dairy products (buttermilk, yogurt, and sour cream

- Chocolate

- Caffeine (coffee, tea, and cola drinks), white wine, port wines, distilled spirits

- Soy sauce, miso, peanuts, almonds

- Beef or chicken liver, herring, meat tenderizer, MSG (Accent)

- Pickles, pumpkin seeds

I offer more suggestions on cachexia in the video on my blog post at ConnersClinic.com/cancer-and-cachexia

Integrative Cancer Treatment FAQ[186]

What is the Definition of an "Integrative Treatment" for Cancer?

The definition for "integrative cancer treatment" that most practitioners use is "the attempt to 'marry' alternative, non-mainstream treatment to the patient's current medical care *for the best interest of the patient*." Generally, these are treatments which are **not** taught to doctors in medical schools (thus not understood by most traditional doctors), **not** advertised in medical journals, and **not** recommended by most physicians to their patients. They are also generally **not** covered by health insurance. None of this, however, means they are not effective. In fact, they often have a much higher documented efficacy than conventional treatments.

Why are Alternative, Non-Toxic Approaches to Cancer so Often More Effective Than Conventional Cancer Treatments?

The answer to this question can be found in the "non-toxic" nature of alternative treatments. All alternative cancer treatment approaches are non-toxic when used correctly. On the other hand, the mainstream medical establishment is committed to chemotherapy drugs and other procedures such as radiation that are toxic by nature. The long-term track records of numerous successful alternative approaches show that cancer can be most effectively overcome by using a non-toxic approach, and I believe this is because of two reasons:

---

[186] Adapted from Protocel.com

1. Non-Toxic Approaches Allow for "Continual" Administration

Toxic conventional approaches cannot be administered in a "continual" way because they are so toxic that continual use would kill the patient before the cancer could. Because of this, toxic approaches are always administered with doses or treatments spaced out in some way. Spacing out treatments, however, is not an effective way to battle cancer because cancer's best attribute is its ability to grow new cells fast. This means that, in-between the toxic treatments while your body is recovery from the treatment, the cancer cells may also recover somewhat from the treatment. And those cells that grow back the fastest are the cells that have some amount of resistance to the treatment. As a result, due to the toxic treatment itself, many cancer patients eventually have to deal with multi-drug-resistant (or MDR) cancer cells in their bodies that are even more difficult to get rid of than the original cancer cells were.

In other words, when a cancer patient needs a few days or weeks for their body to recover from the toxic treatment being given to them, the MDR cancer cells and cancer stem cells may also start to recover during this time. The cancer may even start to grow faster than before due to the body's immune system having been weakened by the toxic treatment. Eventually, a person's body may not be able to recover at all because the immune system and vital organs have been too weakened by the treatment itself.

With non-toxic treatment, however, this vicious cycle is avoided. People using a non-toxic approach can safely do that approach every day for months or even years without any detriment to their body. For example, people using Rife, Protocel, Burzynski's antineoplastons, Dr. Gonzalez's enzymes, Hoxsey's herbal remedy, Cesium High pH therapy, etc. can use these treatment approaches 24/7 for as long as they need to until their cancer is suppressed. Moreover, once a cancer patient using a non-toxic method is pronounced in remission, they can often keep using their approach on a maintenance level, if they choose, to ensure that their cancer will never re-develop. This *continual use* aspect of non-toxic treatments makes them much more effective at combating something as fast replicating as cancer.

2. Lack of Life-Threatening Side-Effects

Toxic conventional treatments can cause extremely serious negative side effects, such as damage to the liver, kidneys, and heart, to the point where the side effects themselves may kill the patient! Many, many people have died from chemotherapy and/or radiation that were used to treat their cancer. Radiation to areas of the chest for breast or lung cancer can cause severe heart damage and the patient may subsequently die from heart failure. Chemotherapy can bring about kidney or liver failure, heart attack, or may promote a fatal infection or blood clot. Then why do conventional doctors keep using it? All I can think of for the answer to that one is that "follow the money."

Moreover, both chemotherapy and radiation can cause secondary cancers to develop later on. (Yes, many conventional cancer treatments are actually carcinogenic!) Thus, even if a cancer patient goes into remission as a result of their toxic conventional treatment, they may either die of a heart attack or other organ failure a few years later, or they may develop a new life-threatening cancer that could kill them. Two of the most common types of secondary cancers caused by conventional treatment are liver cancer and leukemia. Thus, with toxic conventional approaches to cancer, the treatment itself can very often kill the patient.

What Are the Most Common Misconceptions About Alternative Cancer Treatments?

There are many widespread misconceptions, but the three most common ones are:

1. Unscientific, Developed/Administered by Quacks

I for one would rather be a "quack" and a "medical heretic" than bind myself to the pharmaceutical machine that deems it necessary to destroy its perceived competition while it "owns" the right to kill people for money. In my mind, a "quack" that helps people get better beats a "respected oncologist" who kills people for money any day!

2. Simply Eat Organic and Take Supplements

Obviously from this book, you've learned that there is much more.

3. If They Worked, MDs Would Use Them

I think we've addressed what I feel about this.

Do any Experts Endorse Alternative Cancer Treatments?

Yes, plenty! Some alternative approaches today are actually administered by highly acclaimed physicians in very professional settings. But physicians in most U.S. states are not legally allowed to prescribe alternative cancer treatments to their patients. Nor are they allowed to publicly endorse any treatment not approved by the FDA. So, the laws in our country have their hands tied. However, over the decades, numerous books and articles endorsing alternative cancer treatments have been written by certain physicians, Nobel Prize-winning scientists, physicists, and other respected cancer researchers.

The Fellowship program that I just graduated from is taught by leading MD's and cancer researchers from MD Anderson and Yale. Regardless of the criticism out there against conventional medical treatment, there are plenty of great MD's who really care about their patients and are willing to learn and try new things because they truly desire to see the patient succeed. This is **not** a battle against your MD or your oncologist; even if they are extremely antagonistic. This is a battle against ignorance and financially biased organizations that have a **huge** financial interest in protecting the status quo.

Are There Any Alternative Treatments for Cancer That are Bogus?

There can be unscrupulous practitioners in any area of medicine, conventional or alternative. People should be very discerning when it comes to choosing a cancer treatment approach or practitioner. It is important to be diligent and find a particular method, practitioner, or clinic that has a genuine positive track record. Whenever possible, contacting other cancer patients who succeeded with that particular treatment or doctor is recommended. I know a number of books that claim _____ is the cause of **all** cancers; whatever they are claiming may actually be the cause of **some** cancer, but "all" is a pretty strong word. There are many reasons you could get cancer, and everyone is different; care is never a one size fits all approach.

Be careful of anyone claiming the ability to **cure** anything, not just cancer! I would even add that you should be careful of anyone stating that they **treat** cancer, because this very philosophy doesn't make sense. Again, one needs to improve the patient, every aspect, if the disease is ever going to be "cured" by the patient's own body. I don't treat cancer, and I don't fight cancer; I suggest you take the same stance. Work on "causes"; work on achieving homeostasis; work on balancing the body, and I think your outcome will be better!

Why Is It So Important for People to Know About Alternative Treatments for Cancer?

Statistics show that approximately 1 in 3 Americans will develop life-threatening cancer some time in their life (some researchers believe this reality is closer to 1 in 2 Americans.) Unfortunately, the conventional treatments for cancer (which include surgery, radiation, chemotherapy, hormone therapy, and a handful of other recent drug therapies) offer a dismally low chance for "real" recovery if not coupled with some lifestyle changes. Conventional cancer medicine, on the other hand, defines "cured" as merely "alive 5 years after diagnosis." Thus, in most cases, conventional doctors don't even expect to be able to bring a cancer patient back to a normal state.

The sad reality is that most people with cancer will not survive their disease if treated through conventional medicine alone. On the other hand, many people today believe that certain alternative treatments for cancer have historically been much more successful than current conventional treatments, and still offer better track records for "real" recoveries. It is vitally important that anyone dealing with a life-threatening disease be told of the *most* effective options available to them; and this must include lifestyle changes.

How is "Cure" Defined When Dealing with Cancer?

You would think that the term "cure" would be defined the

484

same way in all circles. But, as mentioned in the above answer, that is not the case. The American Cancer Society, the FDA, the National Cancer Institute, and all other mainstream organizations involved with recording or publishing cancer statistics define a cancer cure as "alive 5 years after diagnosis." Thus, if a cancer patient courageously struggles through debilitating surgery, chemotherapy, and radiation, and eventually dies a miserable death, full of cancer, 5 years and two weeks after they were diagnosed, that person will be listed in official statistics as "cured" simply because they were alive five years after diagnosis! By using this strange definition of "cure," official cancer cure rates put out by the American Cancer Society and other organizations make conventional medical approaches look much more successful than they really are.

Here's a really sad statistic: They main reason the medical establishment is pushing for early detection is that the chance of the patient living for five years increases and they can boast of their treatment "cure." How can they be so evil? Most people will disbelieve me on this point because they just cannot grasp that an establishment would operate solely to manipulate statistics for financial gain. There is a fitting quote that states, "I love capitalism, but certainly not every capitalist."

In truth, this strange re-defining of the term "cure" is not only criminal deception, but it also proves that conventional medicine (really the pharmaceutical machine that uses doctors like puppets) has such a poor ability to bring about real cancer recoveries that they must resort to this sort of tactic to make themselves look better. And this is only one of many questionable tactics used to fudge and manipulate conventional cancer statistics to make them look better and mislead the public.

In the field of alternative therapies for cancer, practitioners tend to avoid the word "cure" and "treat" altogether because they will get in trouble with organized medicine if they claim they can do either. So, they tend to use words like, "control" cancer, or "long-term recovery rates." The truth is, however, that if you look into all of the alternative cancer treatments that have been effective over the decades, they historically had great track records in bringing about "real" cures. This means that when people using alternative cancer treatments are referred to as cured, they are typically truly cancer-free and no longer suffering from the disease.

I've stated over and over that we do not treat cancer. I legally can't! My medical doctor friends that I graduated with from the Integrative Cancer Therapy Fellowship can't treat cancer either! We are all confined by the FDA and state boards to leave cancer treatment to Oncologists. That's perfectly okay with me; I have **no** desire to treat cancer, it's futile! I will gladly remain solidly at my post to point people in the right direction. There is little success in treating cancer; there is great success in cleaning the environment that allowed it to grow.

If Alternative Treatments for Cancer Are So Successful, Why Aren't Oncologists and Cancer Clinics Recommending Them?

Most conventional doctors and cancer clinics do not recommend alternative treatments for cancer for a variety of reasons. The primary reason is that, in most U.S. states, doctors are not legally allowed to recommend any treatments for cancer that the FDA has not approved. Since the FDA refuses to even consider approving any treatment that does not bring big profits to the pharmaceutical companies and other large industries they are associated with, any treatment not approved by the FDA is automatically called "alternative." It can be a very serious legal transgression for most doctors if they try to recommend an alternative cancer treatment, even if they know that treatment could give their patient the best possible chance for recovery. Many highly respected doctors have tried to practice alternative approaches and lost their medical licenses as a result or were even thrown in jail. Two of the most liberal states in the U.S., where many of the alternative therapies are being practiced today, are Nevada and Arizona. Numerous physicians who wish to practice alternative cancer medicine have moved to one of these states.

Another reason is that most conventional doctors don't have an adequate understanding of alternative treatments for cancer because they have never been educated about them and there are virtually no references to alternative medicine in their medical school training or their medical journals. These, too, are controlled by pharmaceutical companies. Things are changing though; I trained with many other like-minded MD's wishing to add alternative therapies to their practices.

One more issue that can be problematic is that some doctors might know about alternative treatments but feel emotionally threatened by them. Especially for oncologists, acknowledging that other techniques probably would have worked better for their terminally ill patients than the methods they have been using can be quite painful. It may be easier for an oncologist or other type of doctor to simply deny this reality than to acknowledge that many of the patients he or she treated could have lived rather than died. I recently had a patient that survived 5 years after diagnosis and brought lunch into everyone in our office to celebrate. She had kept in a relationship with her oncologist so she could still receive regular CT scans to monitor her progress and visited him right before her 5-year anniversary. He proceeded to tell her that the other patients who had started with her (and were in a support group with her) had all died; she was the lone survivor! She already knew that information and she was the only one who refused the chemo treatment and had gone an alternate

487

route. So, when the oncologist shared that she was the lone survivor, she proceeded to tell him what she had done differently to achieve such a great outcome. Surprisingly, the oncologist stopped her immediately saying that if she wanted to remain in relation with him that he didn't want to hear anything!

It is utterly appalling! If you were the doctor that had **all** your patient **die** of your treatment, would you want to figure out if there is another way!? It's **sick**! **That** is **not** a doctor, that's a murderer for hire! He gets paid (a lot more than I or other alternative practitioners do) to **kill people** and doesn't even want to know a better way! I can't even think about this without getting mad, so let's move on.

Lastly, many doctors also suffer from the "disbelief factor" so common throughout the public. This disbelief factor tends to be expressed by everyday people in the statement, "If these treatments really work, why aren't all doctors using them?" Many doctors may feel the same way and express their disbelief as, "If these treatments really work, why wasn't I taught them in medical school and why aren't I reading about them in my medical journals?"

Why Can Alternative Treatments for Cancer Have Better Track Records Than Conventional Cancer Treatments?

To be honest, not all do. Understand, I have my foot in alternative and traditional therapies, but I am not against **all** types of chemotherapy. Some alternative therapies **do** have documented cure rates that are better than conventional treatments, and others offer multiple case stories of people who had conventional treatment fail them and then went on to use that alternative approach to achieve a complete recovery or at least some help. We are never legally speaking of a cure; we speak of treating the patient to allow the body to heal itself.

The simple answer is that alternative treatments, in general, deal with the true causes of sickness and with the cancer patient's whole body in a non-toxic way. This can be a much more effective way to completely rid a person of cancer than conventional medical treatments, which involve toxic approaches and only target the "symptoms" of cancer (the tumors themselves.)

What Causes Cancer?

This question is really too big to answer here but I think we've hit on several points in this book. Please refer to my book on Autoimmune Disease, "*Help, My Body is Killing Me*," and one of my favorite books on Cancer, "*Outsmart Your Cancer*," which address this question in depth. Chapter 2 gives an overview of this issue, but each treatment chapter provides an even more in-depth understanding of what causes cancer on the cellular level.

Some People Think That By the Time They Get Cancer the Medical Establishment Will Have Found a Cure. Is This a Reasonable Expectation?

I cannot predict the future, but I would say to those people, "Don't hold your breath!" The mainstream medical establishment has been claiming to be actively searching for a cure since the 1940's or so, and they have been predicting a cure right around the corner; and ever since while they've successfully squashed real success. The problem is that conventional medicine has been looking for a cure in the wrong places. They're looking for things that can be patented and therefore financially marketed; therefore they focus on drugs that are toxic to tumors and, since these drugs are also toxic to the rest of the body, it is impossible to use enough of the drug to get rid of every last cancer cell in a patient without killing them first. It is well-known that, in most cases, if a doctor were to prescribe enough chemotherapy or radiation to a patient to kill every cancer cell in a person's body, the cancer would be gone but so would the patient.

The biggest problem is that organized medicine is governed by the power of the big pharmaceutical companies. The pharmaceutical companies fund most of the cancer research being done, even that performed at universities, yet they will only fund the type of research that could possibly result in patented drugs that can bring them huge profits. Their goal is to make money, **not** to test whatever works; and sad to say, **not** to cure cancer. Since the FDA is intricately involved with and controlled by the pharmaceutical companies, it has now become a watchdog and strong arm of Big Pharma, rather than a protector of the American public as it was intended to be. So, while the pharmaceutical industry searches for profitable "silver bullets" to treat cancer, they are actively and knowingly ignoring the arsenal of alternative cancer treatments that already exist and have been proven effective because they **can't make any money from them**.

Is There a "Conspiracy" to Suppress Alternative Cancer Treatments?

"Conspiracy" is probably not the best word to use here. Money and power are behind the very real suppression that has been going on for decades, but it may not be so organized as to warrant the term "conspiracy." Behind most of the suppression lies the power of the pharmaceutical companies and their far-reaching influence. Some very enlightening books have exposed the documented details of how this has happened, including "*World Without Cancer*," by G. Edward

Griffin, and *"The Cancer Industry,"* by Dr. Ralph Moss.

We all know that there are big industries in existence today that pollute our air and water. Yet, that does not mean those corporations are operating under a "conspiracy" to pollute our environment. They are just doing what corporations do best: protecting their profits. In the cancer industry as well, corporations protect their profits. Unfortunately, this pursuit can involve unscrupulous methods as well as influencing laws. But it involves many different people in positions of power in many different organizations, and probably the better way to describe the cancer treatment suppression would be to say that various people and organizations are in "collusion" to keep alternative approaches that threaten Big Pharma profits suppressed.

Unfortunately, the way the whole medical approval system is set up for testing and accepting new treatments for cancer also supports this suppression. The process not only requires hundreds of millions of dollars, it is only set up for short-term testing of toxic drugs. Any approach that does **not** fit that mold will not be tested effectively. What would have happened if, before airplanes were developed, all scientific organizations had determined that a flying machine **must** have wings that flap like birds? Orville and Wilbur Wright's machine would not have fit that mold and would not have passed the testing that was set up for flapping wing contraptions. We might not be flying the friendly skies today if that had been the case!

If the Mainstream Cancer Industry Has Effectively Suppressed Alternative Cancer Treatments Before, What Will Keep Them from Continuing to Do So?

There is no doubt that they are certainly still trying to suppress effective alternative cancer treatments. Read the book, *The*

491

Burzynski Breakthrough, to find out just how recently the FDA has tried to stop non-toxic anti-neoplaston therapy for cancer. But I do believe that the internet, which has only been available to the public in a widespread way for just over a decade, will save us. As long as nothing can stop people from sharing information over the internet, we now have a chance to stop this deadly suppression by sharing information amongst ourselves!

I also think that the general public is becoming more and more ready to utilize their power to change legislation and to re-claim their right to medical freedom. The FDA, in particular, has strayed from its intended role of protecting the consumer public from unsafe treatments to becoming a "watchdog" and advocate for the pharmaceutical companies. It is up to us to become aware of what is happening and to change this situation. We have the power if we choose to use it!

If I Want to Use an Alternative Cancer Treatment Approach, Should I Still Consult with a Conventional Oncologist First?

Yes. That's my legal opinion; you should always consult with a qualified oncologist. Not for the purpose of asking the oncologist what he or she thinks of the alternative treatment you are considering, but for other reasons: I'm not an Oncologist. As already mentioned, conventional surgery alone may be necessary for some cases and that might be an attractive option for certain people. And, in some cases where a person's cancer is already very advanced when they are first diagnosed, sometimes short-term radiation or short-term chemotherapy may be necessary to give the patient time for an alternative approach to work.

In consulting with a conventional oncologist, it is also very

492

important to ask as many questions as possible. In Chapter 21 of the book, "*Outsmart Your Cancer*," the author presents a list of important questions you can ask to clarify your chances for recovery using the treatment course your oncologist is recommending. By doing so, you are giving yourself the best chance for understanding your options. In all cases, a combination of conventional **and** alternative treatment may be your best choice.

Last but not least, establishing a relationship with a conventional doctor is generally necessary at some point for assessing your progress. Even people using alternative approaches need diagnostic tests at various intervals for the purpose of assessing how they are doing or for any related problems that may occur.

Thus, conventional medical experts should always be consulted. And every cancer patient should be as open to evaluating what they have to offer as they are when it comes to evaluating what alternative medicine has to offer. However, the approach you decide to use for treating your cancer is **your** decision. By being as informed as possible, you will be giving yourself the best chance for making the best possible decision.

Can I Use a Conventional Approach Along with an Alternative Approach at the Same Time?

As mentioned above, usually that is the best choice. You must do your homework and be as informed as possible. This involves finding out, as best you can, which approaches will offer you the best chance for recovery and also finding out what all the possible damaging side effects of the conventional treatment might be. You don't want to add a conventional approach that might in itself threaten your life if you already have an alternative approach you believe can help you.

493

A "Ten Step Protocol" For You and Your Doctor

I've probably given you too much information in this book already. Originally, I promised myself to keep it under one hundred pages to make it more "readable" but there is so much more stuff that I had to leave out to keep from going even longer. So, this section is to summarize everything in 10 easy steps for both you and your doctor. I pray that you find someone that can help you walk through this; someone that will not only guide you but hold your hand and love you. We can possess all information and wisdom, but without love we are just a loud, noisy gong.[187]

In order to derive the greatest potential benefit from any regimen, both patients and physicians must respect and address as many of the facets of each individual's unique cancer. Sadly, the mainstream medical establishment treats the majority of cancer cases (as well as any other disease) with a "one size fits all" strategy that may deprive many patients of a greater chance of successful care.

My hope is that this summary will:

- Aid you and your physician in determining which therapies are most likely to be effective for your unique condition. Since I understand that **not** everyone could possibly come and see me **and** I am not going to live forever (at least not on earth), you may **not** be able to find a competent doctor to perform Kinesiology to "test you" on the supplements that are perfect for you. So, you and your doctor may use this summary as a template.

- Help you and your doctor target multiple biochemical pathways known to be aberrant in many cancers.

---

[187] 1 Corinthians 13:1

- Provide you a more thorough prognostic analysis (reason why) that can help you and your physician make informed decisions about how to proceed.

- Educate everyone about some potential side effects associated with conventional cancer treatment options, and what they can do to minimize risk.

My Ten Step Protocol for Evaluating Someone with a Diagnosis of Cancer

1. Start at the ***beginning***: some homework for your doctor
2. Evaluate for the possible "cancer killers": their use in particular cases
3. Rife Light Frequency Technology: an absolute ***must***
4. Assume that you ***have*** circulating tumor cells
5. Inhibiting the cyclooxygenase Enzymes (COX-1 & COX-2)
6. Suppress Ras oncogene expression
7. Maintain bone integrity
8. Inhibit angiogenesis
9. Inhibit the 5-lipoxygenase (5-LOX) enzyme
10. Inhibit cancer metastasis

Of critical importance to treatment-naïve patients is implementing as many of these ten critical steps as can safely be done concurrently with conventional therapy. In newly diagnosed patients who have not yet been treated, the objective is to eradicate the primary tumor and metastatic cells with a multi-pronged "first strike therapy" so that residual tumor cells are not given an opportunity to evolve survival mechanisms that make them resistant to further treatments.

Step One: Start at the *Beginning*

The "beginning" is really for your doctor but there is much you can do on your own: it means to start every patient just as you would any other, regardless of their previous diagnosis.

- **Identify a possible autoimmune disorder**: do **not** let your doctor skip this step and dismiss this possibility. As stated in greater detail previously, most cancer patients are Th2 dominant autoimmune (and most have **no** idea and have never been diagnosed as such.) Hidden, subclinical autoimmune disorders haunt the patient!

- **HCL**: get tested for, and correct, hypochlorhydria. A decrease in stomach acid production is quite possibly the most common condition known to man.

- **Anemia**: get checked for, and properly treat, Iron Deficiency Anemia, Folic Acid Anemia (if this exists, do **not** just take regular folic acid; you **must** use 5-Methyltetrahydrofolate), Pernicious Anemia, B12 Anemia. Note: we **never** recommend methylated supplements as they have the potential to *turn off* tumor suppressor genes. In the case of anemia, follow our Iron-Artemisinin Protocol found on our blog at ConnersClinic.com/ferritin-iron-and-cancer

- **Vitamin B12**: if needed, use Hydroxocobalamin instead of a methylated cobalamin.

- **Heal the gut**: intestinal permeability issues (leaky gut) is just about a guaranteed condition if you have cancer! Treat it!

- **Nutrient deficiencies**: treat these

- **Metabolic pathway blockages and Liver Detoxification pathway blockages**: run an Organic Acid Profile and correct this and follow my 7 Phases of detox.

- **Identify and correct antigens**
    - Heavy Metal Toxicity issues
    - Food sensitivities
    - Parasites (most are subclinical)
    - Other Biotoxins (mold, fungus, etc. If you are not checking for these, you may be **completely** missing the boat as to the **cause**!!)
    - Other Chemical toxicities (environmental toxicities are rampant)

- **Check and modulate Th1/Th2 balance**: add appropriate nutrition/diet to deal with the antigen

- **Run appropriate Functional Medicine tests**: if necessary

Step Two: Evaluating for the Possible "Cancer Killers"

There are multiple reasons that cancer starts and flourishes, therefore there are numerous possible ways to attack it. The variety of nutraceuticals that I have previously discussed in this book is what we want to address in Step Two. Unfortunately, I do not know of any way other than using Kinesiology (a muscle testing procedure) from a very competent and experienced practitioner, but let's try to work through this.

We know to consider:

- Tumor-promoting genes (oncogenes that may be upregulated)

497

- Tumor suppressor genes (that may be downregulated)

- Receptors or docking sites on the cell membrane where communication with proteins occur to aid the cell to undergo apoptosis (that may be blocked)

- Cellular differentiation: the degree of aggressiveness of the cancer cell (poorly differentiated cancer cells are more aggressive, while highly differentiated cells are less aggressive)

- Inflammatory processes at the site of tumor

- Th2 dominance at the site of tumor

- Toxicity systemically and at the site of tumor growth

- Hypoxic conditions in the milieu

These individual variations (the unique biology of the cancer cell) help to explain why a particular therapy may be highly effective for some cancer patients but fail others.

People typically think of their disease based on the organ it affects (e.g. lung cancer or colon cancer.) The problem with that rationale is that not all cancers are the same, even if they affect the same organ. With the advent of advanced molecular diagnostic profiling, the specific strengths and vulnerabilities of each patient's cancer can be identified in order to design an individually tailored treatment program.

I have stated repeatedly that one cannot be **dogmatic** about treating **any** disorder. Every person is unique as is their condition. If I am going to be a doctor that requires my patients to fit into **my** box instead of fitting a program around them, my percent of failure will rise. Don't let this happen to you!

When a person has cancer, the physician confronts a chain of pressing questions: What type of cancer is it? Where did it originate? Is it a hormonally driven cancer? Which treatments are most likely to be effective?

Cancers have traditionally been treated as follows: if one therapy proves ineffective, then try another until a successful therapy is found or all options are exhausted. Kinesiology (properly performed) helps to eliminate the need for this trial-and-error method by providing individualized information to help determine the optimal therapy before initiating treatment.

However, here are some basic guidelines to help determine a course of action:

- If you have any hormonal cancer, HER1/2 positive, and/or ER or PR positive cancer: consider a fermented soy product like Sano Gastril (Allergy Research Group) or Haelin 951 and definitely add DIM, and Estro Clear that we spoke about in Chapter 2

- If you have Prostate, Breast, or Colon Cancer: consider Protocel, Evolv Immun, Black Salve Bloodroot, Medicinal Mushrooms, IP6

- If you have any of the skin cancers: consider my special mixture that we call Curcumin Cream; use liberally as an ointment everyday

- If you have a Brain Cancer: consider glutamate lowering products like Benagene and Glutamate Scavenger 2 as well as anti-inflammatory products like Curcu Clear, Clear Inflam, our BAM product, and Turmero Clear. Also consider Burzynski's Antineoplastons, Protocel, Arginine, and Medicinal Mushrooms

- If you have Pancreatic Cancer: consider High Dose Enzyme therapy, Mushrooms, Black Salve Bloodroot, and IP6

- If you have Liver Cancer: consider Evolv Immun, Black Salve Bloodroot, High Dose Enzymes, Beta Glucans, IP6, Poly-MVA, and Medicinal Mushrooms

- If you have Blood-born cancers or Bone Cancers: consider Laetrile and Green Tea extract

- With any cancer you can consider some of the less expensive products like Vitamin D3, Essiac Tea, Hoxsey, IP6, Beta Glucan, and Medicinal Mushrooms

I have **such** a difficult time writing this portion of the book because **this** is the biggest hurdle for a patient to overcome: there is **so** much to consider, where do I start and what should I take?

How to Implement Step Two

If you **cannot** determine with a reasonable degree of inner peace which of the above nutraceuticals to take, don't take any. It's **okay**. Do everything else in these ten steps and you've covered 90% of your bases.

If you have the ability to get tested for particular products, do so. My favorites are easy to see: Medicinal Mushrooms, Beta Glucans, Green Tea, Vitamin D3, Curcumin, Modified Citrus Pectin; you just cannot go wrong with these.

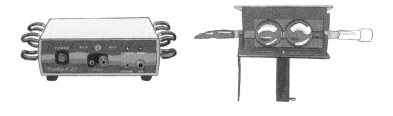

Step Three: Rife Light Frequency Technology

This is **not** a step to omit! I honestly believe that you would not be reading this book if it were not for Rife technology, because I wouldn't have written it. I have seen **way** too many miracles from patients who were complete skeptics to dismiss the overwhelming evidence of its efficacy. As stated previously, you cannot take shortcuts; you need to get a good unit. Every patient that comes to me for care goes home with a Rife unit. We program it specifically for them based on three parameters:

1. Diagnosis from the oncologist (typically, this is from the pathology report)
2. What I find in my examination
3. What we find on the scan we perform
4. What we find with testing

The programs that we create are in several timed components. I require patients to sleep with an overnight bulb so every patient will have at least one set of seven *overnight sets* labeled Sunday through Saturday. This way, a person can get ready for bed, open the Rife program on their laptop computer connected to the Rife machine, select the appropriate night set and hit *run*. They then snuggle into bed with their night tube and get their treatment all night long. Snuggle up to your significant other and they too get the benefits of an increased pH and a healthier body; it's a win-win!

We also will create some specific daytime programs that can help a person overcome the secondary effects of radiation, chemotherapy, and/or surgery if they are going the traditional route as well. Secondary programs for other conditions are often created depending on the patient's particular circumstance.

As previously mentioned, a Rife machine is included in all of our care plans.

How to Implement Step Three

Find a doctor who knows as much about what I've discussed in this section as possible that will be able to guide you through this path.

Step Four: Assume You Have Circulating Tumor Cells

Circulating Tumor Cells (CTCs) can be tested and there are more precise testing methods developed every year. However, just assume that if you have had a previous diagnosis of cancer that you have CTCs. CTCs are the "seeds" that break away from the primary site of cancer and spread to other parts of the body, trying to set up a home and raise a family. Understanding circulating tumor cells is critically important since it is the primary way that cancer spreads to other parts of the body and is very often responsible for the death of a person with cancer.

Historically, medical science has been focused on the primary tumor, attempting to destroy the growing mass. They assume that if they can kill the cancer, they've won the battle. In my opinion, this assumption is foolish at best. Why did the tumor take hold and grow in the first place? Was it just aberrant cells in **that** specific spot or is there an imbalance in the cellular milieu that predisposed you to the process that could predispose you to a similar process elsewhere in your body if not corrected? Let's just use a little common sense here!

You **must** treat your cancer as a **systemic** condition!!

In an illuminating study conducted with metastatic breast cancer patients, researchers compared the genetic composition of the cancer cells that had formed distant metastasis to the genetic composition of the corresponding cancer cells in the primary breast tumor. The findings were alarming: in 31% of the comparisons, the genetic composition of the metastatic cancer cells differed almost completely from that of the primary breast tumors.[188]

Amazingly, further analysis revealed that none of the pairs of primary breast tumors with its corresponding metastatic cancer were identical. Based on these findings, the authors remarked that *"because metastatic cells often have a completely different genetic composition, their phenotype (biological behavior), including aggressiveness and therapy responsiveness, may also vary substantially from that seen in the primary tumors,"* leading to their conclusion that *"the resulting heterogeneity (genetic variability) of metastatic breast cancer may underlie its poor responsiveness to therapy..."* To further support the evidence that metastatic cancer cells can vary genetically from the primary tumor, two additional studies with breast cancer patients have demonstrated that CTC can be HER2 positive while the primary breast tumor can be HER2 negative.[189] [190]

---

[188] Kuukasjärvi et al. 1997
[189] Meng et al. 2004
[190] Wülfing et al. 2006

This as well as other research suggests that directing treatment solely towards the cancer cells of the primary tumor can, in some cases, be "barking up the wrong tree." Standard medical treatments (chemo, surgery, radiation) designed to attack the primary tumor always fail to destroy the circulating tumor cells.

Please allow me to scream here: Treat the **_person_**, not the cancer!!

There are several natural supplements that have shown to be great _binders_ to CTCs and help stop growth of new tumor sites.

See below:

How to Implement Step Four

The following three novel compounds have shown efficacy in inhibiting several mechanisms that contribute to cancer metastasis. It is especially important to consider these compounds during the perioperative period (period before and after surgery), because a known consequence of surgery is an enhanced proclivity for metastasis. I highly recommend:

- **Modified Citrus Pectin**: 15 grams daily, in three divided doses. Continue with at least 5 grams daily throughout your life after you've beat the first round. I use the product Pectasol from EcoEugenics. It comes in a powdered form (I suggest you mix it into a small amount of juice or add it to a smoothie) or capsules.

- **Cimetidine**: 800mg daily, in two divided doses (I don't recommend this, but research proves its benefits)

- **Coriolus Versicolor, Standardized Extract**: 1,200-3,600mg daily. Coriolus versicolor is a mushroom that I love (but I like all the Asian mushrooms.) Different nutrients, polysaccharide K (PSK) and polysaccharide-peptide (PSP), are being studied as possible complementary cancer treatments. I use a mixture of this and several other mushrooms.

- **IP6**: consider taking 2-6 capsules per day (I use the product from Hope Science). IP6 has been shown to help decrease adhesion properties of CTCs.

Bottom line: ***always*** assume you have cancer attempting to go crazy inside of you and you'll better manage it and keep it at bay for your lifetime.

Step Five: Inhibiting the Cyclooxygenase Enzymes: COX-1 & COX-2 Inflammatory Pathways

Controlling inflammation plays a pivotal role in inhibiting growth both at the primary site and possible metastatic areas. There are many inflammatory pathways in the body, but the cyclooxygenase (COX-2) enzyme is a particular inflammatory pathway that has been the focus of research in the realm of oncology.

Initially, scientists believed COX-2 was merely an inducible response to inflammation but it is now thought that the COX-2 pathway performs biological functions in the body, particularly in the brain and kidneys as well as the immune system. Understand that there needs to be a balance between pro- and anti-inflammatory activities in the body.

COX-2 becomes troublesome when upregulated (sometimes 10- to 80-fold) by pro-inflammatory stimuli (subclinical autoimmune disorders, interleukin-1, growth factors, tumor necrosis factor, and endotoxins.) When over-expressed, COX-2 participates in various pathways that could promote cancer (e.g. angiogenesis), cell proliferation, and the production of inflammatory prostaglandins (Sears 1995; Newmark 2000; Chakraborti AK 2010.) This is why Step One is so important!

You **must** deal with hidden autoimmune conditions, anemias, heavy metal toxicities, mold issues, etc.

A growing body of research has documented the relationship between COX-2 and cancer:

- An article in the journal *Cancer Research* showed that COX-2 levels in pancreatic cancer cells are 60 times greater than in adjacent normal tissue.[191]

- Solid tumors contain oxygen-deficient or hypoxic areas (a reduced oxygen supply to a tissue below physiological levels.) Hypoxia promotes up-regulation of COX-2 and angiogenesis and establishes resistance to ionizing radiation.[192]

- Within the nonsteroidal anti-inflammatory drug (NSAIDs) class is a subclass referred to as COX-2 inhibitors (cyclooxygenase inhibitors.) COX-2 inhibitors were popularly prescribed to relieve pain but now have found a place in oncology. It began when scientists recognized that people who regularly take NSAIDs lowered their risk of colon cancer by as much as 50%.[193]

- *JAMA* reported that a 9.4 year epidemiological study showed that COX-2 upregulation was related to more advanced tumor stage, tumor size, and lymph node metastasis as well as diminished survival rates among colorectal cancer patients.[194] With more regular use of aspirin (a COX-2 inhibitor), the risk of dying from the disease decreased.[195] [196] The journal *Gastroenterology*

---

[191] Tucker et al. 1999
[192] Gately 2000
[193] Reddy et al. 2000
[194] Sheehan et al. 1999
[195] Brody 1991
[196] Knorr 2000

reported additional encouragement, showing that three different colon cell lines underwent apoptosis (cell death) when deprived of COX-2; when lovastatin was added to the COX-2 inhibitor the kill rate increased another five-fold.[197] The benefits observed with COX-2 inhibitors extend beyond colon protection to the cardiovascular system, where they help sustain endothelial cell function.[198]

- A groundbreaking study published in 2009 revealed that breast cancer patients treated with COX-2 inhibitors had a greatly reduced risk of bone metastases. In this investigation, the incidence of bone metastases was recorded in breast cancer patients who were not treated with a COX-2 inhibitor, as well as in individuals who received a COX-2 inhibitor for at least 6 months following the diagnosis of breast cancer. The findings were astounding: those who were treated with a COX-2 inhibitor were 90% less likely to develop bone metastases than those who were not treated with a COX-2 inhibitor.[199]

- 134 patients with advanced lung cancer were treated with chemotherapy alone or combined with celebrex® (a COX-2 inhibitor.) For those patients with cancers expressing increased amounts of COX-2, treatment with celebrex dramatically prolonged survival.[200]

- Celebrex® slowed cancer progression in men with recurrent prostate cancer.[201] [202]

---

[197] Agarwal et al. 1999
[198] Tsujii et al. 1998
[199] Valsecchi ME 2009
[200] Edelman 2008
[201] Pruthi et al. 2006
[202] Manola et al. 2006

- Celebrex® prevented weight loss and improved quality of life in individuals with head and neck cancers.[203]

- Regular intake of OTC NSAIDs produced highly significant composite risk reductions of 43% for colon cancer, 25% for breast cancer, 28% for lung cancer, and 27% for prostate cancer. Furthermore, in a series of case control studies, daily use of a selective COX-2 inhibitor, either celecoxib or rofecoxib, significantly reduced the risk for each of these malignancies. The evidence is compelling that anti-inflammatory agents with selective or non-selective activity against cyclooxygenase- 2 (COX-2) have strong potential for the chemoprevention of cancers of the colon, breast, prostate and lung. Results confirming that COX-2 blockade is effective for cancer prevention have been tempered by observations that some selective COX-2 inhibitors pose a risk to the cardiovascular system.[204]

This step addresses a natural approach to inhibit COX-2 in the cancer and though the above studies concentrated on use of medications, the side effects of Celebrex and NSAIDs is simply unnecessary when there are natural methods to perform the same task. The risks associated with traditional NSAIDs include gastrointestinal perforation, ulceration and bleeding, and renal and liver damage, so let's be smart about this.

A study published in *The Journal of Ethnopharmacology* in 2002 revealed that inhibitors of prostaglandin biosynthesis and nitric oxide production have been considered as potential anti-inflammatory and cancer chemo-preventive agents. In this study, "we evaluated approximately 170 methanol extracts of natural products including Korean herbal medicines for the

---

[203] Lai et al. 2008
[204] Harris RE 2009

inhibition of prostaglandin E_2 production (for COX-2 inhibitors) and nitric oxide formation (for iNOS inhibitors) in lipopolysaccharide (LPS)-induced mouse macrophages RAW264.7 cells. As a result, several extracts such as *Aristolochia debilis, Cinnamomum cassia, Cinnamomum loureirii, Curcuma zedoaria, Eugenia caryophyllata, Pterocarpus santalius, Rehmania glutinosa* and *Tribulus terrestris* showed potent inhibition of COX-2 activity (>80% inhibition at the test concentration of 10 µg/ml.) In addition, the extracts of *A. debilis, Caesalpinia sappan, Curcuma longa, C. zedoaria, Daphne genkwa* and *Morus alba* were also considered as potential inhibitors of iNOS activity (>70% inhibition at the test concentration of 10 µg/ml.) These active extracts mediating COX-2 and iNOS inhibitory activities are warranted for further elucidation of active principles for development of new cancer chemopreventive and/or anti-inflammatory agents."

These novel agents (mainly herbal formulas) prove beneficial in blocking both Cox pathways and iNOS pathways. For this as well as other beneficial reasons to add these nutrients, I commonly recommend these herbs along with Medicinal Mushrooms. There's another fascinating study that showed the benefits of blocking these pathways in skin tumors: *"Reduction of UV-induced skin tumors in hairless mice by selective COX-2 inhibition."*[205]

How to Implement Step Five

Take PEOs (Parent Essential Oils) each day, (I previously discussed the benefits of these, you may obtain the same PEOs I use, Professional Health Product's Fatty Acid Liquescence through our store on our website); and think about:

- **Medicinal Mushrooms**: I use a combination of several that are ***also*** combined with:

---

[205] Carcinogenesis(1999) 20 (10):1939-1944.doi: 10.1093/carcin/20.10.1939

       o Lentinula edodes (Shiitake), Grifola frondosa (Maitake), Ganoderma lucidum (Reishi), Agaricus blazei (Himematsutake), Coriolus versicolor (Turkey Tail), and Inonotus obliquus (Chaga)

       o Evolv Immun's polysaccharide product

- Elderberry Aronia & Bilberry Extracts; **and**
- AHCC; **and**
- Magnolia Officinalis Bark; **and**
- Moringa Oleifera Leaf Powder
- A few others…I use a proprietary blend of all of the above that works great!

Step Six: Suppressing Ras Oncogene Expression

The family of proteins known as "Ras" and "Raf" play a central role in the regulation of cell growth; in cancer they suppress or slow growth. They fulfill this fundamental role by integrating the regulatory signals that govern the cell cycle and proliferation, something grossly out of balance in a growing tumor. This means that Ras oncogenes help *turn on* normal cell death.

Defects in the Ras-Raf pathway can result in uncontrolled cancerous growth. Mutant Ras genes were among the first oncogenes identified for their ability to transform cells into a cancerous phenotype (e.g. a cell observably altered because of distorted gene expression.) Mutations in one of three genes (H, N, or K-Ras) encoding Ras proteins are associated with upregulated (increasing) cell proliferation (growth) and are found in an estimated 30-40% of all human cancers. The highest incidences of Ras mutations are found in cancers of the pancreas (80%), colon (50%), thyroid (50%), lung (40%), liver

(30%), melanoma (30%), and myeloid leukemia (30%).[206] [207] [208] [209] [210] [211] [212] [213]

The differences between oncogenes and normal genes can be slight. The mutant protein that an oncogene ultimately creates may differ from the healthy version by only a single amino acid, but this subtle variation can radically alter the protein's functionality. Remember, proteins are just a long chain of amino acids; one seemingly small change changes everything. The Ras-Raf pathway is used by human cells to transmit signals from the cell surface (the membrane) to the cell nucleus. Such signals direct cells to divide, differentiate, or even undergo programmed cell death (apoptosis), therefore the *signals are important*.

A Ras gene usually behaves as a relay switch within the signal pathway that instructs the cell to divide. In response to stimuli transmitted to the cell from outside, cell-signaling pathways are *turned on*. In the absence of stimulus, the Ras protein remains in the *off* position. A mutated Ras protein gene behaves like a switch stuck in the *on* position, continuously misinforming the cell, instructing it to divide when the cycle should be *turned off*[214] [215] So, the question is: How do you turn this switch *off*?

When we understand the physiology behind your body's making Ras genes, we can begin to understand how to manipulate them. The events resulting in maturation of Ras genes take place in three steps, the most critical being the first,

---

[206] Duursma 2003

[207] Minamoto 2000

[208] Vachtenheim 1997

[209] Bartram 1988

[210] Bos 1989

[211] Minamoto 2000

[212] Hsieh JS 2005

[213] Däbritz J 2009

[214] Gibbs et al. 1996

[215] Oliff et al. 1996

referred to as the *farnesylation step*. A specific enzyme, farnesyl-protein transferase (FPTase), speeds up the reaction. One strategy for blocking Ras protein activity has been to inhibit FPTase. Inhibitors of this enzyme block the maturation of Ras protein and reverse the cancerous transformation induced by mutant Ras genes.[216]

A number of natural substances impact the activity of Ras oncogenes. For example, limonene is a substance found in the essential oils of citrus products. Limonene has been shown to act as a farnesyl transferase inhibitor (e.g., it turns off the switch.) Administering high doses of limonene to cancer-bearing animals blocks the farnesylation of Ras, thus inhibiting cell replication.[217] [218] Curcumin also inhibited the farnesylation of RAS and caused cell death in breast cancer cells expressing RAS mutations.[219] [220]

Japanese researchers examined the effects of Vitamin E on the presence of K-Ras mutations in mice with lung cancer. Prior to treatment with Vitamin E, K-Ras mutations were present in 64% of the mice. After treatment with Vitamin E, only 18% of the mice expressed K-Ras mutations.[221] Vitamin E decreased levels of H-Ras proteins in cultured melanoma cells. [222] A study conducted at Mercy Hospital of Pittsburgh also showed that diallyl disulfide, a naturally occurring organosulfide from garlic, inhibits p21 H-Ras oncogenes, displaying a significant restraining effect on tumor growth.[223]

Researchers at Rutgers University investigated the ability of different green and black tea polyphenols to inhibit H-Ras oncogenes. The Rutgers team found that all the major

---

[216] Oliff et al. 1996
[217] Bland 2001
[218] Asamoto et al. 2002
[219] Kim et al. 2001
[220] Chen et al. 1997
[221] Yano et al. 1997
[222] Prasad et al. 1990
[223] Singh et al. 2000

polyphenols contained in green and black tea except epicatechin showed strong inhibition of cell growth.[224] Investigators at Texas A&M University also found that fish oil decreased colonic Ras membrane localization and reduced tumor formation in rats. In view of the central role of oncogenic Ras in the development of colon cancer, the finding that essential fatty acids modulate Ras activation could explain why good omegas protect against colon cancer.[225]

How to Implement Step Six

Consider the following to inhibit the activity of Ras oncogenes:

- **Curcumin**: about 2.5g/day either taken with a fat (use coconut oil) or pre-emulsified in a fat. Studies also show greater benefits if taken with black pepper

- **Magnolia Officinalis Bark**

- **PEOs**: 3-12/day with meals

- **Green Tea Extract**: I use Premier Research Labs liquid formula, 3tsp/day; or use a standardized extract: 725 to 1,450mg of EGCG daily

- **Aged Garlic Extract or Whole Garlic Cloves**: 2,400mg daily with meals

- **Vitamin E**: it *must* be whole food, containing *all* the tocopherols *and* tocotrienols!

- **Citrus Oil Extracts**: grapefruit seed, lemon, etc.

- *Stop Eating Dairy*

---

[224] Chung et al. 1999
[225] Collett et al. 2001

Step Seven: Maintaining Bone Integrity

Understand that some types of cancer (e.g. breast, prostate, and multiple myeloma) have a proclivity to metastasize to the bone. The result may be bone pain and weakening of the bone with an increased risk of fractures. This usually starts with bone inflammation and osteoclastic activity (bone breakdown.)

Patients with breast and prostate cancer have been found to have a very high incidence of osteoporosis or osteopenia even before the use of therapies that lower hormone levels (a usual approach from medical circles.) If excessive bone loss is occurring (even in patients without cancer), there is a release of bone-derived growth factors, such as TGF-beta-1, due in part to high levels of cytokine IL-6 (a Th2, pro-inflammatory cytokine.) Prostate cancer cells can produce interleukin-6 (IL-6), which in itself affects the further breakdown of bone.[226] [227] Thus, a vicious cycle results: bone breakdown, the stimulation of cancer cell growth, and the production of interleukin IL -6 and other cell products, which leads to further bone breakdown. Ugh!

Recent studies reveal that Green Tea polyphenols are essential in inhibiting IL-6 levels and are an absolute **must** for nearly **every** cancer patient, regardless of type. A study in the *Journal of Clinical Oncology* [228] reveals:

"Epigallocatechin gallate (EGCG) is the predominant polyphenolic constituent of green tea leaves that possesses antitumor, anti-inflammatory, and antioxidant activity. EGCG exerts its effects through potentially multiple mechanisms including inhibition of growth factor receptor signaling. The compound is currently under investigation in a

---

[226] Cafagna et al. 1997
[227] Mousa 2002
[228] 2007 ASCO Annual Meeting Proceedings Part I. Vol 25, No. 18S (June 20 Supplement), 2007: 8114

phase I/II clinical trial for treatment of patients with early stage chronic lymphocytic leukemia at Mayo Clinic."

The results were impressive:

"EGCG inhibited the *in vitro* growth of human myeloma cell lines by inducing cell death in a time and dose-dependent manner. IC_{50} concentrations were between 12,5 µM and 50 µM. IL-6 mediated growth of INA-6 cells was inhibited at similar doses. The addition of excess amounts of IL-6 could not protect from EGCG induced cytotoxicity."

The authors further stated, "EGCG has growth inhibitory activity on myeloma cells. Specific inhibition of signaling pathways that regulate expression of anti-apoptotic proteins could be one mechanism how EGCG exerts its activity."

Another study published in the *Journal of American Science*,[229] revealed the benefits of caffeine added to green tea (hint, hint…coffee enemas) even improved IL-6, TNF-alpha (tumor necrosis factor), and CRP levels:

"The addition of caffeine to EGCG after 5 weeks showed enhancement of the effect on TNF-α, IL-6 and CRP…"

How to Implement Step Seven

To support bone integrity, the use of bone-supporting nutrients is highly recommended:

- **Green Tea Extract**: we use US Enzyme's Teavigo

- **Coffee Enemas**: help clear the liver and decrease cytokine levels

---

[229] 2011;7(8)

- **Complete Mineral Complex**: from an organic, whole-food source that is properly chelated. I use our product called Clear Multi Min Plus

Step Eight: Inhibiting Angiogenesis (Blood Supply to the Cancer)

Angiogenesis, the growth of new blood vessels, is critical during fetal development but occurs minimally in healthy adults. Exceptions occur during wound healing, inflammation, following a myocardial infarction (which is desired), in female reproductive organs, and in pathologic conditions such as cancer.

Angiogenesis is a strictly controlled process in the healthy adult human body, a process regulated by endogenous angiogenic promoters and inhibitors. Dr. Judah Folkman, the father of the angiogenesis theory of cancer stated, *"Blood vessel growth is controlled by a balancing of opposing factors. A tilt in favor of stimulators over inhibitors might be what trips the lever and begins the process of tumor angiogenesis."*[230]

Technically, solid tumors cannot grow beyond the size of a pinhead (about one million cells) without inducing the formation of new blood vessels to supply the nutritional needs of the tumor.[231] Since rapid vascularization and tumor growth appear to occur concurrently, interrupting the formation of new blood vessels is paramount to overcoming the malignancy, essentially cutting off the nutrient supply-lines.

Tumor angiogenesis results from a number of cellular processes initiated by the release of specific angiogenic growth factors. At a critical phase in the growth of a cancer, signal molecules are secreted from the cancer cells to nearby endothelial cells in an attempt to activate new blood vessel

---

[230] Cooke 2001
[231] Folkman J 1971

growth and a stronger supply-line. These angiogenic growth factors are chemical signals that diffuse in the direction of preexisting blood vessels, encouraging the formation of new blood vessel growth. VEGF (vascular endothelial growth factor) and basic fibroblast growth factors are expressed by many tumors and appear to be particularly important for angiogenesis.

A number of natural substances, such as Curcumin, green tea, N-acetyl-cysteine (NAC), resveratrol, grape seed-skin extract, and Vitamin D have anti-angiogenic properties. FDA has approved an anti-angiogenesis drug called Avastin® (bevacizumab), but it has demonstrated such severe side effects and often only mediocre efficacy. Again, if there are natural substances that do a better job, the only reason to use the pharmaceutical would be…well I guess there really isn't any reason to use the drug.

How to Implement Step Eight

Several nutrients have demonstrated potential anti-angiogenesis effects and should be considered:

- **Green Tea Extract**: in dosage stated in steps above. I use 1-3/day of the US Enzyme Teavigo

- **Curcumin**: in dosage stated in steps above. 1-5 grams per day, 1-5/day of our Curcu Clear

- **Vitamin D**: 5,000-20,000 IU daily (depending on blood levels on testing)

- **Grape Extract (seed and skin)**: 150-300mg daily

- **N-Acetyl Cysteine (NAC)**: 600-1,200mg daily

Step Nine: Inhibiting the 5-lipoxygenase (5-LOX) Enzyme

As discussed above regarding the Cyclooxygenase-2 (COX-2) Enzyme, inflammation plays a pivotal role in the formation and progression of cancer. The 5-lipoxygenase (5-LOX) enzyme is another inflammatory enzyme that can contribute to the formation and progression of cancer. Arachidonic acid (AA)--a saturated fat found in high concentrations in meat and dairy products—promotes elevation of the 5-LOX enzyme. But remember, most every study revealing the negative effects of AA was performed with processed (non-organic, pasteurized) AA which is caustic to your cells. This type of arachidonic acid is metabolized by 5-LOX to 5-HETE, a potent survival factor that prostate cancer cells utilize to escape destruction.[232] [233]

In response to poor quality fat overload, the body increases its production of enzymes like 5-lipooxygenase (5-LOX) to degrade them and rid them from your body. Not only does 5-LOX directly stimulate cancer cell propagation,[234] but the breakdown products that 5-LOX produces from poor quality fat overload (such as leukotriene B4, 5-HETE, and hydroxylated fatty acids) causes tissue destruction, chronic inflammation, and increased resistance of tumor cells to apoptosis (programmed cell destruction.) [235]

Specific extracts from the boswellia plant selectively inhibit 5-lipoxygenase (5-LOX).[236] In several well-controlled human

---

[232] Matsuyama et al. 2004; Sundaram et al. 2006; Myers et al. 1999

[233] Nakao-Hayashi et al. 1992; Cohen et al. 1991

[234] Ghosh 2003; Jiang et al. 2006; Yoshimura et al. 2004; Zhang et al. 2006; Soumaoro et al. 2006; Hayashi et al. 2006; Matsuyama et al. 2004; Hoque et al. 2005; Hennig et al. 2002; Ding et al. 1999; Matsuyama et al. 2005

[235] Hassan 2006; Sundaram 2006; Zhi 2003; Penglis 2000; Rubinsztajn 2003; Subbarao 2004; Laufer 2003

[236] Safayhi 1997; Safayhi 1995

studies, boswellia has been shown to be effective in alleviating various chronic inflammatory disorders.[237] Scientists have discovered that the specific constituent in boswellia responsible for suppressing 5-LOX is AKBA (3-O-acetyl-11-keto-B-boswellic acid.) Boswellia-derived AKBA binds directly to 5-LOX and inhibits its activity.70 Other boswellic acids only partially and incompletely inhibit 5-LOX.[238]

How to Implement Step Nine

Decrease the consumption of poor-quality fats such as grain-fed meats and pasteurized dairy products, along with high-glycemic carbohydrates (mainly grains and white potatoes.)

Consider supplementing with the following nutrients to suppress 5-LOX enzyme activity:

- **Boswelia Complex**: I use our Clear Inflam capsules, 2-6 daily

- **Curcumin**: again, I use our Curcu Clear or Turmero Clear

Step Ten: Inhibiting Cancer Metastasis

I know this step is really a duplication of step four, but I don't care; it's that important! The surgical removal of the primary tumor has been the cornerstone of treatment for the great majority of cancers. The rationale for this approach is straightforward: if you can get rid of the cancer by simply removing it from the body, then a cure can likely be achieved. Unfortunately, this approach does not take into account that

---

[237] Kimmatkar 2003; Ammon 2002; Wallace 2002; Gupta 2001; Gerhardt 2001; Gupta 1998; Kulkarni 1991; Park 2002; Liu 2002; Syrovets 2000
[238] Safayhi 1995; Sailer 1996

after surgery the cancer will frequently metastasize (spread to different organs.) Quite often, the metastatic recurrence is far more serious than the original tumor. In fact, for many cancers, it is the metastatic recurrence, and not the primary tumor, that ultimately proves to be fatal.[239]

One mechanism by which surgery increases the risk of metastasis is by enhancing cancer cell adhesion.[240] Cancer cells that have broken away from the primary tumor utilize adhesion to boost their ability to form metastases in distant organs. These cancer cells like to be able to clump together and form colonies that can expand and grow; basically, they desire to travel together as a team. It is unlikely that a single cancer cell will form a metastatic tumor, just as one person is unlikely to form a thriving community. Cancer cells use adhesion molecules, such as *galectin-3*, to facilitate their ability to clump together. Present on the surface of cancer cells, these molecules act like Velcro by allowing free-standing cancer cells to adhere to each other.[241] These free-standing cancer cells are called circulating tumor cells (CTCs) when they are looking for a home.

CTCs in the bloodstream also make use of galectin-3 surface adhesion molecules to latch onto the lining of blood vessels. The adherence of CTCs to the blood vessel walls is an essential step for the process of metastasis for if a cancer cell cannot adhere to the blood vessel wall, they wander through the blood stream incapable of forming metastases. They'd become like ships without a port, eventually destroyed by white blood cells. If the CTC's successfully bind to the blood vessel wall and burrow their way through the basement membrane, they will then utilize galectin-3 adhesion molecules to adhere to the organ to form a new metastatic cancer.[241]

---

[239] Bird 2006
[240] Dowdall 2002
[241] Raz 1987

Regrettably, though sometimes necessary, research has shown that cancer surgery increases tumor cell adhesion. Therefore, it is critically important for the person undergoing cancer surgery to take measures that can help to neutralize the surgery-induced increase in cancer cell adhesion. I list several ways below.

Fortunately, a natural compound called modified citrus pectin (MCP) can do just that. Citrus pectin, a type of dietary fiber, is not well absorbed in the intestine. However, modified citrus pectin has been altered so that it can be easily absorbed into the blood and exert its anti-cancer effects throughout the body. The mechanism by which modified citrus pectin inhibits cancer cell adhesion is by binding to galectin-3 adhesion molecules on the surface of cancer cells, thereby preventing cancer cells from sticking together and forming a cluster.[242]

MCP essentially chelates the CTCs. It can also inhibit circulating tumor cells from latching onto the lining of blood vessels. This was demonstrated by an experiment in which modified citrus pectin blocked the adhesion of galectin-3 to the lining of blood vessels by an astounding 95%. Modified citrus pectin also substantially decreased the adhesion of breast cancer cells to the blood vessel walls in other experiments.[242] Why doesn't every oncologist recommend MCP? I don't know, ask yours! It's relatively inexpensive and even little babies can take it.

One cancer trial took 10 men with recurrent prostate cancer giving them modified citrus pectin (14.4g per day.) After one year, a considerable improvement in cancer progression was noted, as determined by a reduction of the rate at which the prostate-specific antigen (PSA) level increased.[243] This was followed by a study in which 49 men with prostate cancer of various types were given modified citrus pectin for a four-week cycle. After two cycles of treatment with modified citrus pectin,

---

[242] Nangia-Makker 2002
[243] Guess 2003

22% of the men experienced a stabilization of their disease or improved quality of life; 12% had stable disease for more than 24 weeks. The authors of the study concluded:

"MCP (modified citrus pectin) seems to have positive impacts especially regarding clinical benefit and life quality for patients with far advanced solid tumor."[244]

In addition to modified citrus pectin, a well-known over-the-counter medication can also play a pivotal role in reducing cancer cell adhesion. Cimetidine, commonly known as Tagamet®, is a drug historically used to alleviate heartburn. A growing body of scientific evidence has revealed that cimetidine also possesses potent anti-cancer activity.

Cimetidine inhibits cancer cell adhesion by blocking the expression of an adhesive molecule, called *E-selectin,* on the surface of cells lining blood vessels.[245] Cancers cells latch onto E-selectin in order to adhere to the lining of blood vessels. By preventing the expression of E-selectin, cimetidine significantly limits the ability of cancer cell adherence to the blood vessel walls. This effect is analogous to removing the velcro from the blood vessels walls that would normally enable circulating tumor cells to bind.

Another major contributor to cancer metastasis is a diminished immune function; primarily that which occurs immediately following a surgical procedure such as removal of a primary tumor or after chemo/radiation destroy the immune response. Specifically, surgery suppresses the number of specialized immune cells called natural killer (NK) cells, which are a type of white blood cell tasked with seeking out and destroying cancer cells.

To illustrate the importance of NK cell activity in fighting cancer, a study published in the journal *Breast Cancer Research*

---

[244] Jackson 2007
[245] Eichbaum 2011

and Treatment examined NK cell activity in women shortly after surgery for breast cancer. The researchers reported that low levels of NK cell activity were associated with an increased risk of death from breast cancer. In fact, reduced NK cell activity was a better predictor of survival than the actual stage of the cancer! In another alarming study, individuals with reduced NK cell activity before surgery for colon cancer had a 350% increased risk of metastasis during the following 31 months![246] Yikes! If you are planning on surgery, you better follow this step below.

One fantastic natural compound that can increase NK cell activity is PSK (*protein-bound polysaccharide K*), a specially prepared extract from the mushroom *Coriolus versicolor* as well as properly processed polysaccharides from aloe in *Evolv Immun* (personally, this is exactly what I take.)

PSK has been shown to enhance NK cell activity in multiple studies.[247] PSK's ability to enhance NK cell activity helps to explain why it has been shown to dramatically improve survival in cancer patients. For example, 225 patients with lung cancer received radiation therapy with or without PSK (I recommend 3-6 per day of either of the above products.)

For those with more advanced Stage 3 cancers, more than three times as many individuals taking PSK were alive after five years (26%), compared to those not taking PSK (8%.) PSK more than doubled five-year survival in those individuals with less advanced Stage 1 or 2 disease (39% vs.17%).[248]

In a 2008 study, a group of colon cancer patients were randomized to receive chemotherapy alone or chemotherapy plus PSK, which was taken for two years. The group receiving PSK had an exceptional 10-year survival of 82%. Sadly, the group receiving chemotherapy alone had a 10-year survival of

---

[246] Koda 1997
[247] Fisher 2002; Garcia-Lora 2001
[248] Hayakawa 1997

only 51% (Sakai 2008.) In a similar trial reported in the *British Journal of Cancer*, colon cancer patients received chemotherapy alone or combined with PSK (3 grams per day) for two years. In the group with a more dangerous Stage 3 colon cancer, the five-year survival was 75% in the PSK group. This compared to a five-year survival of only 46% in the group receiving chemotherapy alone.[249]

Additional research has shown that PSK improves survival in cancers of the breast, stomach, esophagus, and uterus as well.[250] I like to use the *whole food* form of PSK in the mushroom itself (Coriolus versicolor.) I have a lot of this in my Medicinal Mushroom blend as well!

How to Implement Step Ten

The following novel compounds have shown efficacy in inhibiting several mechanisms that contribute to cancer metastasis. It is especially important to consider these compounds during the perioperative period (period before and after surgery), because a known consequence of surgery is an enhanced proclivity for metastasis:

- **Modified Citrus Pectin**: 5-15 grams daily, in three divided doses if possible

- **Cimetidine**: 800mg daily, in two divided doses

- **Coriolus Versicolor, Standardized Extract**: 1,200-3,600mg daily *or* Evolv Immun, 3/day, *or* our Medicinal Mushroom blend, 1-3 teaspoons per day

- **IP6**: has been shown help decrease adhesion properties of CTCs; consider taking 2-6 capsules per day (I use the product from Hope Science)

---

[249] Ohwada 2004
[250] Okazaki 1986; Nakazato 1994; Toi 1992

Summary

When you look at everything as a whole, these ten steps aren't really that confusing. Many of the nutrients cross between steps and have a double or triple purpose. I am **not** in favor of giving huge numbers of nutrients; utilizing a technique like kinesiology can help cut down on things that your body just doesn't need right now. When I teach doctors about taking care of people with a cancer diagnosis, I try to give them the big picture, similar to what I've attempted here. I believe it's great to know how and why things work as well as making every attempt to simplify things that can become complex.

Walk through these steps with a qualified healthcare professional, educate yourself and you'll feel more equipped at taking care of yourself, and learn as much as you can so you can take the fear out of your disease and remain in the driver's seat; don't become the victim.

Don't let it go to your head but knowing the above ten steps just might make you smarter than your doctor. Use your knowledge wisely.

Never Give Up, *Always* Give In

"Then I heard what sounded like a great multitude, like the roar of rushing waters and like loud peals of thunder, shouting: "Hallelujah! For our Lord God Almighty reigns." – Revelation 19:5-7

I make no apologies for my spiritual belief, for this is why I wrote this book. You do not need to agree with everything I say, but no book on such grave a subject as cancer should omit the eternal perspective. I am a Christian with a strong belief that there is only one way to heaven as well as any true joy in this life, and that is through Jesus Christ.

I believe that God is sovereign; that means He allows things in my life for reasons I may never understand this side of heaven. He is my heavenly Father who loves me beyond my understanding and sent His Son to die in place of what I deserved. He called me, made me His son, and I have given myself to Him and in so doing, should He allow me to "get cancer" as He has, I must logically seek possible reasons He did so.

Does He desire for me to be healed and be a witness of His power? Does He desire me to find answers that may help thousands of other to suffer less? Does He desire me to be a witness of His grace and mercy throughout my struggles? Is He calling me home and using cancer to do so?

There are a million possible questions that a believer may have, many spoken in frustration, some in anger and confusion, but most whispered silently, ultimately accepting the will of the One in whom we place our trust. God doesn't answer all our questions because, in truth, we can't handle the answers. Our job is to walk in faith.

Every person sick with cancer or seemingly springing with health should contemplate such thoughts. It's only human to ask, "Why me, why do I have to get cancer," even when the more appropriate question may be, "Why *not* me?"

I want *all* that God has for me and I am mature enough in my faith to understand that it's **not** the temporal things He's concerned about. He desires me, He loves me, He wants me by His side forever and ever and I give Him permission (though He doesn't need it) to mold me and shape me, be it ever so painful, more into the image of His Son. The temporal sliver of time we spend on earth pales in comparison to eternity.

I am not a doctor who believes that God desires to heal all our wounds or cure every cancer patient. We all will die, some from car accidents, some from old age, and others from cancer. Where we go after we die is of most concern. We must surrender to the fact that God is God and we are not. This doesn't mean we should allow the world and its evils to beat us down; we keep fighting the fight while surrendering to God.

My prayer for you is this: that when seemingly all that you've ever held dearly is slipping through your fingers, you let go, give up, and fall on your knees before your Creator and admit something like, "Dear Father, I'm lost and need You to find me, I'm broken and need You to heal me, I'm hopeless and confused, tired of trying and unable to fight on my own any longer. I need *you*. Forgive me; change me; make me Your child. Renew me; for You are my only hope."

This is when the healing begins. This is when the peace that passes all human understanding can fill you, comfort you, and snuggle you with warmth through the chill of despair. This is my prayer for you; not that your cancer goes away but that your cancer drives you to a relationship with your Father that is new, refreshed, real and eternal.

I pray for faith to heal my doubt,
To understand You work it out.
To cleanse my heart of selfish sin,
To purify me deep within.

To stop pretending, stop the games,
Stop praising self and God the same.
To see the dungeons of my soul,
That Christ my only hope I'd know

I pray for able that I am,
To stand alone for God's own lamb.
That 'til the very end of breath,
My trust remains in Jesus' death.

I pray through all I may see clear,
Oh, that I may, Lord, persevere.

Should you desire to read more on this subject, dare to read my book, *"Cancer Can't Kill You"* available as a ***free download*** on our website at ConnersClinic.com/books or on Amazon.com

Know that I'll pray for you always!

Final Remarks

Regardless of what you choose about healthcare, I pray that you make wise, rational decisions based on facts (though often hidden) and not fear. You need to take responsibility and not hand it over to any practitioner, conventional or alternative. Get advice from many, weigh it all against their biases, and pray for peace about your decisions.

– Dr. Kevin Conners